Natural Products in Photodynamic Therapy

Natural Products in Photodynamic Therapy

Guest Editors

Renato Sonchini Gonçalves
Gustavo Braga

MDPI

Basel • Beijing • Wuhan • Barcelona • Belgrade • Novi Sad • Cluj • Manchester

Guest Editors
Renato Sonchini Gonçalves
Department of Chemistry
Federal University of
Maranhão
São Luís
Brazil

Gustavo Braga
Department of Chemistry
Federal University of
Maranhão
São Luís
Brazil

Editorial Office
MDPI AG
Grosspeteranlage 5
4052 Basel, Switzerland

This is a reprint of the Special Issue, published open access by the journal *Pharmaceutics* (ISSN 1999-4923), freely accessible at: https://www.mdpi.com/journal/pharmaceutics/special_issues/94LCD6421Q.

For citation purposes, cite each article independently as indicated on the article page online and as indicated below:

Lastname, A.A.; Lastname, B.B. Article Title. *Journal Name* **Year**, *Volume Number*, Page Range.

ISBN 978-3-7258-6468-3 (Hbk)
ISBN 978-3-7258-6469-0 (PDF)
https://doi.org/10.3390/books978-3-7258-6469-0

Contents

About the Editors

Renato Sonchini Gonçalves

Renato Sonchini Gonçalves is a Professor of Organic Chemistry at the Department of Chemistry, Federal University of Maranhão, São Luís, Brazil. His scientific work encompasses natural products chemistry, photodynamic therapy, pharmaceutical nanotechnology, and the development of sustainable strategies grounded in green chemistry and bioeconomy principles. His research focuses on the isolation, structural characterization, and photoreactivity of bioactive plant-derived compounds, as well as the design of nanostructured delivery systems that enhance photosensitizer stability, biological transport, and therapeutic performance. He has contributed to advances in supramolecular organization, polymeric nanogels, and photophysical mechanisms relevant to antimicrobial and antitumor applications. He has authored more than 60 scientific publications across these areas, including interdisciplinary collaborations. His recent work emphasizes eco-friendly formulations for daylight photodynamic therapy, targeting both neglected tropical diseases and cancer treatment. He collaborates actively with research groups from diverse scientific fields across strategic regions of Brazil and with international partners, integrating chemistry, molecular biology, sustainability frameworks, and innovative formulation.

Gustavo Braga

Gustavo Braga is a faculty member in Basic, Technical, and Technological Education at the University College (COLUN) of the Federal University of Maranhão (UFMA), Brazil, where he leads research and outreach programs, supervises undergraduate students through the Institutional Program of Scientific Initiation Scholarships for High School Students (PIBIC-EM), and serves on scientific and advisory committees. Dr. Braga's research focuses on colloidal and polymeric materials, with particular emphasis on the physicochemical and thermodynamic interactions of photoactive drugs within polymeric and colloidal systems. His work encompasses photophysics, photodynamic therapy, nanotechnology, and the development of advanced materials for biomedical and technological applications.He has a comprehensive academic background culminating in a Ph.D. in Science from the State University of Maringá (UEM), Brazil, where he focused on the interdisciplinary fields of Physical Chemistry, Inorganic Chemistry, and Materials Science and Engineering.

Preface

This Reprint brings together recent scientific contributions that explore the role of natural photosensitizers in photodynamic therapy, emphasizing their chemical diversity, photophysical behavior, and therapeutic potential. The scope of this Reprint extends from fundamental molecular mechanisms to applied research in oncology, infectious diseases, and nanotechnology, reflecting the interdisciplinary nature of this rapidly advancing field. Our aim was to assemble studies that demonstrate how natural compounds can serve as effective agents for controlled light activation, generating selective and potent biological responses. The motivation for organizing this Reprint arose from the growing interest in sustainable, biocompatible, and mechanistically versatile photosensitizers that align with current challenges in global health. This Reprint is intended for researchers, clinicians, and students interested in photodynamic therapy, natural products, molecular photobiology, and advanced formulation strategies, offering an updated reference on the state of the art and future directions for natural-product-based photodynamic interventions.

Renato Sonchini Gonçalves and Gustavo Braga
Guest Editors

pharmaceutics

MDPI

Article

Photodynamic Therapy with Natural Photosensitizers: Bridging Oncology, Infectious Diseases, and Global Health

Renato Sonchini Gonçalves [1,*] and Gustavo Braga [2]

[1] Laboratory of Chemistry of Natural Products, Department of Chemistry, Federal University of Maranhão (UFMA), São Luís 65080-805, Brazil
[2] University College (COLUN), Federal University of Maranhã (UFMA), São Luís 65080-805, Brazil; gustavo.braga@ufma.br
* Correspondence: renato.sg@ufma.br; Tel.: +55-98-985-149-235

1. Introduction

Photodynamic therapy (PDT) has undergone a remarkable transformation since its inception more than a century ago, evolving from a niche experimental technique into a versatile biomedical platform with wide-ranging therapeutic applications [1,2]. At its core, PDT relies on three interconnected components: a photosensitizer, a light source, and molecular oxygen to generate reactive oxygen species (ROS) that exert cytotoxic, antimicrobial, or immunomodulatory effects [3–5]. What distinguishes PDT from many conventional therapies is its spatio-temporal selectivity, the possibility of repeated administration without cumulative toxicity, and its ability to act through multimodal mechanisms that include direct cell death, vascular damage, and immune system activation [6–9].

In recent decades, the refinement of light sources, the discovery of novel photosensitizers, and the advent of nanotechnology have considerably expanded the therapeutic window of PDT [10–12]. Parallel advances in molecular and cellular biology have revealed that PDT is not only a destructive therapy, but also a powerful modulator of tumor microenvironments, microbial biofilms, and host immune responses [13–15]. In this context, natural photosensitizers have gained attention as sustainable and biocompatible alternatives to synthetic compounds, offering lower toxicity, chemical diversity, and alignment with green chemistry principles. Identification of natural photosensitizers such as hypericin, riboflavin, curcumin, and anthraquinones has further aligned PDT with the principles of sustainability and green chemistry, while simultaneously broadening its chemical and mechanistic diversity [16–20].

These innovations coincide with urgent global health needs. In oncology, PDT provides alternatives for tumors resistant to conventional therapies [21]; in infectious diseases, it emerges as a strategy against antimicrobial resistance [22,23]; and in dentistry and dermatology, it offers minimally invasive approaches for biofilm control, wound healing, and periimplantitis [24]. In particular, PDT shows promise for neglected tropical diseases such as leishmaniasis, where accessible treatments remain scarce [25,26].

This Special Issue of *Pharmaceutics* reflects these advances through studies on molecular mechanisms, translational research, nanotechnology, and systematic reviews. Collectively, the contributions underscore the cytotoxic, immunomodulatory, and antimicrobial potential of PDT, strengthening its evolution into an integrative, patient-centered modality. By situating PDT at the intersection of chemistry, nanotechnology, immunology, and clinical science, this Special Issue demonstrates a paradigm shift. PDT is no longer a peripheral drug, but a rapidly maturing therapeutic strategy to tackle pressing biomedical challenges.

2. Overview of Published Work

The articles collected in this Special Issue provide a broad and multifaceted perspective on the potential of PDT, encompassing mechanistic, translational, and clinical viewpoints.

At the cellular and molecular level, Olek et al. provided compelling evidence for the immunomodulatory effects of hypericin-mediated PDT in oral cancer cells [18]. Their findings demonstrate not only direct cytotoxicity but also the activation of immune-related pathways, suggesting that PDT can act as a bridge between local tumor ablation and systemic immune engagement. Extending these observations, Krupka-Olek et al. confirmed the dual cytotoxic and immunomodulatory role of hypericin in skin cell cultures, reinforcing the relevance of this natural compound as a clinically translatable photosensitizer for dermatological malignancies [27].

In the context of infectious diseases, Jeong and Hwang revealed that natural phytochemicals combined with visible light irradiation display a potent synergistic antibacterial activity against *Staphylococcus aureus* [21]. This contribution is particularly relevant in the era of antimicrobial resistance, as it demonstrates that PDT can bypass classical resistance mechanisms and expand the therapeutic arsenal against multidrug-resistant pathogens. In addition, Marioni et al. highlighted the antifungal potential of natural anthraquinone parietin, showing its ability to disrupt Candida tropicalis biofilms through photodynamic mechanisms [23]. These results broaden the chemical diversity of natural photosensitizers and support the applicability of PDT in fungal infections, a field traditionally limited in therapeutic options.

Three systematic reviews strengthened the translational scope of this Special Issue. Łopaciński, et al. analyzed riboflavin- and hypericin-mediated PDT for oral candidiasis, integrating preclinical and clinical data to demonstrate promising efficacy in the management of opportunistic fungal infections [28]. Fiegler-Rudol et al. evaluated the role of riboflavin-mediated PDT in periodontology, critically assessing its benefits for periodontal regeneration and biofilm control [20]. Warakomska et al. extended these insights to periimplantitis, systematically demonstrating how PDT, mediated by natural photosensitizers, can reduce microbial burden and inflammation while preserving implant integrity [24]. Together, these reviews underscore the consolidation of PDT as an evidence-based adjunct in oral medicine and dentistry.

From a nanotechnological and translational point of view, Campos et al. introduced an innovative nanogel formulation coencapsulating curcumin and essential oil *Pectis brevipedunculata*, designed for daylight-mediated PDT against leishmaniasis [25]. This study exemplifies how nanostructured delivery systems can enhance the solubility, stability, and synergistic activity of natural products, while addressing neglected tropical diseases that disproportionately affect low-resource regions. Beyond its biomedical implications, the work also highlights the importance of integrating sustainability and accessibility in the innovation of PDT.

Taken together, the contributions in this Special Issue highlight the breadth and dynamism of PDT research. They collectively reveal how natural products, nanotechnology, and systematic clinical evaluation are converging to redefine PDT as a clinically relevant, sustainable, and patient-centered therapeutic strategy. Table 1 provides a consolidated overview of the natural photosensitizers discussed in the articles published in this Special Issue, summarizing their biological sources, irradiation parameters, and therapeutic applications. It is not intended as an exhaustive list of all photosensitizers employed in photodynamic therapy.

Table 1. Summary of natural photosensitizers included in the articles published in this Special Issue, their biological sources, irradiation parameters, and therapeutic applications in photodynamic therapy (PDT).

Photosensitizers (Concentration)	Natural Source	Wavelength Range (nm)	Application/Carrier Medium
Hypericin (0.25–1.0 µM) Immunomodulation; cytotoxicity [18].	*Hypericum perforatum*	580–720	Oral carcinoma/DMSO solution
Hypericin (0.1–1.0 µM) Reduced inflammation; apoptosis [27].	*Hypericum perforatum*	450–720	Inflammatory dermatoses/DMSO solution
Plant extracts (31–500 µg/mL) Synergistic antibacterial effect [21].	*Sophora officinalis, Ulmus davidiana, Cimicifuga simplex, Glycyrrhiza uralensis*	465–625	Antibacterial therapy/Aqueous extract
Parietin (0.98 µg/mL) Biofilm disruption via ROS [23].	*Teloschistes nodulifer*	428	Antifungal therapy/Hydroalcoholic sol. (1%)
Riboflavin and Hypericin (0.25–320 µM) Biofilm inactivation; antifungal synergy [28].	*Aspergillus gossypii, Hypericum perforatum*	365–750	Oral candidiasis/Micelles (P123)–lipid carriers
Riboflavin (10–100 µg/mL) Adjunct antimicrobial action [20].	*Aspergillus gossypii, Bacillus subtilis, Arabidopsis thaliana*	390–670	Periodontology/Hydrogel–NP dispersion
Curcumin, Riboflavin, 5-ALA, Hypericin (0.1–0.5%) Reduced microbial load and inflammation [24].	*Curcuma longa, Aspergillus gossypii, Bacillus subtilis, Hypericum perforatum*	390–810	Peri-implantitis/ Nanogels–biopolymers
Curcumin (2–18 µg/mL) Anti-*Leishmania* effect; synergistic PDT [25].	*Curcuma longa* and *Pectis brevipedunculata*	Daylight	Antileishmanial therapy/Pluronic F127–Carbopol 974P

3. Future Perspectives

The insights from this Special Issue highlight both the remarkable achievements and the persisting gaps that will shape the trajectory of photodynamic therapy (PDT) in the coming decade. Collectively, the contributions emphasize that PDT is transitioning from an experimental or adjunctive technique to a mainstream therapeutic strategy, supported by strong preclinical evidence, growing clinical validation, and innovative technological platforms. Nevertheless, for PDT to achieve its full translational and societal impact, several priorities must be pursued.

1. Clinical Standardization and Protocol Harmonization: The field urgently requires harmonized preclinical and clinical protocols to improve reproducibility and facilitate regulatory approval. Establishing standardized parameters for light dosimetry, photosensitizer concentration, and treatment regimens will enhance cross-study comparability and accelerate clinical translation.
2. Nano- and Bioengineered Photosensitizer Platforms: Advances in nanotechnology—such as stimuli-responsive nanogels, hybrid lipid-polymeric carriers, and bioinspired delivery systems—should be leveraged to improve selectivity, tissue penetration, and pharmacokinetics. Theranostic nanoplatforms capable of combining imaging, controlled release, and therapeutic action represent a frontier for precision PDT.
3. Integration with Immunotherapy and Host Modulation: PDT's ability to induce immunogenic cell death and release danger-associated molecular patterns (DAMPs) positions it as a synergistic partner to immune checkpoint inhibitors and vaccines. Exploring PDT as a bridge between local ablation and systemic immunity could redefine its role in oncology and infectious disease management.
4. Applications in Neglected and Emerging Diseases: The promising results against Leishmania parasites and fungal biofilms point to the potential of PDT in neglected tropical diseases and hard-to-treat infections. Future research should emphasize low-cost, daylight-mediated PDT approaches adaptable to resource-limited settings, reinforcing the alignment with global health equity.

5. Green Chemistry and Sustainable Development: The increasing reliance on natural products as photosensitizers highlights the relevance of sustainability. Bioprospecting guided by ethnopharmacology, combined with scalable green extraction and synthetic biology approaches, can ensure eco-friendly and socially responsible production of next-generation photosensitizers.
6. Artificial Intelligence and Predictive Modeling: The incorporation of artificial intelligence and systems biology into PDT research holds promise for optimizing treatment planning, predicting patient-specific responses, and designing adaptive protocols. These tools can also accelerate the rational design of novel photosensitizers with improved photophysical and pharmacological profiles.

Author Contributions: Conceptualization, R.S.G. and G.B.; writing—original draft preparation, R.S.G.; writing—review and editing, R.S.G. and G.B. All authors have read and agreed to the published version of the manuscript.

Funding: This editorial received no external funding.

Conflicts of Interest: The authors declare no conflicts of interest.

References

1. Alvarez, N.; Sevilla, A. Current Advances in Photodynamic Therapy (PDT) and the Future Potential of PDT-Combinatorial Cancer Therapies. *Int. J. Mol. Sci.* **2024**, *25*, 1023. [CrossRef] [PubMed]
2. El-Sadek, M.Z.; El-Aziz, M.K.A.; Shaaban, A.H.; Mostafa, S.A.; Wadan, A.-H.S. Advancements and Emerging Trends in Photodynamic Therapy: Innovations in Cancer Treatment and Beyond. *Photochem. Photobiol. Sci.* **2025**, *24*, 1489–1511. [CrossRef] [PubMed]
3. Allison, R.R.; Moghissi, K. Photodynamic Therapy (PDT): PDT Mechanisms. *Clin. Endosc.* **2013**, *46*, 24–29. [CrossRef]
4. Castano, A.P.; Demidova, T.N.; Hamblin, M.R. Mechanisms in Photodynamic Therapy: Part One—Photosensitizers, Photochemistry and Cellular Localization. *Photodiagn. Photodyn. Ther.* **2004**, *1*, 279–293. [CrossRef] [PubMed]
5. Rkein, A.M.; Ozog, D.M. Photodynamic Therapy. *Dermatol. Clin.* **2014**, *32*, 415–425. [CrossRef]
6. Ortenzio, M.P.; Anand, S.; Travers, J.B.; Maytin, E.V.; Rohan, C.A. Immunomodulatory Effects of Photodynamic Therapy for Skin Cancer: Potential Strategies to Improve Treatment Efficacy and Tolerability. *Photochem. Photobiol.* 2025, *in press*. [CrossRef]
7. Selbo, P.K.; Korbelik, M. Enhancing Antitumour Immunity with Photodynamic Therapy. *Photochem. Photobiol. Sci.* **2025**, *24*, 227–234. [CrossRef]
8. Chen, L.; Lin, Y.; Ding, S.; Huang, M.; Jiang, L. Recent Advances in Clinically Used and Trialed Photosensitizers for Antitumor Photodynamic Therapy. *Mol. Pharm.* **2025**, *22*, 3530–3541. [CrossRef]
9. Jiang, W.; Liang, M.; Lei, Q.; Li, G.; Wu, S. The Current Status of Photodynamic Therapy in Cancer Treatment. *Cancers* **2023**, *15*, 585. [CrossRef]
10. Aebisher, D.; Szpara, J.; Bartusik-Aebisher, D. Advances in Medicine: Photodynamic Therapy. *Int. J. Mol. Sci.* **2024**, *25*, 8258. [CrossRef]
11. Ji, B.; Wei, M.; Yang, B. Recent Advances in Nanomedicines for Photodynamic Therapy (PDT)-Driven Cancer Immunotherapy. *Theranostics* **2022**, *12*, 434–458. [CrossRef]
12. Nasir, A.; Rehman, M.U.; Khan, T.; Husn, M.; Khan, M.; Khan, A.; Nuh, A.M.; Jiang, W.; Farooqi, H.M.U.; Bai, Q. Advances in Nanotechnology-Assisted Photodynamic Therapy for Neurological Disorders: A Comprehensive Review. *Artif. Cells Nanomed. Biotechnol.* **2024**, *52*, 84–103. [CrossRef]
13. Sorrin, A.J.; Kemal Ruhi, M.; Ferlic, N.A.; Karimnia, V.; Polacheck, W.J.; Celli, J.P.; Huang, H.C.; Rizvi, I. Photodynamic Therapy and the Biophysics of the Tumor Microenvironment. *Photochem. Photobiol.* **2020**, *96*, 232–259. [CrossRef]
14. Wang, X.; Luo, D.; Basilion, J.P. Photodynamic Therapy: Targeting Cancer Biomarkers for the Treatment of Cancers. *Cancers* **2021**, *13*, 2992. [CrossRef]
15. Aebisher, D.; Czech, S.; Dynarowicz, K.; Misiołek, M.; Komosińska-Vassev, K.; Kawczyk-Krupka, A.; Bartusik-Aebisher, D. Photodynamic Therapy: Past, Current, and Future. *Int. J. Mol. Sci.* **2024**, *25*, 11325. [CrossRef]
16. Kubrak, T.P.; Kołodziej, P.; Sawicki, J.; Mazur, A.; Koziorowska, K.; Aebisher, D. Some Natural Photosensitizers and Their Medicinal Properties for Use in Photodynamic Therapy. *Molecules* **2022**, *27*, 1192. [CrossRef] [PubMed]
17. Imaizumi, U.; Inaba, K.; Kurahashi, A.; Kuroda, H.; Sanuki, T.; Yoshida, A.; Yoshino, F.; Hamada, N. Effectiveness of Curcumin-Based Antimicrobial Photodynamic Therapy against *Staphylococcus aureus*. *J. Oral Sci.* **2023**, *65*, 270–274. [CrossRef] [PubMed]

18. Olek, M.; Machorowska-Pieniążek, A.; Czuba, Z.P.; Cieślar, G.; Kawczyk-Krupka, A. Immunomodulatory Effect of Hypericin-Mediated Photodynamic Therapy on Oral Cancer Cells. *Pharmaceutics* **2023**, *16*, 42. [CrossRef] [PubMed]
19. de Oliveira, A.C.V.; de Morais, F.A.P.; Campanholi, K.D.S.S.; Bidóia, D.L.; Balbinot, R.B.; Nakamura, C.V.; Caetano, W.; Hioka, N.; Monteiro, O.D.S.; da Rocha, C.Q.; et al. Melanoma-Targeted Photodynamic Therapy Based on Hypericin-Loaded Multifunctional P123-Spermine/Folate Micelles. *Photodiagn. Photodyn. Ther.* **2022**, *40*, 103103. [CrossRef]
20. Fiegler-Rudol, J.; Łopaciński, M.; Los, A.; Skaba, D.; Wiench, R. Riboflavin-Mediated Photodynamic Therapy in Periodontology: A Systematic Review of Applications and Outcomes. *Pharmaceutics* **2025**, *17*, 217. [CrossRef]
21. Jeong, J.-Y.; Hwang, Y.-J. Natural Phytochemical and Visible Light at Different Wavelengths Show Synergistic Antibacterial Activity against *Staphylococcus aureus*. *Pharmaceutics* **2024**, *16*, 612. [CrossRef] [PubMed]
22. Cieplik, F.; Deng, D.; Crielaard, W.; Buchalla, W.; Hellwig, E.; Al-Ahmad, A.; Maisch, T. Antimicrobial Photodynamic Therapy—What We Know and What We Don't. *Crit. Rev. Microbiol.* **2018**, *44*, 571–589. [CrossRef]
23. Marioni, J.; Romero, B.C.; Mugas, M.L.; Martinez, F.; Gómez, T.I.; Morales, J.M.N.; Konigheim, B.S.; Borsarelli, C.D.; Nuñez-Montoya, S.C. The Natural Anthraquinone Parietin Inactivates *Candida tropicalis* Biofilm by Photodynamic Mechanisms. *Pharmaceutics* **2025**, *17*, 548. [CrossRef]
24. Warakomska, A.; Fiegler-Rudol, J.; Kubizna, M.; Skaba, D.; Wiench, R. The Role of Photodynamic Therapy Mediated by Natural Photosensitisers in the Management of Peri-Implantitis: A Systematic Review. *Pharmaceutics* **2025**, *17*, 443. [CrossRef]
25. Campos, L.M.O.; Marques, E.M.; Lera-Nonose, D.S.S.L.; Gonçalves, M.J.S.; Lonardoni, M.V.C.; Nunes, G.C.d.S.; Braga, G.; Gonçalves, R.S. Enhanced Nanogel Formulation Combining the Natural Photosensitizer Curcumin and *Pectis brevipedunculata* (Asteraceae) Essential Oil for Synergistic Daylight Photodynamic Therapy in Leishmaniasis Treatment. *Pharmaceutics* **2025**, *17*, 286. [CrossRef]
26. Najm, M.; Pourhajibagher, M.; Badirzadeh, A.; Razmjou, E.; Alipour, M.; Khoshmirsafa, M.; Bahador, A.; Hadighi, R. Photodynamic Therapy Using Toluidine Blue O (TBO) Dye as a Photosensitizer against *Leishmania major*. *Iran. J. Public Health* **2021**, *50*, 2111–2120. [CrossRef] [PubMed]
27. Krupka-Olek, M.; Bożek, A.; Czuba, Z.P.; Kłósek, M.; Cieślar, G.; Kawczyk-Krupka, A. Cytotoxic and Immunomodulatory Effects of *Hypericin* as a Photosensitizer in Photodynamic Therapy Used on Skin Cell Cultures. *Pharmaceutics* **2024**, *16*, 696. [CrossRef] [PubMed]
28. Łopaciński, M.; Fiegler-Rudol, J.; Niemczyk, W.; Skaba, D.; Wiench, R. Riboflavin- and Hypericin-Mediated Antimicrobial Photodynamic Therapy as Alternative Treatments for Oral Candidiasis: A Systematic Review. *Pharmaceutics* **2025**, *17*, 33. [CrossRef] [PubMed]

pharmaceutics

MDPI

Article

Immunomodulatory Effect of Hypericin-Mediated Photodynamic Therapy on Oral Cancer Cells

Marcin Olek [1,2,*], Agnieszka Machorowska-Pieniążek [2], Zenon P. Czuba [3], Grzegorz Cieślar [4] and Aleksandra Kawczyk-Krupka [4,*]

[1] Doctoral School of Medical University of Silesia, 40-055 Katowice, Poland
[2] Department of Orthodontics, Faculty of Medical Sciences in Zabrze, Medical University of Silesia, 40-055 Katowice, Poland; apieniazek@sum.edu.pl
[3] Department of Microbiology and Immunology, Faculty of Medical Sciences in Zabrze, Medical University of Silesia, 40-055 Katowice, Poland; zczuba@sum.edu.pl
[4] Department of Internal Diseases, Angiology and Physical Medicine, Center for Laser Diagnostics and Therapy, Faculty of Medical Sciences in Zabrze, Medical University of Silesia, 40-055 Katowice, Poland; cieslar1@tlen.pl
* Correspondence: d200922@365.sum.edu.pl (M.O.); akawczyk@gmail.com (A.K.-K.)

Abstract: In 2020, there were 377,713 new oral and lip cancer diagnoses and 177,757 deaths. Oral cancer is a malignancy of the head and neck region, and 90% of cases are squamous cell carcinomas (OSCCs). One of the alternative methods of treating pre-cancerous lesions and oral cancer is photodynamic therapy (PDT). In addition to the cytotoxic effect, an important mechanism of PDT action is the immunomodulatory effect. This study used the OSCC (SCC-25) cell line and the healthy gingival fibroblast (HGF-1) line. A compound of natural origin—hypericin (HY)—was used as the photosensitizer (PS). The HY concentrations of 0–1 μM were used. After two hours of incubation with PS, the cells were irradiated with light doses of 0–20 J/cm^2. The MTT test determined sublethal doses of PDT. Cell supernatants subjected to sublethal PDT were assessed for interleukin 6 (IL-6), soluble IL-6 receptor alpha (sIL-6Ralfa), sIL-6Rbeta, IL-8, IL-10, IL-11 IL-20, IL-32, and Pentraxin-3 using the Bio-Plex Pro^{TM} Assay. The phototoxic effect was observed starting with a light dose of 5 J/cm^2 and amplified with increasing HY concentration and a light dose. HY-PDT affected the SCC-25 cell secretion of sIL-6Rbeta, IL-20, and Pentraxin-3. HY alone increased IL-8 secretion. In the case of HGF-1, the effect of HY-PDT on the secretion of IL-8 and IL-32 was found.

Keywords: photodynamic therapy; oral cancer; hypericin; immunomodulatory effect

1. Introduction

Photodynamic therapy (PDT) is a method of treatment in which a photosensitizer (PS) is applied to the desired place, which is then activated by light of the appropriate wavelength and dose. In the presence of oxygen in the tissues, a photodynamic reaction (PDR) occurs [1]. After irradiation, according to the absorption spectrum of PS located inside the cell, a transition occurs from the basic singlet state to the excited singlet state by cause of the absorption of photon energy. Some of the energy is radiated in the form of a fluorescence quantum. The therapeutic form of PS is the excited triplet state, which is formed because of a non-radiative inter-combination transition [2]. As a result of the reaction of the excited photosensitizer with environmental biomolecules, free radicals and anion radicals of the photosensitizer and the substrate are generated. The electrons interact with oxygen to form reactive oxygen species (ROS). This process results in oxidative stress and the death of cancer cells, which is a type I of the PDT mechanism. Type II photodynamic reaction involves a direct transfer of energy from the triplet excited form of PS to an oxygen molecule, resulting in the formation of singlet oxygen, which has a powerful oxidizing effect. It is believed that the most important type of PDT reaction is type II [3]. The percentage of mechanisms involved in the photodynamic reaction depends on many factors, such as the concentration of oxygen in the tissues, the type of photosensitizer, and the pH of the environment. PDT leads to programmed cell death, necrosis, or autophagy, depending on the intracellular location of PS and damage to given cellular structures [4]. PDR also occurs in the blood vessels supplying the tumor, disrupting the vessel walls, aggregating platelets, and, consequently, causing a loss of blood supply to the tumor and its necrosis. A significant role of PDT is the activation of the immune system. Neutrophils and macrophages are activated due to the release of cytokines, inflammatory mediators, and proteins. After phagocytosis of damaged cells, macrophages present antigens to helper CD4 T cells, which activate CD8 cytotoxic T cells [1,5].

In 2020, there were 377,713 new oral and lip cancer diagnoses and 177,757 deaths [6]. Oral cancer is a malignancy of the head and neck region, and 90% of cases are squamous cell carcinomas (OSCCs). Predisposing factors include smoking, chewing betel leaves, alcohol consumption, human papillomavirus infection, and poor oral hygiene [7–9]. The standard treatment method for OSCC is the excision of the tumor within the healthy tissues, which is accompanied by surgery of the lymphatic system of the neck in the case of metastases to the lymph nodes [10]. Adjuvant radiotherapy or chemotherapy is also used depending on the cancer stage and the surgery's radicality [11]. As a result of typical complications after traditional treatment, patients' quality of life decreases [12]. The most frequently observed consequences of the surgical procedure are speech, chewing, and swallowing disorders and aesthetic problems [13]. Radiotherapy is also not indifferent, causing xerostomia, increased susceptibility to caries and periodontitis, tissue fibrosis, and opportunistic infections [14,15]. Because of the above, alternative treatment methods are sought, and PDT is one of them. The use of PDT in precancerous lesions and OSCC is being tested in preclinical and clinical trials with encouraging results [16–19]. One of the important directions of research is to understand the immunomodulatory effect of PDT.

The aim of our study was to evaluate the effect of PDT on the secretory activity of persistent oral squamous cell carcinoma cells and healthy cells that occur in the tumor environment fibroblasts.

2. Materials and Methods

2.1. Chemicals

Hypericin (HY), dimethyl sulfoxide (DMSO), MTT (3-[4,5-dimethylthiazol-2-yl]-2,5-diphenyltetrazolium bromide), and hydrocortisone were purchased from Sigma-Aldrich (St. Louis, MO, USA). Dulbecco's Modified Eagle's Medium (DMEM), DMEM: F-12, inactivated fetal bovine serum (FBS), and trypsin (0.23%)-ethylenediaminetetraacetic acid (EDTA) (0.53 mM) were obtained from ATCC (Manassas, VA, USA). Dulbecco's phosphate-buffered saline (DPBS) without calcium and magnesium ions was obtained from PAA. Bio-Plex Pro™ Assays were obtained from BIO-RAD Laboratories, Inc. (Hercules, CA, USA). All other chemicals were of analytical grade or purer.

2.2. Cell Cultures

Two cell lines were used in this study. The first one is an OSCC obtained from the tongue of a 70-year-old man—SCC-25 (ATCC CRL-1628). The second cell line is healthy gingival fibroblasts from a 28-year-old man—HGF-1 (ATCC CRL-2014). Frozen cell lines were purchased from ATCC (American Type Cell Culture—ATCC LGC Limited, London, UK).

2.3. Preparation of Cell Cultures

After defrosting, the cells were cultured strictly according to the manufacturer's recommendations. DMEM: F12 supplemented with 10% FBS and 400 ng/mL hydrocortisone was used to culture the SCC-25 line. For HGF-1, the culture medium was DMEM supplemented with 10% FBS. Cultures were carried in culture flasks with 25 cm^2 and 75 cm^2 cultivation areas at 37 °C, 5% carbon dioxide, and constant humidity. Culture media were changed 2–3 times a week for both lines. Cell passage was performed when the monolayer did not exceed 80% confluency. A 0.25% trypsin solution with 0.53 mM EDTA was used to harvest the cells. After 5–10 min of trypsinization, the cells were diluted in a culture medium, centrifuged, and resuspended in a culture medium.

2.4. Incubation of Cells with the HY

A 1 mM HY stock solution in DMSO was diluted to final concentrations of 0.25 µM, 0.5 µM, and 1 µM in the appropriate culture medium. The final DMSO concentration did not exceed 0.1%. The cells were suspended in appropriate culture media, HGF in the amount of 1×10^4/mL, and SCC-25 in the amount of 1×10^5/mL. After the cells were seeded on a 96-well plate at 200 µL per well, incubation was carried out for 24 h to obtain adherence. The medium was changed, and HY was added at concentrations of 0 µM, 0.25 µM, 0.5 µM, and 1 µM. After 2 h incubation, the medium was changed again, and the cells were washed with PBS without calcium and magnesium ions to remove unabsorbed PS.

2.5. Fluorescence Microscopy

The presence of HY in the cells was confirmed using the Olympus IX51 (Olympus Inc., Tokyo, Japan) with a color view camera and Cell F version 2.6 software (Soft Imaging System GmbH, Münster, Germany).

2.6. Cell Exposure to Light

The cells were irradiated with a PDT TP1 photodynamic therapy lamp (Cosmedico Medizintechnik GmbH, Stuttgart, Germany). It is an incoherent light source that emits light with wavelengths of 580–720 nm after installing an orange and infrared filter. To avoid the thermal effect, a double water filter was used. With the water filters, the fluence rate was 35 mW/cm^2. Cells were exposed to light at doses of 0 J/cm^2, 1 J/cm^2, 2 J/cm^2, 5 J/cm^2, 10 J/cm^2, and 20 J/cm^2. The exposure time was calculated automatically by the lamp controller. After irradiation, the cells were incubated for 24 h under the same conditions described previously.

2.7. MTT Assay for Cytotoxicity Evaluation

Supernatants were gently collected from above the cell surface. The cells were washed twice with PBS without magnesium and calcium ions. The appropriate culture medium with 0.5 mg/mL MTT was added to the cells. Only living cells can metabolize the yellow-colored soluble MTT into water-insoluble purple formazan crystals. After 4 h of incubation, the culture medium was removed, and the crystals were extracted with DMSO added in a volume of 200 µL. The plates were placed on a shaker for 10 min. Then, 150 µL of the solution was transferred onto a 96-well flat-bottom polypropylene plate. Absorbance at 550 nm was assessed using a microplate reader (ELx 800, Bio-Tek Instruments Inc., Winooski, VT, USA). MTT reduction was calculated as a percentage of the control group.

2.8. Cytokines Secretion Measurement

The measurement of interleukin 6(IL-6), soluble IL-6 receptor alpha (sIL-6Ralfa), sIL-6Rbeta, IL-8, IL-10, IL-11 IL-20, IL-32, and Pentraxin-3 (PTX3) was carried out 24 h after the application of PDT. To determine the level of cytokines, supernatants of cells on which PDT had a sublethal effect were selected, which allows the assessment of the immunomodulatory effect. Previous studies have used this procedure with OSCC and HGF-1 lines [20] and other cell lines [21,22]. Concentrations were assessed in supernatants using the Bio-Plex Pro™ Assay and Bio-Plex® 200 System (BIO-RAD Laboratories, Inc.). The multiplex assay method is commonly used to determine the concentration of cytokines in both clinical and preclinical studies [23,24]. All steps of the procedure were performed following the manufacturer's instructions. The experiments were repeated 4 times (*n* = 4).

2.9. Statistical Analysis

The Shapiro–Wilk test was used to check the normality of distribution. In the case of the MTT test, normality of distribution was obtained, and the percentage of MTT reduction of the study group with the control group was compared using the Student's t-test. Kruskal–Wallis analysis of variance (ANOVA) with post hoc analysis using the multiple comparison test was used for cytokine concentrations. The statistical analysis was performed in Statistica version 13 (TIBCO Software Inc., Palo Alto, CA, USA, 2017), and the charts were prepared using Excel® (Microsoft 365, 2303 version). Values of $p < 0.05$ were considered statistically significant.

3. Results

3.1. Fluorescence Microscopy

Images of cells obtained in a fluorescence microscope with a fluorescein isothiocyanate filter showed no fluorescence for the control group of cells not treated with HY and increasing fluorescence after incubation with PS solutions for both cancer cells and fibroblasts. The results are consistent with those previously published [20].

3.2. MTT Cytotoxicity Assay

MTT reduction was assessed for HY concentrations of 0, 0.25, 0.5, and 1 μM and light doses of 0, 1, 2, 5, 10, and 20 J/cm^2 and compared to a control group of cells not treated with PS or light. In the dark, HY showed no cytotoxic effect on tumor cells. On the other hand, in the case of fibroblasts, HY with the highest concentration significantly reduced MTT reduction (MTT reduction = 82.88% ± 2.84%). In the case of the irradiation of cells with a dose of 1 J/cm^2, a similar result was obtained in the form of HY cytotoxicity of 1 μM against HGF-1 cells (MTT reduction = 90.63% ± 5.06%). Interestingly, for the light dose of 2 J/cm^2, no cytotoxic effect of PDT was demonstrated; however, for the HY concentration of 0.5 μM, a stimulating effect on fibroblasts was demonstrated (MTT reduction = 119.37% ± 10.16%). The repeated MTT study showed that the results were consistent with those previously published. Charts for doses of 0–10 J/cm^2 are included in the Supplementary Material. Starting from a light dose of 5 J/cm^2, PDT showed a cytotoxic effect on SCC-25 and HGF1 cells; the effect was stronger with increasing light dose and PS concentration (Figure 1). Therefore, supernatants of cells treated with 0 J/cm^2, 1 J/cm^2, and 2 J/cm^2 and preincubated with doses of 0 μM, 0.25 μM, and 0.5 μM HY were used for further determinations.

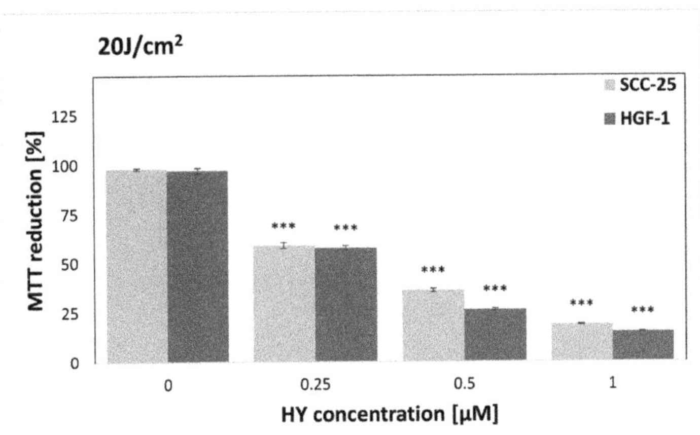

Figure 1. Percentage of MTT reduction by SCC-25 and HGF-1 cells after photodynamic therapy (PDT) using 0–1 μM hypericin (HY) doses and a 20 J/cm^2 light dose. The values represent the means ± standard error (SE). *** $p < 0.01$.

3.3. *Effect of HY-PDT on Secretory Activity: IL-6*

HY-PDT did not affect the secretion of IL-6 in both the SCC-25 and HGF-1 lines (Figures 2 and 3). There was a significantly higher production of IL-6 by fibroblasts compared to cancer cells in the corresponding groups. In the case of cancer cells, the level of IL-6 for the dark control without PS was 1.00 pg/mL ± 0.18 pg/mL. For gingival fibroblasts in the corresponding group, it was 4.60 pg/mL ± 0.23 pg/mL.

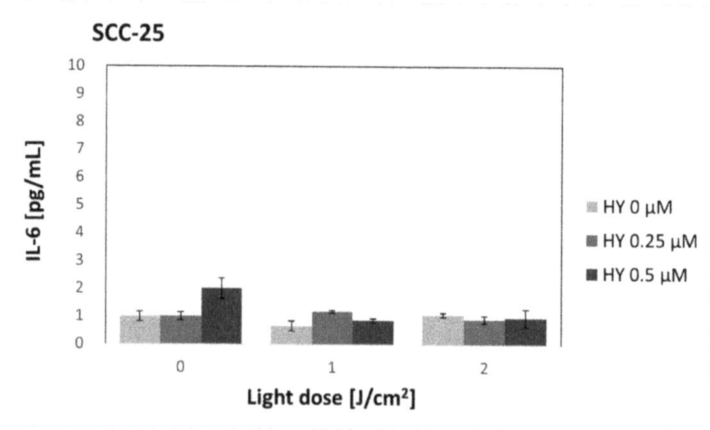

Figure 2. The concentration of interleukin 6 (IL-6) in the supernatants from the oral cancer cell culture SCC-25 line. The values represent the means ± SE.

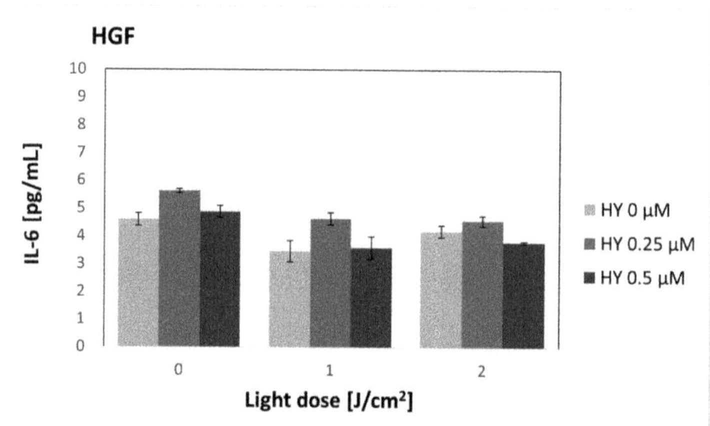

Figure 3. The concentration of IL-6 in the supernatants from the gingival fibroblast HGF-1 line. The values represent the means ± SE.

3.4. *Effect of HY-PDT on Secretory Activity: sIL-6Ralpha*

There were no changes in the secretion of sIL-6Ralpha after the use of HY-PDT in both cancer cells and fibroblasts (Figures 4 and 5). A significantly higher production of sIL-6Ralpha by cancer cells was found compared to fibroblasts in the corresponding groups. For the dark control without PS, in the case of SCC-25 cells, the sIL-6Ralpha level was 194.47 pg/mL ± 6.89 pg/mL, while for the HGF-1 line, it was 6.83 pg/mL.

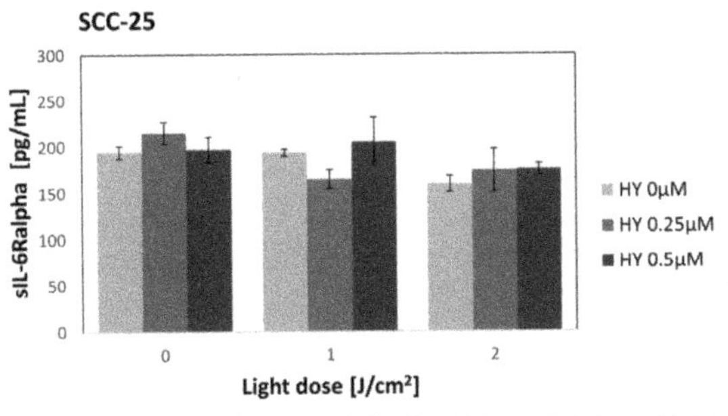

Figure 4. The concentration of sIL-6Ralpha in the supernatants from the oral cancer cell culture SCC-25 line. The values represent the means ± SE.

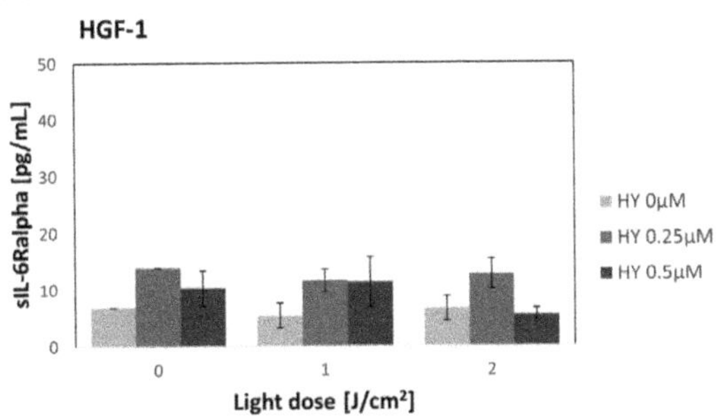

Figure 5. The concentration of sIL-6Ralpha in the supernatants from the gingival fibroblast HGF-1 line. The values represent the means ± SE.

3.5. Effect of HY-PDT on Secretory Activity: sIL-6Rbeta

HY alone did not cause significant changes in sIL-6Rbeta secretion (Figure 6). For the dark control without HY, sIL-6Rbeta production was found to be 32.69 pg/mL ± 4.69 pg/mL. In the case of cancer cells, a statistically significant change was found after applying a light dose of 2 J/cm^2. The sIL-6Rbeta level for 0 μM HY was 24.25 pg/mL ± 1.46 pg/mL, and for 0.5 μM HY, it was 43.73 pg/mL ± 3.64 pg/mL. The level of sIL-6Rbeta did not change after PDT application on fibroblasts (Figure 7). For the dark control, a value of 42.87 pg/mL ± 9.69 was obtained.

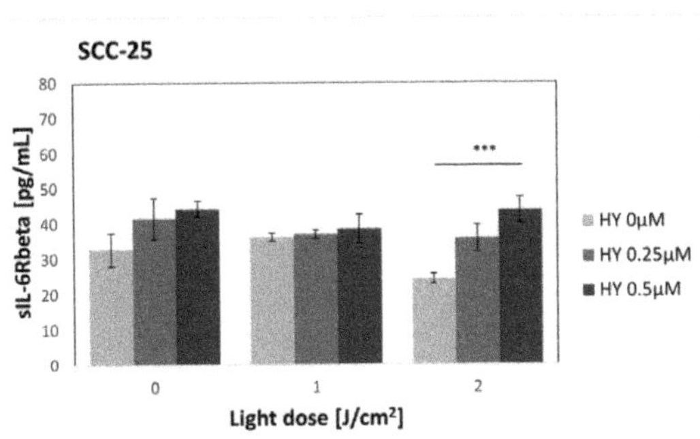

Figure 6. The concentration of sIL-6Rbeta in the supernatants from the oral cancer cell culture SCC-25 line. The values represent the means ± SE. The line over the bars indicates groups that were significantly different (Kruskal–Wallis Test and Dunn's multiple comparisons tests). *** $p < 0.01$.

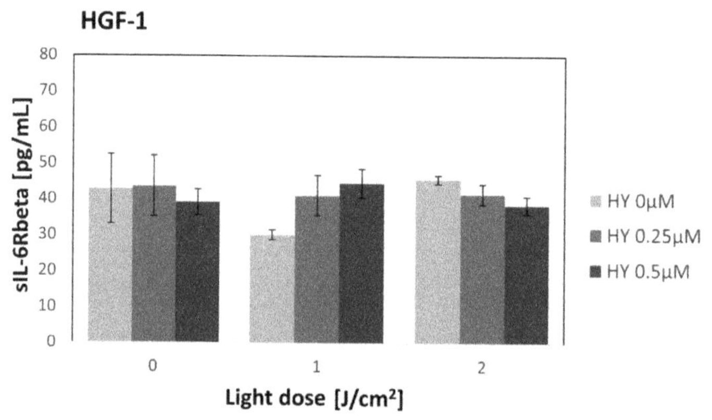

Figure 7. The concentration of sIL-6Rbeta in the supernatants from the gingival fibroblast HGF-1 line. The values represent the means ± SE.

3.6. Effect of HY-PDT on Secretory Activity: IL-8

There was an increase in the concentration of IL-8 for the SCC-25 line (Figure 8) between the control without PS and the 0.25 µM HY dose without irradiation. For the 0 µM dose, the cytokine concentration was 13.35 pg/mL ± 1.04 pg/mL, and for the 0.25 µM dose, it was 20.60 pg/mL ± 2.38 pg/mL. For other doses of the PS and light, no statistically significant differences were found in the case of cancer cells.

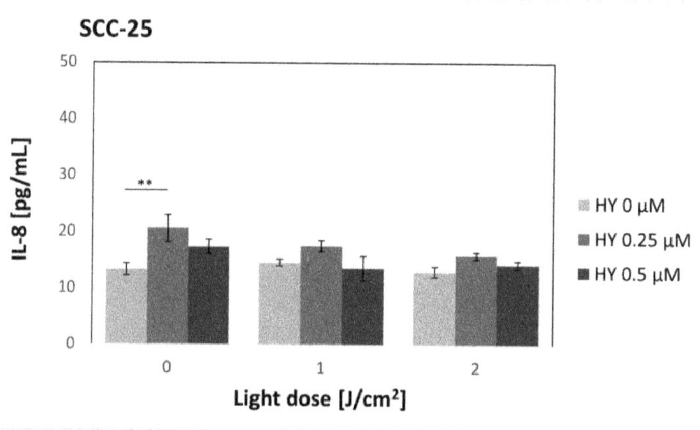

Figure 8. The concentration of IL-8 in the supernatants from the oral cancer cell culture SCC-25 line. The values represent the means ± SE. The line over the bars indicates groups that were significantly different (Kruskal–Wallis Test and Dunn's multiple comparisons tests). ** $p < 0.05$.

As for the HGF-1 line (Figure 9), a statistically significant increase in IL-8 concentration was also demonstrated after using PS alone at a dose of 0.25 µM without the use of light compared to the dose of 0 µM HY; the concentration values were 25.85 pg/mL ± 0.42 pg/mL and 12.88 pg/mL ± 0.81 pg/mL, respectively. A similar picture is visible for the light dose of 1 J/cm^2, where for the dose of 0 µM, the concentration of IL-8 was 8.46 pg/mL ± 0.89 pg/mL, and after PDT, with the use of 0.25 µM HY, it was 19.40 pg/mL ± 1.3 pg/mL. The situation is different at the light dose of 2 J/cm^2, where after irradiation of cells not incubated with PS, there was an increase in the concentration of IL-8 (21.47 pg/mL ± 2.35 pg/mL).

However, it was not a statistically significant increase compared to the dark control. After using HY, the 0.25 μM concentration remained similar (23.16 pg/mL ± 1.29). In the case of cells incubated with 0.5 μM HY, there was a significant decrease in IL-8 concentration (11.43 pg/mL ± 0.74).

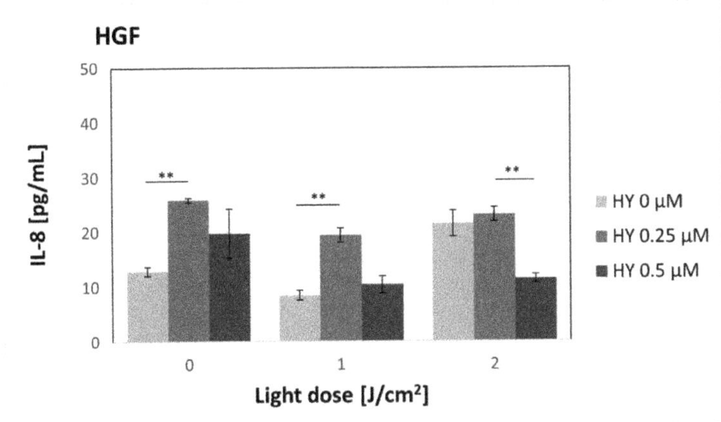

Figure 9. The concentration of IL-8 in the supernatants from the gingival fibroblast HGF-1 line. The values represent the means ± SE. The lines over the bars indicate groups that were significantly different (Kruskal–Wallis Test and Dunn's multiple comparisons tests). ** $p < 0.05$.

3.7. *Effect of HY-PDT on Secretory Activity: IL-10*

In the case of IL-10, no statistically significant differences were demonstrated for both the SCC-25 and HGF-1 cell lines (Figures 10 and 11). In the case of SCC-25, the cytokine level was 4.80 pg/mL ± 1.14 pg/mL, while for HGF-1, it was 6.84 pg/mL ± 1.74 pg/mL.

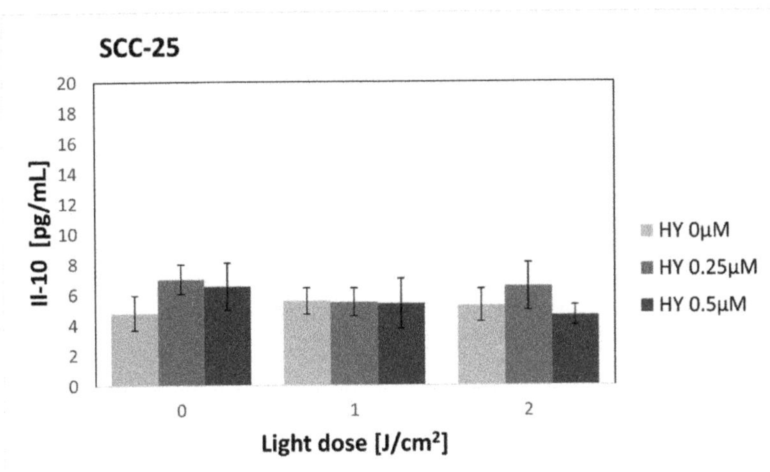

Figure 10. The concentration of IL-10 in the supernatants from the oral cancer cell culture SCC-25 line. The values represent the means ± SE.

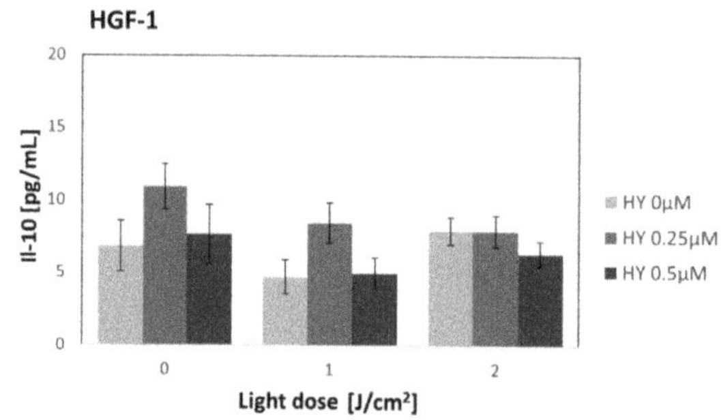

Figure 11. The concentration of IL-10 in the supernatants from the gingival fibroblast HGF-1 line. The values represent the means ± SE.

3.8. *Effect of HY-PDT on Secretory Activity: IL-11*

There were no changes in the concentration of IL-11 after using PDT in the case of the SCC-25 line (Figure 12). In the control group, the secretion reached 106.67 pg/mL ± 4.19. For HGF-1 (Figure 13), an increase in cytokine concentration was noted after using 0.25 μM HY alone (169.60 pg/mL ± 14.19 pg/mL) and 2 J/cm^2 irradiation alone (153.75 pg/mL ± 26.66 pg/mL) compared to the control group (119.91 pg/mL ± 4.24 pg/mL). Those differences, however, were not statistically significant.

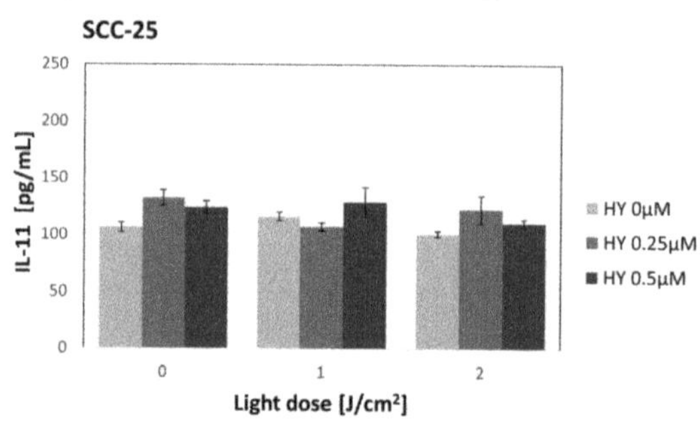

Figure 12. The concentration of IL-11 in the supernatants from the oral cancer cell culture SCC-25 line. The values represent the means ± SE.

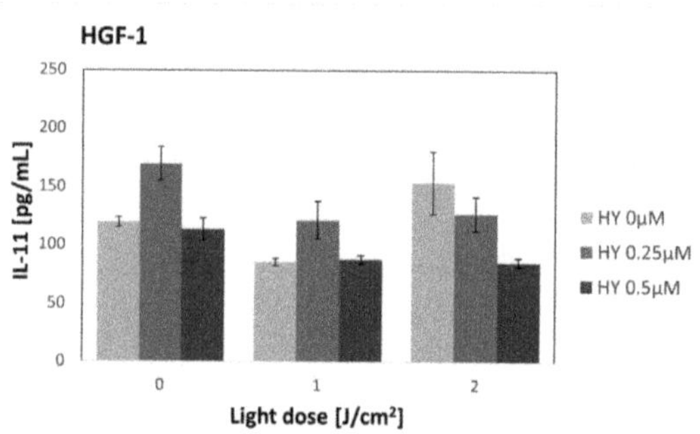

Figure 13. The concentration of IL-11 in the supernatants from the gingival fibroblast HGF-1 line. The values represent the means ± SE.

3.9. Effect of HY-PDT on Secretory Activity: IL-20

The use of HY in doses of 0.25 μM and 0.5 μM increased the secretion of IL-20 compared to the control group of SCC-25 (8.54 pg/mL ± 1.40 pg/mL) (Figure 14). However, it was not statistically significant. After using PDT, the secretion of IL-20 significantly increased for cancer cells incubated with 0.5 μM HY and irradiated with 1 J/cm^2 (18.67 pg/mL ± 1.75 pg/mL). In the case of a light dose of 2 J/cm^2, a statistically significant increase in the secretion of this cytokine was found for both 0.25 μM HY (20.18 pg/mL ± 1.73 pg/mL) and 0.5 μM HY (18.68 pg/mL ± 0.66 pg/mL). In the case of HGF-1 cells, no secretion of this cytokine was found.

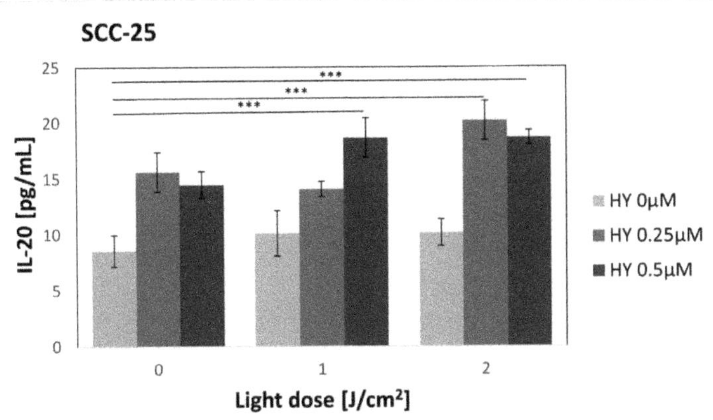

Figure 14. The concentration of IL-20 in the supernatants from the oral cancer cell culture SCC-25 line. The values represent the means ± SE. The lines over the bars indicate groups that were significantly different (Kruskal–Wallis Test and Dunn's multiple comparisons tests). *** $p < 0.01$.

3.10. Effect of HY-PDT on Secretory Activity: IL-32

There was no change in IL-32 secretion after applying PDT to SCC-25 cells (Figure 15). In the control group, the concentration was 244.89 pg/mL ± 10.35 pg/mL. In the case of fibroblasts (Figure 16), there was a statistically significant decrease in the cytokine concentration after applying PDT at a dose of 2 J/cm^2 and 0.25 μM HY compared to the control group. The values were 215.55 pg/mL ± 11.10 pg/mL and 291.51 pg/mL ± 10.63 pg/mL, respectively.

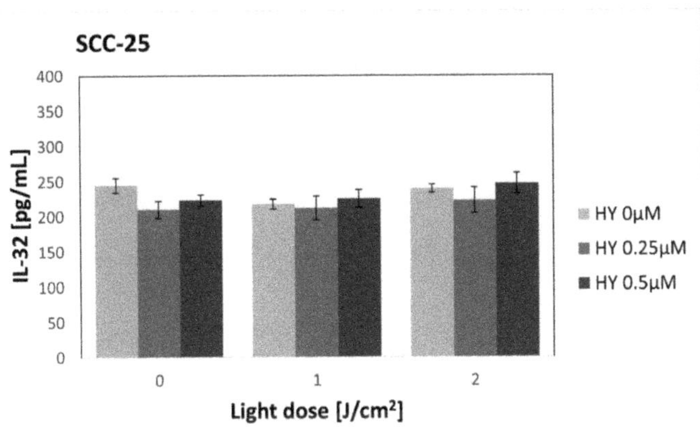

Figure 15. The concentration of IL-32 in the supernatants from the oral cancer cell culture SCC-25 line. The values represent the means ± SE.

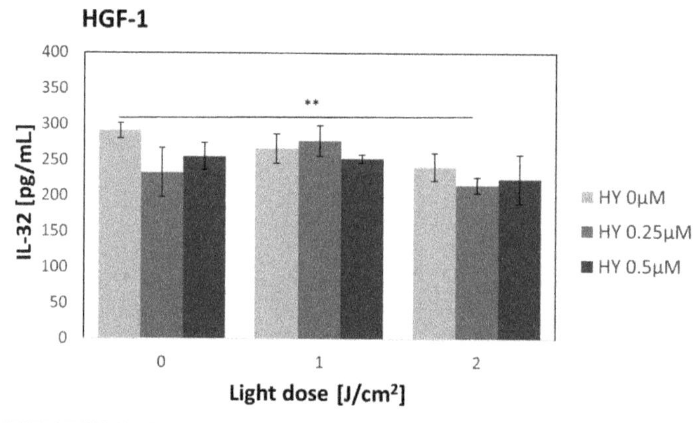

Figure 16. The concentration of IL-32 in the supernatants from the gingival fibroblast HGF-1 line. The values represent the means ± SE. The line over the bars indicates groups that were significantly different (Kruskal–Wallis Test and Dunn's multiple comparisons tests). ** $p < 0.05$.

3.11. Effect of HY-PDT on Secretory Activity: PTX3

The SCC-25 control group had a PTX3 secretion of 356.23 pg/mL ± 10.21 pg/mL. After HY alone, there was an insignificant increase in PTX3 secretion for both 0.25 µM HY (516.66 pg/mL ± 36.00 pg/mL) and 0.5 µM HY (458.04 pg/mL ± 46.78 pg/mL). After using HY-PDT, the PTX3 secretion decreased again. In the group with 0.5 µM HY and 2 J/cm^2, the level was 180.91 pg/mL ± 26.36 pg/mL. However, there was no significant difference compared to the control group (p = 0.073) (Figure 17). There were statistical differences between the remaining groups but without any visible dependence on the dose of light or PS used. Therefore, this was not placed on the graph so as not to limit its readability. The level of the PTX3 secreted by the HGF-1 line was below the quantifiable value.

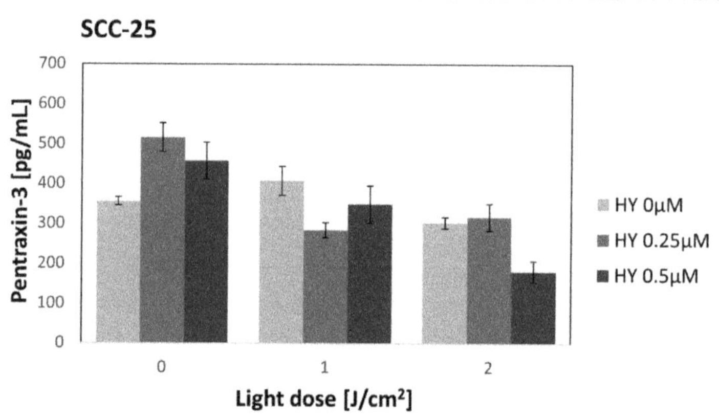

Figure 17. The concentration of PTX3 in the supernatants from the oral cancer cell culture SCC-25 line. The values represent the means ± SE.

4. Discussion

The effect of HY-PDT on the secretion of selected cytokines by persistent OSCC cells was assessed. The tumor microenvironment (TME) of oral cancer is complex, consisting of cellular components and an extracellular matrix. Cellular components include immune cells and stromal cells. The main group of stromal cells are cancer-associated fibroblasts (CAF). Fibroblasts located in the TME may secrete cytokines, influencing tumor progression, metastasis, or escape from the immune system [25]. For this reason, the authors chose oral cancer cell lines (SCC-25) and fibroblasts (HGF-1) for this study.

Immune, healthy, and malignant cells are in a close relationship during cancer development. A cancer's distinctive characteristic is its ability to combat the immune system. Cytokines play a key role in intercellular interactions in a tumor environment. They have concentration-dependent and multidirectional effects due to the multitude of cells that secrete them, the presence of diverse receptors, and signaling pathways. Therefore, the cytokine can be responsible for the initiation, progression, and, even further, the inhibition of tumor development [26].

Cancer cells can be characterized by overexpression of certain cytokines groups, e.g., IL-6 or IL-11. These act in an autocrine manner, leading to increased proliferation, stimulation of migration, inhibition of apoptosis, and further production of cytokines, e.g., IL-8. IL-8, among others, that is secreted by the tumor may promote an immunosuppressive tumor environment by recruiting polymorphonuclear leukocytes [27]. Il-6 and Il-8 are considered oncogenic cytokines because they are associated with epithelial-mesenchymal transition, disrupting intercellular interactions, hindering macrophage function, and promoting cancer cell invasion. Increased levels of these cytokines were found in patients with OSCC [28].

Unlike many soluble interleukin receptors, which act antagonistically when bound to interleukin, the Il-6/sIl-6R complex acts agonistically and will broaden the spectrum of the cells it acts on via membrane-bound gp130. This complex influences cell proliferation, differentiation, and regulation of plan-state mediators and also extends the half-life of Il-6. IL-11 also signals through gp130 and therefore has an overlapping effect with the mentioned complex and may mimic the stimulatory properties of Il-6/sIl-6R [29,30].

In the tumor microenvironment, IL-10 has a pleiotropic effect. It can both activate cytotoxic T lymphocytes and have an immunosuppressive effect, inhibiting the secretion of IL-12 and the inflammatory process [27]. Immunosuppressive cytokines may have a bidirectional effect, inhibiting the pro-inflammatory effects leading to tumor progression, or may reduce the anti-tumor immune response. Also, the concentration of IL-10 may be increased in patients with OSCC, and its increased expression is associated with a more aggressive type of OSCC [28]. IL-20 has a tumor growth-promoting effect by inducing programmed cell death protein [27].

Fibroblasts participate in the immune response that involves the secretion of pro-inflammatory cytokines and the presentation of antigens to T lymphocytes. The secretion of cytokines by fibroblasts depends on the stimulating factor. It is controlled at the level of transcription, translation, and post-translational processing, among others [31]. CAFs play a key role in cancer development. They can induce tumor immunosuppression through the secretion of, for instance, IL-6 and IL-32 [32,33].

Determining cytokine secretion after PDT can allow for a better understanding of the mechanisms of the therapy's immunomodulatory effect.

The use of PDT in the treatment of pre-cancerous lesions as well as OSCC is extensively studied in in vitro preclinical studies [17], an animal model [16], and clinical trials [34]. The results of these studies encourage further study of the mechanisms of PDT action and the search for the most effective procedure for a given type of cancer. In addition to the direct cytotoxic effect, an important mechanism is an immunomodulatory effect [1]. Our study used HY as a PS and an incoherent light source for photodynamic action. Such a procedure has been reported previously in studies on colorectal cancer cells [35] and our earlier OSCC studies [20]. Using sublethal doses, we demonstrated the immunomodulatory effect of PDT and changes in the secretion of cytokines such as sIL-6Rbeta, IL-8, IL-20, IL-32, and PTX3.

According to the authors' best knowledge, this is the first study using Hypericin in PDT of OSCC and assessing its effect on the secretion of the cytokines mentioned above by cancer cells and fibroblasts potentially located in the TME. The cytokines were selected based on their previously described effects on cancer development and their interactions.

In our study, we repeated the MTT cytotoxicity test, and the results were consistent with those obtained in the previous study. Due to the reproducibility of HY-PDT cytotoxicity results, we refer readers to the Supplemental Material and the authors' earlier studies for detailed results [20]. In our study, we found no cytotoxic effect of HY in the dark, except for the highest dose of PS applied to fibroblasts. A similar effect was found for a light dose of 1 J/cm^2. The cytotoxic effect of HY has already been observed in the dark at higher concentrations [36]. In the case of light irradiation of 2 J/cm^2, a stimulating effect on HGF-1 cells was found when 0.5 μM HY was used; moreover, no phototoxic effect of 1 μM HY was observed as in the case of lower light doses. Authors suspect that this result is related to the photobiomodulating effect of subthreshold doses of light. Etemadi et al. demonstrated the stimulating effect of low light doses on healthy gingival fibroblasts [37]. Starting from 5 J/cm^2, we found increasing cytotoxicity of PDT against both the SCC-25 and HGF-1 lines, with increasing light and PS doses. A linear increase in HY cytotoxicity with increasing concentration towards HNSCC cells was also observed by Bublik et al. [38].

The cytotoxic effect was observed both against cancer cells and healthy gingival fibroblasts, which indicates the lack of selectivity of HY towards cancer cells. This also indicates the need to target the cancer cells to avoid damage to healthy tissues. Similar observations were found in a study of leukemic and healthy bone marrow cells [39] In the case of studies on 2D monocultures, both cancer and healthy cells have direct contact with PS dissolved in the culture medium; therefore, HY easily enters both groups of cells [40].

It is widely known that cytokines are secreted by immune system cells; they play a vital role in both inhibition and progression of the cancer process. However, in addition to the immune cells, cancer cells themselves can produce cytokines [27]. Only living cells can actively secrete proteins; therefore, to determine the influence of cancer cells on the immunomodulatory effect of PDT, tests were performed for sublethal doses. Moreover, from a clinical point of view, it is important to understand the behavior of residual cancer cells in the event that the treatment is not radical, as well as the response of accompanying healthy cells.

Our previous studies on HY-PDT showed increased secretion of the soluble receptor for tumor necrosis factor alpha by SCC-25 cells after applying sublethal doses of light and PS [20]. Kaleta-Richter et al. showed the effect of sublethal doses of HY-PDT on the secretion of IL-8 depending on the malignancy of the cells. However, they did not show the effect of HY-PDT on the secretion of IL-10 [35]. These results correlate with our results because we also, in our experiments, did not obtain statistically significant differences after using PDT on IL-10 secretion. In the case of IL-8, in our experiment, we noted the stimulating effect of HY alone without light in both the HGF-1 and SCC-25 lines. No such effect was found in the study on colorectal cancer cells. Similar results were obtained by Du et al. on nasopharyngeal cells. They also found an increase in IL-8 production after using HY alone. At the same time, HY-PDT did not affect the production of this cytokine. They did not find any effect of HY and HY-PDT on the level of IL-10 [41].

Barathan et al. used HY-PDT against a human hepatocellular liver carcinoma cell line and found an increase in IL-6 secretion after the therapy. The most significant increase was noted when the cells were preincubated with HY at a concentration of 1.98 μM. Similarly, they found an increase in the secretion of IL-4, IL-10, and IFN-gamma, but at much lower values [42]. Our studies did not find statistically significant differences in the secretion of IL-6 and IL-10. However, the highest dose for which we determined the secretion of cytokines was 0.5 μM HY. In in vitro and in vivo studies on nasopharyngeal carcinoma cells, Du et al. found that the level of IL-6 gene expression and IL-6 secretion after applying HY-PDT depends on the degree of histological differentiation, basal cytokine production, and cell type. Researchers found higher levels of IL-6 in less differentiated cells [43].

IL-6 has two different signaling pathways. It can bind to a membrane receptor (mIL-6R) or a soluble (sIL-6R). The classical pathway is restricted to cells expressing a membrane-bound receptor. Proteolytic cleavage generates sIL-6R, which also can bind IL-6. The IL-6/sIL-6R complex can stimulate cells that do not have a receptor on their surface in the mechanism of the so-called trans-signaling [44]. We have demonstrated the production of sIL-6Ralpha and sIL-6Rbeta by the SCC-25 cells and that using PDT can affect the level of sIL-6Rbeta. Hwang et al. showed that sIL-6R is involved in osteoclast formation stimulated by OSCC [45]. Wang et al., examining samples from patients with OSCC, found a significantly higher expression of IL-6R and IL-6 mRNA transcripts in tumor tissue compared to healthy tissue. Receptor overexpression was associated with more histologically advanced and more extensive tumors [46].

We found increased IL-20 secretion by the SCC-25 cells after applying HY-PDT. IL-20 belongs to the IL-10 family and is a pro-inflammatory cytokine that plays an essential role in developing inflammatory diseases, such as psoriasis and rheumatoid arthritis [47]. Hsu et al. showed a higher expression of IL-20 and its receptors in the tumor tissue of patients with OSCC. The level correlated with the advancement of the tumor, which may indicate the involvement of this cytokine in the pathogenesis of OSCC. In in vitro studies, they found that IL-20 caused increased tumor cell proliferation and ROS production. In turn, administering an IL-20 inhibitor reduced proliferation and ROS production. Incubation of the OSCC cells with IL-20 increased expression of the pro-inflammatory cytokines TNF-α, IL-1β, and MCP-1, but not IL-6, IL-8, matrix metalloproteinase-2 (MMP-2), MMP-7, and MMP-9. In addition, IL-20 promoted tumor cell colony formation on agar, and a monoclonal antibody to IL-20 inhibited tumor growth in vivo. A possible cause of increased IL-20 secretion by cells is hypoxia [48]. Chen et al. found an increase in the production of IL-20 by HaCaT cells, keratinocytes, renal epithelial cells, monocytes, and chondrocytes in a hypoxic environment and increased levels of the cytokine after experimental ischemic stroke in a rat [49].

The function of IL-32 is not fully understood in cancer development. Studies indicate that it affects proliferation and metastasis by affecting the NF-κB pathway, STAT3, and MAPK signaling [50]. Guenina et al., in a study of OSCC patients, found that IL-32 overexpression was associated with reduced patient survival due to a potential role in metastasis [51]. Our study found that HY-PDT did not significantly affect IL-32 production by SCC-25 but decreased IL-32 production by HGF-1 cells. Wen et al. showed in their study on cancer-associated fibroblast (CAF) that IL-32-secreting fibroblasts promoted invasion and metastasis of breast cancer. They found that IL-32, interacting with β3 integrin, plays a significant role in the invasiveness of breast cancer. CAF-derived IL-32 bound to β3 integrin activating the MAPK pathway. This signaling resulted in the overexpression of fibronectin, N-cadherin, and vimentin. The knockdown of IL-32, β3 integrin, and blockade of MAPK signaling reduced the invasiveness of breast cancer [33].

PTX3 plays a key role in innate immunity. It can be overexpressed in many types of cancer and act as a prognostic factor. Its diverse activity in oncogenesis can play anti-cancer and pro-cancer roles [52]. Chang et al. found that malignant and metastatic HNSCC cells overexpress the PTX3 gene. EGF-induced PTX3 expression followed the PI3K/Akt and NF-κB pathways. Autocrine secretion of PTX3 increased the production of fibronectin and MMP-9, which promoted metastasis [53]. Chan et al. found that oleate increased PTX3 expression and secretion by activating the Akt/NF-κB pathway in HNSCC cells. Depleting PTX3 and inhibiting NF-κB reduced migration and invasiveness of HNSCC cells. PTX3 depletion also reduced the oleate-induced epithelial-mesenchymal transition markers vimentin and MMP-3. In addition, after PTX3 depletion, the researchers found that lung metastasis was blocked in mice [54]. In a study of cervical cancer, Ying et al. found that increased PTX3 expression was associated with tumor progression, and PTX3 knockdown resulted in reduced tumor cell viability, impaired colony formation, cell cycle arrest in the G2/M phase, and inhibition of MMP-2, MMP-9, and urokinase plasminogen activator. Blockade of PTX3 resulted in reduced carcinogenicity in mice and potential for lung metastasis [55].

There is evidence that HY can act on cells independently without irradiation. Our study demonstrated the cytotoxic effect of HY on HGF-1 cells at a concentration of 1 μM, while Besic Gyenge et al. demonstrated the cytotoxic effect of HY also on HSCC cells in the dark [36]. Huntosova et al. studied the effect of light-independent HY on glioma cells and benign endothelial cells. It showed faster uptake of HY by malignant cells, which was explained by the likely faster proliferation and metabolism of malignant cells. HY caused hyperpolarization of the mitochondrion and increased reactive oxygen species (ROS), but this was at a lower level than that induced by PDT. Moreover, HY caused an increase in the share of glycolysis in the cellular metabolism of malignant cells, indicating the PS's ability to slow down the metabolism. HY in the dark showed a cytotoxic effect, and a higher level of toxicity was noted for endothelial cells than for glioblastoma [56]. Martínez-Poveda et al. showed on endothelial cells that HY not activated by light had an IC50 of 10 μM, while it had an IC50 of 13 nM when activated by light. In addition, HY in the dark inhibited endothelial tube formation on Matrigel, reduced urokinase production, and had an inhibitory effect on the wound healing assay [57].

HY exhibits absorption of electromagnetic radiation with a wavelength of 500 to 620 with a maximum at 595 nm [58]. Light of the mentioned length is characterized by poor penetration into tissues; therefore, in clinical conditions, it would enable the therapy of superficial precancerous lesions and the initial stages of cancer development [59]. The PS used is characterized by poor solubility in water, which requires modification with other ingredients before use [58].

A limitation of our experiment is that the study was conducted on a monolayer of cells. Such a model does not reflect the actual structure of the tumor or tissues. There is no extracellular matrix and proper intercellular interaction. The above-mentioned factors can affect cell proliferation, viability, and secretory activity, including cytokine secretion. In addition, the cultured cells have unlimited access to nutrients and oxygen, but also to the ingredients being tested [40,60]. In fact, the tumor structure is complex and there are other cells in the tumor environment, so what is important in determining the immunomodulatory effect of therapy is to see whether there are cells of the immune system. Among the immunomodulatory effects are those on the tumor microenvironment and intercellular interactions, where both cancer cells and immune cells coexist. Therefore, confirming the research results achieved with monolayer-cultured cells in spheroid studies with co-culture of immune cells, animal studies, and preferably in clinical trials is vital.

5. Conclusions

We confirmed the cytotoxic effect of HY-PDT on oral cancer cells and fibroblasts. We showed the immunomodulatory effect of sublethal doses of PDT and the possible effect of HY alone without irradiation. HY-PDT affected the SCC-25 cell secretion of sIL-6Rbeta, IL-20. HY alone increased the IL-8 secretion. In the case of HGF-1, the effect of HY-PDT on the secretion of IL-8 and IL-32 was found. There were no statistically significant differences in the secretion of IL-6, sIL-6Ralpha, IL-10, IL-11, or Pentraxin-3. However, no dependence on the change in the secretion of the above-mentioned cytokines on the increase in the dose of light or hypericin was observed.

Supplementary Materials: The following supporting information can be downloaded at: https://www.mdpi.com/article/10.3390/pharmaceutics16010042/s1, Figure S1: Images of SCC-25 cells taken using an inverted fluorescence microscope. (A) Control group without PS. (B) PS absorption after incubation with 0.25 μM HY. (C) PS absorption after incubation with 0.5 μM HY. (D) PS absorption after incubation with 1 μM HY; Figure S2: Images of HGF-1 cells taken using an inverted fluorescence microscope. (A) Control group without PS. (B) PS absorption after incubation with 0.25 μM HY. (C) PS absorption after incubation with 0.5 μM HY. (D) PS absorption after incubation with 1 μM HY; Figure S3: Percentage of MTT reduction by SCC-25 and HGF-1 cells after PDT using 0–1 μM HY doses and a 0 J/cm^2 light dose. The values represent the means ± SE. *** $p < 0.01$; Figure S4: Percentage of MTT reduction by SCC-25 and HGF-1 cells after PDT using 0–1 μM HY doses and a 1 J/cm^2 light dose. The values represent the means ± SE. ** $p < 0.05$; Figure S5: Percentage of MTT reduction by SCC-25 and HGF-1 cells after PDT using 0–1 μM HY doses and a 2 J/cm^2 light dose. The values represent the means ± SE. *** $p < 0.01$; Figure S6: Percentage of MTT reduction by SCC-25 and HGF-1 cells after PDT using 0–1 µM HY doses and a 5 J/cm^2 light dose. The values represent the means ± SE. ** $p < 0.05$, *** $p < 0.01$; Figure S7: Percentage of MTT reduction by SCC-25 and HGF-1 cells after PDT using 0–1 µM HY doses and a 10 J/cm^2 light dose. The values represent the means ± SE. *** $p < 0.01$.

Author Contributions: Conceptualization, M.O., A.K.-K. and A.M.-P.; methodology, Z.P.C. and A.K.-K.; validation, G.C.; formal analysis: Z.P.C. and A.M.-P.; data curation, M.O.; writing—original draft preparation, M.O., A.M.-P. and A.K.-K.; writing—review and editing, M.O., A.M.-P. and A.K.-K.; visualization, M.O.; supervision, A.M.-P., A.K.-K. and Z.P.C. All authors have read and agreed to the published version of the manuscript.

Funding: This research was funded by the Medical University of Silesia, Katowice, grant number PCN-2-089/N/1/K.

Institutional Review Board Statement: Not applicable.

Informed Consent Statement: Not applicable.

Data Availability Statement: The data can be shared up on request.

Conflicts of Interest: The authors declare no conflicts of interest.

References

1. Allison, R.R.; Moghissi, K. Photodynamic Therapy (PDT): PDT Mechanisms. *Clin. Endosc.* **2013**, *46*, 24–29. [CrossRef] [PubMed]
2. Robertson, C.A.; Evans, D.H.; Abrahamse, H. Photodynamic therapy (PDT): A short review on cellular mechanisms and cancer research applications for PDT. *J. Photochem. Photobiol. B* **2009**, *96*, 1–8. [CrossRef] [PubMed]
3. Plaetzer, K.; Krammer, B.; Berlanda, J.; Berr, F.; Kiesslich, T. Photophysics and photochemistry of photodynamic therapy: Fundamental aspects. *Lasers Med. Sci.* **2009**, *24*, 259–268. [CrossRef] [PubMed]
4. Kwiatkowski, S.; Knap, B.; Przystupski, D.; Saczko, J.; Kędzierska, E.; Knap-Czop, K.; Kotlińska, J.; Michel, O.; Kotowski, K.; Kulbacka, J. Photodynamic therap -mechanisms, photosensitizers and combinations. *Biomed. Pharmacother.* **2018**, *106*, 1098–1107. [CrossRef] [PubMed]
5. Dougherty, T.J.; Gomer, C.J.; Henderson, B.W.; Jori, G.; Kessel, D.; Korbelik, M.; Moan, J.; Peng, Q. Photodynamic therapy. *J. Natl. Cancer Inst.* **1998**, *90*, 889–905. [CrossRef] [PubMed]
6. WHO International Agency for Research on Cancer. Available online: https://gco.iarc.fr/ (accessed on 26 June 2023).
7. Chamoli, A.; Gosavi, A.S.; Shirwadkar, U.P.; Wangdale, K.V.; Behera, S.K.; Kurrey, N.K.; Kalia, K.; Mandoli, A. Overview of oral cavity squamous cell carcinoma: Risk factors, mechanisms, and diagnostics. *Oral Oncol.* **2021**, *121*, 105451. [CrossRef] [PubMed]
8. Paver, E.C.; Currie, A.M.; Gupta, R.; Dahlstrom, J.E. Human papilloma virus related squamous cell carcinomas of the head and neck: Diagnosis, clinical implications and detection of HPV. *Pathology* **2020**, *52*, 179–191. [CrossRef]
9. Singh, S.; Singh, A.K. Porphyromonas gingivalis in oral squamous cell carcinoma: A review. *Microbes Infect.* **2022**, *24*, 104925. [CrossRef]
10. Omura, K. Current status of oral cancer treatment strategies: Surgical treatments for oral squamous cell carcinoma. *Int. J. Clin. Oncol.* **2014**, *19*, 423–430. [CrossRef]
11. Philips, R.; Martin, D.; Eskander, A.; Schord, J.; Brown, N.; Zhao, S.; Brock, G.; Kumar, B.; Carrau, R.; Ozer, E.; et al. Effect of adjuvant radiotherapy treatment center volume on overall survival. *Oral Oncol.* **2018**, *78*, 46–51. [CrossRef]
12. Mücke, T.; Koschinski, J.; Wolff, K.D.; Kanatas, A.; Mitchell, D.A.; Loeffelbein, D.J.; Deppe, H.; Rau, A. Quality of life after different oncologic interventions in head and neck cancer patients. *J. Cranio-Maxillofac. Surg.* **2015**, *43*, 1895–1898. [CrossRef] [PubMed]
13. Gellrich, N.C.; Schimming, R.; Schramm, A.; Schmalohr, D.; Bremerich, A.; Kugler, J. Pain, function, and psychologic outcome before, during, and after intraoral tumor resection. *J. Oral Maxillofac. Surg.* **2002**, *60*, 772–777. [CrossRef] [PubMed]
14. Kakoei, S.; Haghdoost, A.A.; Rad, M.; Mohammadalizadeh, S.; Pourdamghan, N.; Nakhaei, M.; Bahador, M. Xerostomia after radiotherapy and its effect on quality of life in head and neck cancer patients. *Arch. Iran. Med.* **2012**, *15*, 214–218. [PubMed]
15. Sroussi, H.Y.; Epstein, J.B.; Bensadoun, R.J.; Saunders, D.P.; Lalla, R.V.; Migliorati, C.A.; Heaivilin, N.; Zumsteg, Z.S. Common oral complications of head and neck cancer radiation therapy: Mucositis, infections, saliva change, fibrosis, sensory dysfunctions, dental caries, periodontal disease, and osteoradionecrosis. *Cancer Med.* **2017**, *6*, 2918–2931. [CrossRef] [PubMed]
16. Olek, M.; Machorowska-Pieniążek, A.; Olek, K.; Cieślar, G.; Kawczyk-Krupka, A. Photodynamic therapy in the treatment of oral squamous cell carcinoma—The state of the art in preclinical research on the animal model. *Photodiagnosis Photodyn. Ther.* **2021**, *34*, 102236. [CrossRef]
17. Olek, M.; Kasperski, J.; Skaba, D.; Wiench, R.; Cieślar, G.; Kawczyk-Krupka, A. Photodynamic therapy for the treatment of oral squamous carcinoma-Clinical implications resulting from in vitro research. *Photodiagnosis Photodyn. Ther.* **2019**, *27*, 255–267. [CrossRef]

18. Volgger, V.; Betz, C.S. Photodynamic therapy in the upper aerodigestive tract. Overview and outlook. *J. Biophotonics* **2016**, *9*, 1302–1313. [CrossRef]
19. Meulemans, J.; Delaere, P.; Vander Poorten, V. Photodynamic therapy in head and neck cancer: Indications, outcomes, and future prospects. *Curr. Opin. Otolaryngol. Head Neck Surg.* **2019**, *27*, 136–141. [CrossRef]
20. Olek, M.; Machorowska-Pieniążek, A.; Czuba, Z.P.; Cieślar, G.; Kawczyk-Krupka, A. Effect of Hypericin-Mediated Photodynamic Therapy on the Secretion of Soluble TNF Receptors by Oral Cancer Cells. *Pharmaceutics* **2023**, *15*, 1279. [CrossRef]
21. Wei, L.H.; Baumann, H.; Tracy, E.; Wang, Y.; Hutson, A.; Rose-John, S.; Henderson, B.W. Interleukin-6 trans signalling enhances photodynamic therapy by modulating cell cycling. *Br. J. Cancer* **2007**, *97*, 1513–1522. [CrossRef]
22. Dorst, D.N.; van Caam, A.P.M.; Vitters, E.L.; Walgreen, B.; Helsen, M.M.A.; Klein, C.; Gudi, S.; Wubs, T.; Kumari, J.; Vonk, M.C.; et al. Fibroblast Activation Protein Targeted Photodynamic Therapy Selectively Kills Activated Skin Fibroblasts from Systemic Sclerosis Patients and Prevents Tissue Contraction. *Int. J. Mol. Sci.* **2021**, *22*, 12681. [CrossRef] [PubMed]
23. Feurino, L.W.; Zhang, Y.; Bharadwaj, U.; Zhang, R.; Li, F.; Fisher, W.E.; Brunicardi, F.C.; Chen, C.; Yao, Q.; Min, L. IL-6 stimulates Th2 type cytokine secretion and upregulates VEGF and NRP-1 expression in pancreatic cancer cells. *Cancer Biol. Ther.* **2007**, *6*, 1096–1100. [CrossRef] [PubMed]
24. Gabitass, R.F.; Annels, N.E.; Stocken, D.D.; Pandha, H.A.; Middleton, G.W. Elevated myeloid-derived suppressor cells in pancreatic, esophageal and gastric cancer are an independent prognostic factor and are associated with significant elevation of the Th2 cytokine interleukin-13. *Cancer Immunol. Immunother.* **2011**, *60*, 1419–1430. [CrossRef]
25. Liu, C.; Wang, M.; Zhang, H.; Li, C.; Zhang, T.; Liu, H.; Zhu, S.; Chen, J. Tumor microenvironment and immunotherapy of oral cancer. *Eur. J. Med. Res.* **2022**, *27*, 198. [CrossRef] [PubMed]
26. Samadi, M.; Kamrani, A.; Nasiri, H.; Shomali, N.; Heris, J.A.; Shahabi, P.; Ghahremanzadeh, K.; Mohammadinasab, R.; Sadeghi, M.; Sadeghvand, S.; et al. Cancer immunotherapy focusing on the role of interleukins: A comprehensive and updated study. *Pathol. Res. Pract.* **2023**, *249*, 154732. [CrossRef]
27. Briukhovetska, D.; Dörr, J.; Endres, S.; Libby, P.; Dinarello, C.A.; Kobold, S. Interleukins in cancer: From biology to therapy. *Nat. Rev. Cancer* **2021**, *21*, 481–499. [CrossRef]
28. Niklander, S.E. Inflammatory Mediators in Oral Cancer: Pathogenic Mechanisms and Diagnostic Potential. *Front. Oral Health* **2021**, *2*, 642238. [CrossRef]
29. Chalaris, A.; Garbers, C.; Rabe, B.; Rose-John, S.; Scheller, J. The soluble Interleukin 6 receptor: Generation and role in inflammation and cancer. *Eur. J. Cell Biol.* **2011**, *90*, 484–494. [CrossRef]
30. Jones, S.A.; Horiuchi, S.; Topley, N.; Yamamoto, N.; Fuller, G.M. The soluble interleukin 6 receptor: Mechanisms of production and implications in disease. *FASEB J.* **2001**, *15*, 43–58. [CrossRef]
31. Apte, R.N. Mechanisms of cytokine production by fibroblasts-implications for normal connective tissue homeostasis and pathological conditions. *Folia Microbiol.* **1995**, *40*, 392–404. [CrossRef]
32. Nishiwaki, N.; Noma, K.; Ohara, T.; Kunitomo, T.; Kawasaki, K.; Akai, M.; Kobayashi, T.; Narusaka, T.; Kashima, H.; Sato, H.; et al. Overcoming cancer-associated fibroblast-induced immunosuppression by anti-interleukin-6 receptor antibody. *Cancer Immunol. Immunother.* **2023**, *72*, 2029–2044. [CrossRef] [PubMed]
33. Wen, S.; Hou, Y.; Fu, L.; Xi, L.; Yang, D.; Zhao, M.; Qin, Y.; Sun, K.; Teng, Y.; Liu, M. Cancer-associated fibroblast (CAF)-derived IL32 promotes breast cancer cell invasion and metastasis via integrin β3-p38 MAPK signalling. *Cancer Lett.* **2019**, *442*, 320–332. [CrossRef] [PubMed]
34. Mosaddad, S.A.; Namanloo, R.A.; Aghili, S.S.; Maskani, P.; Alam, M.; Abbasi, K.; Nouri, F.; Tahmasebi, E.; Yazdanian, M.; Tebyaniyan, H. Photodynamic therapy in oral cancer: A review of clinical studies. *Med. Oncol.* **2023**, *40*, 91. [CrossRef] [PubMed]
35. Kaleta-Richter, M.; Aebisher, D.; Jaworska, D.; Czuba, Z.; Cieślar, G.; Kawczyk-Krupka, A. The Influence of Hypericin-Mediated Photodynamic Therapy on Interleukin-8 and -10 Secretion in Colon Cancer Cells. *Integr. Cancer Ther.* **2020**, *19*, 1534735420918931. [CrossRef] [PubMed]
36. Besic Gyenge, E.; Forny, P.; Lüscher, D.; Laass, A.; Walt, H.; Maake, C. Effects of hypericin and a chlorin based photosensitizer alone or in combination in squamous cell carcinoma cells in the dark. *Photodiagnosis Photodyn. Ther.* **2012**, *9*, 321–331. [CrossRef] [PubMed]
37. Etemadi, A.; Sadatmansouri, S.; Sodeif, F.; Jalalishirazi, F.; Chiniforush, N. Photobiomodulation Effect of Different Diode Wavelengths on the Proliferation of Human Gingival Fibroblast Cells. *Photochem. Photobiol.* **2021**, *97*, 1123–1128. [CrossRef] [PubMed]
38. Bublik, M.; Head, C.; Benharash, P.; Paiva, M.; Eshraghi, A.; Kim, T.; Saxton, R. Hypericin and pulsed laser therapy of squamous cell cancer in vitro. *Photomed. Laser Surg.* **2006**, *24*, 341–347. [CrossRef]
39. Kapsokalyvas, D.; Dimitriou, H.; Skalkos, D.; Konstantoudakis, G.; Filippidis, G.; Stiakaki, E.; Papazoglou, T.; Kalmanti, M. Does Hypericum perforatum L. extract show any specificity as photosensitizer for HL-60 leukemic cells and cord blood hemopoietic progenitors during photodynamic therapy? *J. Photochem. Photobiol. B* **2005**, *80*, 208–216. [CrossRef]
40. Kapałczyńska, M.; Kolenda, T.; Przybyła, W.; Zajączkowska, M.; Teresiak, A.; Filas, V.; Ibbs, M.; Bliźniak, R.; Łuczewski, Ł.; Lamperska, K. 2D and 3D cell cultures—A comparison of different types of cancer cell cultures. *Arch. Med. Sci.* **2018**, *14*, 910–919. [CrossRef]
41. Du, H.; Bay, B.H.; Mahendran, R.; Olivo, M. Endogenous expression of interleukin-8 and interleukin-10 in nasopharyngeal carcinoma cells and the effect of photodynamic therapy. *Int. J. Mol. Med.* **2002**, *10*, 73–76. [CrossRef]

42. Barathan, M.; Mariappan, V.; Shankar, E.M.; Abdullah, B.J.; Goh, K.L.; Vadivelu, J. Hypericin-photodynamic therapy leads to interleukin-6 secretion by HepG2 cells and their apoptosis via recruitment of BH3 interacting-domain death agonist and caspases. *Cell Death Dis.* **2013**, *4*, e697. [CrossRef] [PubMed]
43. Du, H.; Bay, B.H.; Mahendran, R.; Olivo, M. Hypericin-mediated photodynamic therapy elicits differential interleukin-6 response in nasopharyngeal cancer. *Cancer Lett.* **2006**, *235*, 202–208. [CrossRef] [PubMed]
44. Rose-John, S.; Waetzig, G.H.; Scheller, J.; Grötzinger, J.; Seegert, D. The IL-6/sIL-6R complex as a novel target for therapeutic approaches. *Expert Opin. Ther. Targets* **2007**, *11*, 613–624. [CrossRef] [PubMed]
45. Hwang, Y.S.; Lee, S.K.; Park, K.K.; Chung, W.Y. Secretion of IL-6 and IL-8 from lysophosphatidic acid-stimulated oral squamous cell carcinoma promotes osteoclastogenesis and bone resorption. *Oral Oncol.* **2012**, *48*, 40–48. [CrossRef] [PubMed]
46. Wang, Y.F.; Chang, S.Y.; Tai, S.K.; Li, W.Y.; Wang, L.S. Clinical significance of interleukin-6 and interleukin-6 receptor expressions in oral squamous cell carcinoma. *Head Neck* **2002**, *24*, 850–858. [CrossRef] [PubMed]
47. Blumberg, H.; Conklin, D.; Xu, W.F.; Grossmann, A.; Brender, T.; Carollo, S.; Eagan, M.; Foster, D.; Haldeman, B.A.; Hammond, A.; et al. Interleukin 20: Discovery, receptor identification, and role in epidermal function. *Cell* **2001**, *104*, 9–19. [CrossRef] [PubMed]
48. Hsu, Y.H.; Chang, M.S. Interleukin-20 antibody is a potential therapeutic agent for experimental arthritis. *Arthritis Rheum.* **2010**, *62*, 3311–3321. [CrossRef]
49. Chen, W.Y.; Chang, M.S. IL-20 is regulated by hypoxia-inducible factor and up-regulated after experimental ischemic stroke. *J. Immunol.* **2009**, *182*, 5003–5012. [CrossRef]
50. Hong, J.T.; Son, D.J.; Lee, C.K.; Yoon, D.Y.; Lee, D.H.; Park, M.H. Interleukin 32, inflammation and cancer. *Pharmacol. Ther.* **2017**, *174*, 127–137. [CrossRef]
51. Guenin, S.; Mouallif, M.; Hubert, P.; Jacobs, N.; Krusy, N.; Duray, A.; Ennaji, M.M.; Saussez, S.; Delvenne, P. Interleukin-32 expression is associated with a poorer prognosis in head and neck squamous cell carcinoma. *Mol. Carcinog.* **2014**, *53*, 667–673. [CrossRef]
52. Zhang, H.; Wang, R.; Wang, Z.; Wu, W.; Zhang, N.; Zhang, L.; Hu, J.; Luo, P.; Zhang, J.; Liu, Z.; et al. Molecular insight into pentraxin-3: Update advances in innate immunity, inflammation, tissue remodeling, diseases, and drug role. *Biomed. Pharmacother.* **2022**, *156*, 113783. [CrossRef]
53. Chang, W.C.; Wu, S.L.; Huang, W.C.; Hsu, J.Y.; Chan, S.H.; Wang, J.M.; Tsai, J.P.; Chen, B.K. PTX3 gene activation in EGF-induced head and neck cancer cell metastasis. *Oncotarget* **2015**, *6*, 7741–7757. [CrossRef] [PubMed]
54. Chan, S.H.; Tsai, J.P.; Shen, C.J.; Liao, Y.H.; Chen, B.K. Oleate-induced PTX3 promotes head and neck squamous cell carcinoma metastasis through the up-regulation of vimentin. *Oncotarget* **2017**, *8*, 41364–41378. [CrossRef] [PubMed]
55. Ying, T.H.; Lee, C.H.; Chiou, H.L.; Yang, S.F.; Lin, C.L.; Hung, C.H.; Tsai, J.P.; Hsieh, Y.H. Knockdown of Pentraxin 3 suppresses tumorigenicity and metastasis of human cervical cancer cells. *Sci. Rep.* **2016**, *6*, 29385. [CrossRef] [PubMed]
56. Huntosova, V.; Novotova, M.; Nichtova, Z.; Balogova, L.; Maslanakova, M.; Petrovajova, D.; Stroffekova, K. Assessing light-independent effects of hypericin on cell viability, ultrastructure and metabolism in human glioma and endothelial cells. *Toxicol. In Vitro* **2017**, *40*, 184–195. [CrossRef] [PubMed]
57. Martínez-Poveda, B.; Quesada, A.R.; Medina, M.A. Hypericin in the dark inhibits key steps of angiogenesis in vitro. *Eur. J. Pharmacol.* **2005**, *516*, 97–103. [CrossRef] [PubMed]
58. Wu, J.J.; Zhang, J.; Xia, C.Y.; Ding, K.; Li, X.X.; Pan, X.G.; Xu, J.K.; He, J.; Zhang, W.K. Hypericin: A natural anthraquinone as promising therapeutic agent. *Phytomedicine* **2023**, *111*, 154654. [CrossRef]
59. Ash, C.; Dubec, M.; Donne, K.; Bashford, T. Effect of wavelength and beam width on penetration in light-tissue interaction using computational methods. *Lasers Med. Sci.* **2017**, *32*, 1909–1918. [CrossRef]
60. Martinez-Pacheco, S.; O'Driscoll, L. Pre-Clinical In Vitro Models Used in Cancer Research: Results of a Worldwide Survey. *Cancers* **2021**, *13*, 6033. [CrossRef]

pharmaceutics

MDPI

Article

Natural Phytochemical and Visible Light at Different Wavelengths Show Synergistic Antibacterial Activity against *Staphylococcus aureus*

Jae-Young Jeong [1] and You-Jin Hwang [1,2,*]

1 Department of Biohealth & Medical Engineering, College of IT Convergence, Gachon University, Seongnam 13120, Republic of Korea; jini656565@gachon.ac.kr
2 Department of Biomedical Engineering, College of IT Convergence, Gachon University, Seongnam 13120, Republic of Korea
* Correspondence: gene@gachon.ac.kr

Abstract: As the risk of antibiotic-resistant bacteria increases, interest in non-antibiotic treatment is also increasing. Among the methods used in non-antibiotic therapy, natural antibiotics such as essential oils have disadvantages such as low efficiency. In the case of phototherapy, the light used for antibacterial activities has low penetration into the human body because of its short wavelength, making it of low medical utility. To solve this problem, this study aimed to determine conditions for enhancing the antibacterial activity of natural phytochemicals and visible light. Four natural phytochemical extracts that showed high antibacterial properties in previous studies were analyzed. Synergistic effects on antibacterial activity and cytotoxicity were determined when natural phytochemical extracts and visible light were simultaneously used. As a result, it was confirmed that the antibacterial activity increased by four times when *Sanguisorba officinalis* L. was irradiated with 465 nm for 10 min and 520 nm for 40 min, and *Uncaria gambir* Roxb. was irradiated with 465 nm for 10 min and 520 nm for 60 min compared to when *Sanguisorba officinalis* L. and *Uncaria gambir* Roxb. were used alone. The synergistic effect on antibacterial activity was independent of the absorption peak of the natural phytochemical extracts. In addition, in the case of natural phytochemical extracts with improved antibacterial activity, it was confirmed that the improvement of antibacterial activity was increased in inverse proportion to the light irradiation wavelength and in proportion to the light irradiation time. The antibacterial activity was enhanced regardless of antibiotic resistance. In the case of cytotoxicity, it was confirmed that there was no toxicity to A549 cells when treated with 465 nm, the shortest wavelength among the natural phytochemical extracts. These results show how to replace blue light, which has been underutilized due to its low transmittance and cytotoxicity. They also demonstrate the high medical potential of using natural phytochemical and visible light as a combination therapy.

Keywords: photodynamic therapy; visible light; natural phytochemical; antibacterial activity; *Staphylococcus aureus*; synergistic effect

1. Introduction

Staphylococcus aureus is the most common and deadly pathogen involved in purulent acute bacterial skin and skin structure infections [1,2]. *S. aureus* can lead to various skin diseases such as folliculitis, impetigo, abscesses, furuncles, furunculosis, mastitis, and hidradenitis suppurativa by causing local and systemic infections and producing staphylococcal toxins through the skin [1–3]. More than 2.8 million antibiotic-resistant infections occur annually in the United States, accounting for 35,000 deaths [4]. In Korea, the estimated annual number of antibiotic-resistant infections in 10 hospitals in 2017 was 7979, resulting in about 3280 deaths and socioeconomic losses of USD 294,505,002 [5]. The use of empirical and broad-spectrum antibiotics to eliminate antibiotic-resistant bacteria creates a vicious cycle of generating other antibiotic-resistant bacteria [4]. Therefore, interest in non-antibiotic therapies that can replace antibiotics is increasing.

Methods emerging as non-antibiotic therapies include treatment using natural phytochemical extracts and light-based antibacterial therapy [6,7]. Representative natural phytochemical extracts used for antibacterial therapy include essential oils, which are volatile components made from aromatic plants. About 3000 essential oils are known, of which 300 are certified by the US Food and Drug Administration as generally safe for humans. They are widely used in cosmetics, perfumes, food preservatives, and additives [6,7]. Since these natural phytochemical extracts have low cost, high accessibility, structural diversity, various modes of activation, high biocompatibility, potential anti-biofilm properties, environmental friendliness, and low probability of antibiotic resistance, they are attracting attention as environmentally friendly non-antibiotic therapies [6–9].

Light-based antibacterial therapy, including antibacterial photodynamic therapy (aPDT) and ultraviolet C (UVC) irradiation therapy, is being studied as a method for treating local infection [10]. aPDT essentially requires a photosensitizer (PS), molecular oxygen, and light of a specific wavelength to activate the PS, and for this antibacterial activity to be active, the PS must possess a large amount of singlet oxygen quantum [11]. Regarding the action mechanism for the antibacterial activity of aPDT, it involves reactive oxygen species (ROS) by combining the PS with visible or near-infrared rays, causing cell death [11–15]. The antibacterial activity of UVC occurs by causing DNA damage through various mutagenesis and cytotoxic DNA lesions [16]. Light-based therapy has advantages such as fast antibacterial activity unrelated to antibiotic resistance, high treatment repeatability, fewer side effects, and high compatibility with other treatments [10–12,14,17]. However, in the case of aPDT, there are disadvantages in that a photosensitizer must be separately administered. In addition, it is difficult to have a bacteria-specific antibacterial activity [10,17]. On the other hand, since it can damage host cells, active research on human use has not been conducted in the case of ultraviolet C irradiation [10,16].

Blue light therapy, which appears to compensate for these disadvantages, is receiving a lot of attention because it has an antibacterial effect alone without needing additional photosensitizers. Its antibacterial mechanism remains unclear; a representative hypothesis is that the generation of ROS is induced by photoactivation of the endogenous photosensitive porphyrin possessed by bacteria [7,18–20]. Blue light is known to cause much less damage to host cells than ultraviolet light [10,19]. However, blue light therapy is not useful for medical purposes because it is difficult for blue light to affect the target area due to its low permeability caused by its short wavelength and toxic to some cells [21–25].

To solve these problems, this study aims to confirm the synergy of antibacterial activity through natural phytochemical extracts, previously identified to possess potent antibacterial properties [26], and visible light as a fusion therapy, such as using zinc oxide nanoparticles and essential oil together to increase the antibacterial activity effect [27]. This study assessed their absorbance and the effect of visible light on their antibacterial activity and cytotoxicity.

2. Materials and Methods

2.1. Plant Materials

A total of four species (*Caesalpinia sappan* L., *Glycyrrhiza uralensis* Fisch., *Sanguisorba officinalis* L., *Uncaria gambir* Roxb) of natural phytochemicals that showed high antibacterial activities in previous studies [26] were purchased from Samhong Medicinal Herb Market (Seoul, Republic of Korea).

2.2. Preparation of Plant Extracts

Preparation of plant extracts was carried out using the same method as in the previous study [26]. Plant materials were blended to powder with a grinder and extracted by shaking (110 rpm) in 70% ethanol for 24 h. The ratio of material powder to solvent was 1:10 (w/v). Supernatants were separated from crude extracts by centrifugation at 3000 rpm for 10 min and concentrated through a rotary evaporator WEV-1001V (Daihan Scientific Co., Wonju, Republic of Korea) in a vacuum at 50 °C. The concentrated extract was dissolved in 10% dimethyl sulfoxide (DMSO; Sigma Chemical Co., St. Louis, MO, USA) aqueous solution and finally filtered through a Whatman filter paper No. 2 (Whatman, Kent, UK). All samples were placed into conical tubes, sealed, and stored in a refrigerator at 4 °C until further use.

2.3. Light Source

An experimental device was equipped with a light-emitting diode (LED) (Jin LED, Seoul, Republic of Korea) with peak emission at 465, 520, 590, and 625 nm. Irradiation of each LED was measured by X1-5 optometer (Gigahertz-Optik, Munich, Germany). Specifications of the LED used in the experiment are shown in Table 1.

Table 1. LED specifications used in this study.

Wavelength (nm)	Voltage (V)	Current (mA)	Irradiance (mW/cm^2)	Distance Between Light Source and Solution Surface (mm)
620–625	2–2.2	20	73.29	6
591–593	2–2.2	20	84.17	6
520–522.5	3–3.2	20	71.68	6
465–467.5	3–3.2	20	93.34	6

2.4. Bacteria Culture

S. aureus (ATCC 29213) and MRSA (ATCC 33591) standard strains were used in the present study [26]. These strains were purchased from the American Type Culture Collection (ATCC) (Manassas, VA, USA). MRSA isolates (CI-2 and CI-21) were originally obtained from clinical specimens and identified at Gachon University Gil Medical Center (Incheon, Republic of Korea) [28]. These isolates were preserved in a −80 °C freezer in 20% glycerol (*v*/*v*) until further use. Each strain was initially cultivated on a brain heart infusion (BHI) (Kisan Bio, Seoul, Republic of Korea) plate. A single colony was picked from each plate and pre-cultured in BHI broth at 37 °C for 24 h prior to assays. Bacterial stocks were subcultured every 3–4 weeks to maintain bacterial viability.

2.5. Ultra-Performance Liquid Chromatography (UPLC) Analysis

UPLC analysis was conducted under the same conditions as described in previous studies [29]. UPLC analysis of natural phytochemical extracts (3 mg/mL in 70% ethanol) was performed on an AQUITY UPLC I-Class system (Waters Corporation, Milford, MA, USA) using a BEH C18 1.7 µm column (2.1 × 100 mm) through Korea Plant Extract Bank (KPEB) (Daejeon, Republic of Korea). The sample was separated by a mobile phase consisting of distilled water with 0.1% formic acid (A) and acetonitrile with 0.1% formic acid (B). The column was set at 35 °C and the injection volume was 1 µL. The eluent was program set as follows: 0 min 92% A (8% B), 1.0 min 92% A (8% B), 16.0 min 30% A (70% B), 17.0 min 0% A (100% B), 19.0 min 0% A (100% B), 19.3 min 92% A (8% B), and 22.0 min 92% A (8% B). The flow rate was 0.4 mL/min.

High-resolution electrospray ionization mass spectrometry (HRESIMS) data were obtained on a Waters Vion QTOF/MS spectrometer in a negative/positive electrospray ionization (ESI$^-$/ESI$^+$) mode. MS conditions were as follows: desolvation gas (N_2) flow rate = 800 L/h, desolvation gas temperature = 350 °C, source temperature = 110 °C, capillary voltage = 300 V, cone voltage = 40 V, and *m*/*z* range = 100–1500 Da.

2.6. Absorbance Measurement of Natural Phytochemical Extracts

Absorbance was measured for natural phytochemical extracts to determine the correlation between absorbance and wavelength of a specific component in the extract with a multimode plate reader (Tecan, Infinite™ M200 PRO, Männedorf, Switzerland). Absorbance was measured at 2 nm intervals from 300 nm to 800 nm.

2.7. Determination of Minimum Inhibitory Concentration (MIC)

Minimum inhibitory concentration (MIC) for the combination of medical plant extract and visible light was measured to determine synergistic effect on antibacterial activity against *S. aureus*. MIC was determined using the broth microdilution method according to a previous study [26] with slight modifications. Briefly, 200 μL of samples were inoculated to first columns of 96-well microplates and serially diluted two-fold (ranging from 1 to 1/4 MIC resulting from the previous study [26]). Then, 100 μL of *S. aureus* bacterial suspension (1×10^6 CFU/mL) was inoculated into wells. The total volume was 200 μL per well. The microplate was irradiated with light of a specific wavelength at intervals of 10 min from 0 to 60 min and incubated in BHI broth with shaking (110 rpm) at 37 °C for 24 h. The optical density (OD) was measured at 595 nm with a spectrophotometer (Multiskan FC; Thermo Fisher Scientific, Waltham, MA, USA). MIC was defined as the lowest concentration that inhibited the visible growth of bacteria. The criteria for enhancing antibacterial activity were determined according to the fractional inhibitory concentration (FIC) value. FIC_I was calculated using the following equation: $FIC_I = FIC_E + FIC_V$, where FIC_E was the MIC of the extract in combination/MIC of extract alone and FIC_V was the minimum inhibitory time (MIT) of visible light in combination/MIT of visible light alone. Results were interpreted as follows: synergistic interaction, $FIC_I \leq 0.5$; partial synergy, $0.5 < FIC_I \leq 0.75$; additive interaction, $0.75 < FIC_I \leq 1.0$; indifferent, $1.0 < FIC_I \leq 4.0$; and antagonistic interaction, $FIC_I > 4.0$ [30].

2.8. Measurement of Synergy Effect of Antibacterial Activity against Methichillin-Resistant Staphylococcus aureus (MRSA)

Antibacterial activity for the combination of medical plant extract and visible light was measured to determine synergistic effect on antibacterial activity against MRSA, and MIC was determined using the broth microdilution method according to a previous study [26] with slight modifications. Briefly, 100 μL of 1/4 MIC samples in which synergistic effect on antibacterial activity was found due to visible light irradiation in Materials and Methods 2.7 were inoculated to wells of 96-well microplates. Then 100 μL of each MRSA bacterial suspension (1×10^6 CFU/mL) was inoculated into wells. The total volume was 200 μL per well. The microplate was irradiated with light of a specific wavelength under the same conditions as those when enhanced antibacterial activity against *S. aureus* at 1/4 MIC was found. The optical density (OD) was measured at 595 nm with a spectrophotometer.

2.9. Cell Culture

Human skin keratinocytes (HaCaT; ATCC PCS-200-011) cell line was purchased from American Type Culture Collection (ATCC; Manassas, VA, USA) and human lung carcinoma (A549; KCLB 10185) cell line was purchased from Korean Cell Line Bank (KCLB, Seoul, Republic of Korea). These cells were grown in 25 cm^2 flasks with 4 mL of Roswell Park Memorial Institute Medium (RPMI 1640; Gibco, Grand Island, NY, USA) with 10% fetal bovine serum added (FBS; Gibco) and 1% penicillin and streptomycin (Sigma Chemical Co., St. Louis, MO, USA). They were cultured at 37 °C in a CO_2 cell chamber (MMM Group, Planegg, Germany) with 5% CO_2. When cells fill 80–90% of the bottom of the 25 cm^2 flask, cells were dissociated with 4 mL of trypsin-ethylenediaminetetraacetic acid (Trypsin-EDTA; Gibco) solution. After centrifugation at 500 rpm for 10 min at 4 °C, cells were re-suspended with RPMI 1640 to 2×10^4 cells/mL and plated at 100 μL per well in a 96-well microplate. After incubation for 6 h at 37 °C with 5% CO_2, cell physiological activities were performed using exponential phase cells.

2.10. Measurement of Cell Physiological Activity

Cell physiological activities after treatment with natural phytochemicals and visible light were analyzed using methods of measuring cell proliferation and cell metabolic activity of Rohringer et al. [31] with slight modifications. Briefly, 100 μL of a natural phytochemical extract that showed synergistic effect on antibacterial activity against MRSA strains at 1/2 MIC was inoculated so that the total volume was 200 μL. Afterwards, cell proliferation and cell metabolism were measured at 24 h intervals for 72 h at 37 °C and 5% CO_2 after irradiation with visible light under the same conditions under which the MIC appeared when combined with 1/4 MIC of a natural phytochemical extract. Cell proliferation and toxicity were examined by removing the solution from each well, inoculating 100 μL of 0.05% Trypsin-EDTA solution, and incubating cells for 10 min at 37 °C with 5% CO_2. The separated cell solution was mixed with an equal amount of trypan blue solution (Sigma Chemical Co., St. Louis, MO, USA). After reacting for 5 min at room temperature, the number of viable cells was measured using a hemocytometer. Cytotoxicity was judged to be toxic if the cell viability of the experimental group was less than 70% when comparing the experimental group and the control group. For cell metabolism, 20 μL of 5 mg/mL MTT solution was inoculated per well and reacted for 2 h. After the reaction, the plate was washed with phosphate-buffered saline (PBS; Gibco), inoculated with 200 μL of DMSO, and reacted at room temperature for 15 min. Afterwards, cellular metabolism was determined by measuring absorbance at 595 nm via spectrophotometry.

2.11. Statistical Analysis

Statistical analysis was performed by Microsoft Excel 2016 (Microsoft, Redmond, WA, USA) and SigmaPlot version 12.0 (Systat Software, Palo Alto, CA, USA). Average values were calculated as means and standard deviation (±SD). Statistical differences were assessed by analysis of variance (ANOVA). Results were considered statistically significant if the *p*-value was less than 0.05. All experiments were performed in duplicate three times.

3. Results and Discussion

3.1. Ultra-Performance Liquid Chromatography (UPLC) Analysis

UPLC analysis for each extract and mass spectrum (MS) and UV spectrum for a specific peak were conducted through the Korea Plant Extract Bank (Table 2). In the case of analysis for specific peaks, the structure was predicted through comparative analysis with the existing literature for each natural phytochemical based on results of the MS and UV spectra. As a result of the analysis, for all natural phytochemical extracts, peaks in various areas, not a single peak, appeared in all analysis results. When comparing these results with the existing literature on each natural phytochemical, the main expected effective phytochemicals of each natural phytochemical extract were episappanol; protosappanin C; brazilin; a mixture of protosappanin B, isoprotosappanin B, and sappanol for CS at 280 nm [32]; liquiritin and glycyrrhizin for GU at 254 nm [33]; quercetin and proanthocyanidins for SO at 360 nm [34]; and catechin for UG at 280 nm [35] because of the UPLC in the same UV area. Some of the above components are also expected to create synergy with visible light.

Table 2. Expected effective phytochemical analysis of each natural phytochemical extract [29].

Extracts	RT (min)	Molecular Formula	Molecular Weight (*m*/*z*)	Phytochemical Name
CS	2.98	$C_{16}H_{14}O_5$	285.07	Brazilin
	3.10	$C_{16}H_{16}O_6$	304.30	Protosappanin B
GU	4.35	$C_{26}H_{30}O_{13}$	550.51	Liquiritin apioside
	9.48	$C_{42}H_{62}O_{16}$	822.94	Glycyrrhizin
SO	6.60	$C_{16}H_{10}O_{11}S$	410.31	2,7-*O*-methyl-8-(sulfooxy)ellagic acid
UG	3.07	$C_{15}H_{14}O_6$	290.27	Catechin

CS: *Caesalpinia sappan* L.; GU: *Glycyrrhiza uralensis* Fisch.; SO: *Sanguisorba officinalis* L.; UG: *Uncaria gambir* Roxb.; RT: Retention time.

3.2. Absorbance Measurement of Natural Phytochemical Extracts

The absorption peak of each natural phytochemical extract was measured at 2 nm intervals from 300 nm to 800 nm (Figure 1). CS and SO showed absorption peaks at 440 and

350 nm, respectively. However, GU and UG did not show specific peaks. If the synergistic effect on the antibacterial activity of the natural phytochemicals through photoactivity is correlated with the absorbance peak, it is expected that the synergistic effect on the antibacterial activity of CS will be the highest when irradiated with blue light (465 nm) close to the 440 nm wavelength. However, as a result of measuring the antibacterial activity, CS, which showed an absorption peak at 440 nm with blue light, did not show a synergistic effect on antibacterial activity. Only SO and UG, which did not show absorption peaks, showed a synergistic effect on antibacterial activity at a concentration of one-fourth MIC. It was confirmed that the absorbance peak of the crude extract was not associated with photoactivation.

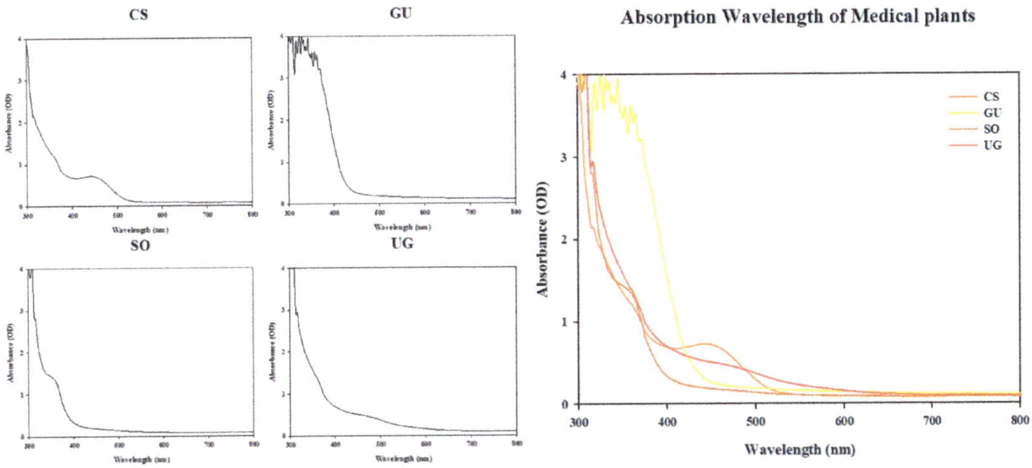

Figure 1. Absorption peaks of natural phytochemical extracts used in the experiment. The absorbance of each natural phytochemical extract at 4 mg/mL was measured. CS is *Caesalpinia sappan* L.; GU is *Glycyrrhiza uralensis* Fisch.; SO is *Sanguisorba officinalis* L.; UG is *Uncaria gambir* Roxb.

3.3. Determination of Minimum Inhibitory Concentration (MIC)

The MIC of each natural phytochemical extract at each wavelength for *S. aureus* was determined by measuring the absorbance at 595 nm using a spectrophotometer (Figure 2a). When BL was irradiated, the minimum inhibition of *S. aureus* was measured from 40 min. When one-fourth MIC of the natural phytochemical extract and BL were simultaneously treated, the minimum inhibition of *S. aureus* was measured from 10 min for SO, 10 min for UG, 40 min for CS, and 50 min for GU. When irradiated with GL, the minimum inhibition of *S. aureus* was not measured up to 60 min when GL was single-treated. When one-fourth MIC of the natural phytochemical extract and GL were simultaneously treated, the minimum inhibition of *S. aureus* was measured from 40 min for SO and 60 min for UG. However, the minimum inhibition was not measured for CS and GU up to 60 min. When irradiated with YL and RL, the minimum inhibition of *S. aureus* was not measured for up to 60 min with either single treatment of light of each wavelength or simultaneously with natural phytochemical extracts of one-fourth MIC. The synergistic effect on antibacterial activity was determined based on the FIC_I according to the FIC_V. When results were analyzed, CS and GU at one-fourth MIC were not found to have any synergistic effects on antibacterial activity at any wavelength. However, SO and UG were found to show synergistic effects on antibacterial activity with BL and GL. For SO and UG at one-fourth MIC, the minimum inhibition time with BL showed a strong synergy because $FIC_I \leq 0.5$ was 10 min, which was equivalent to one-fourth of the BL single processing result at 40 min. In addition, the minimum inhibition time of GL single treatment was not measured up to 60 min, although there was a possibility of synergy because the minimum inhibition time was 40 min for one-fourth MIC SO and 60 min for one-fourth MIC UG, both of which fell in the range of $0.25 \leq FIC_I < 1.25$.

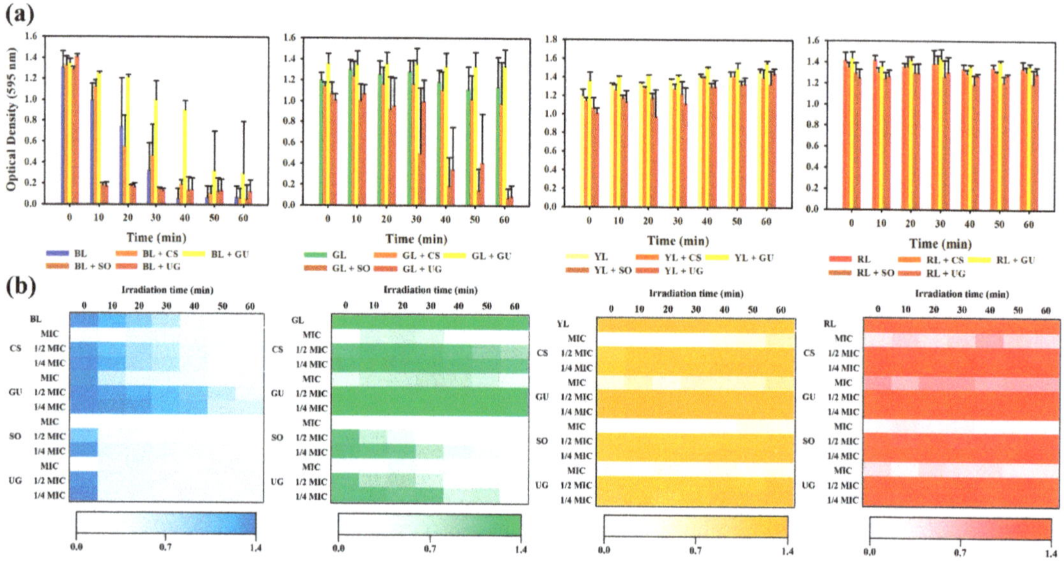

Figure 2. Synergistic effect on natural phytochemical extracts on antibacterial activity. (**a**) One-fourth MIC according to the wavelength of visible light. Antibacterial activity was confirmed by measuring absorbance at 595 nm. BL is 465 nm light, GL is 520 nm light, YL is 590 nm light, and RL is 625 nm light. (**b**) Heat map of enhancement of antibacterial activity according to the concentration of natural phytochemical extract and irradiation time based on visible light wavelength. Antibacterial activity was confirmed by measuring absorbance at 595 nm.

To determine the synergy conditions for antibacterial activity, a heat map was prepared according to the concentration of the natural phytochemical extracts and the irradiation time of visible light (Figure 2b). Natural phytochemical extracts were diluted two-fold from the MIC and measured for *S. aureus* treated with a single extract at one-fourth MIC. Visible light irradiation time was measured from 0 min to 60 min at intervals of 10 min. When BL was used for irradiation and measurement of antibacterial activity was performed at intervals of 10 min, measurement time results of antibacterial activity for half MIC and one-fourth MIC of natural phytochemical extracts were the same. When GL was used for irradiation and when GL single treatment and CS or GU were simultaneously used for treatment, antibacterial activity was not measured up to 60 min. During the simultaneous treatment with GL or SO, the half MIC of SO showed an antibacterial activity from 20 min and the one-fourth MIC of SO showed an antibacterial activity from 40 min. When GL single treatment and CS or GU were simultaneously used for treatment, the antibacterial activity was not measured up to 60 min. During simultaneous treatment with GL or UG, the antibacterial activity was measured from 30 min at half MIC and from 60 min at one-fourth MIC. When irradiated with YL or RL, the antibacterial activity was not measured in any situations up to 60 min.

When comparing single treatment with each of four visible light wavelengths, the shorter the irradiation wavelength and the longer the irradiation time, the higher the antibacterial activity. These results confirmed that antibacterial active ingredients included in the natural phytochemical extract used in this experiment showed a concentration-dependent antibacterial activity. In addition, when the concentration of natural phytochemical extract was the same, antibacterial activity of the natural phytochemical extract had the following trend: BL > GL > YL = RL. Thus, the four natural phytochemical extracts used in this experiment are expected to show synergy in antibacterial activity by specific wavelengths rather than the absorption peaks of the extracts.

3.4. Measurement of Synergy Effect of Antibacterial Activity against Methichillin-Resistant Staphylococcus aureus (MRSA)

Antibacterial activity against MRSA was measured to determine whether the synergistic effect on antibacterial activity works regardless of antibiotic resistance. Antibacterial activity was measured using one MRSA standard strain and two clinically isolated MRSA strains used in a previous study [26] under the same conditions as those in which synergistic effect on antibacterial activity was shown at one-fourth MIC of SO or UG for the *S. aureus* standard strain (Figure 3). Two types of conditions that show synergistic effects on antibacterial activity were targeted: one-fourth MIC of SO or UG with irradiation at 465 nm for 10 min and at 520 nm for 40 min. As a result, under both conditions, all MRSA strains and *S. aureus* showed similar results. Synergistic effect on antibacterial activity compared to control was observed. This results showed that the synergistic effect between visible light and natural phytochemicals used in this study on antibacterial activity occurred regardless of antibiotic resistance.

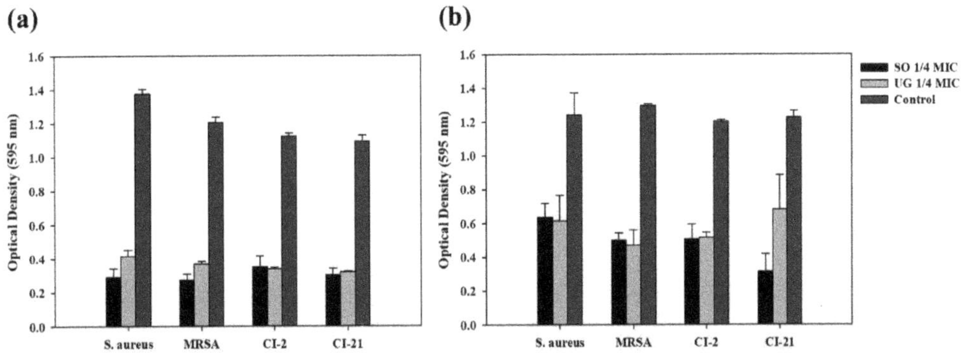

Figure 3. Synergistic effect of antibacterial activity against *S. aureus* and MRSA. (**a**) Optical density against *S. aureus* and MRSA when simultaneously treated with 1/4 MIC of natural phytochemical extract and irradiated at 465 nm for 10 min. (**b**) Optical density against *S. aureus* and MRSA when simultaneously treated with 1/4 MIC of natural phytochemical extract and irradiated at 520 nm for 40 min.

3.5. Measurement of Cell Physiological Activity

When cell proliferation was determined under conditions where antibacterial activity synergy occurred, both A549 cells and HaCaT cells showed a survival rate of less than 10%, indicating a strong cytotoxicity. When single irradiation at each wavelength was performed, 465 nm showed toxicity to both cells, with a survival rate of 16% for A549 cells and 29% for HaCaT cells. However, irradiation at 520 nm resulted in a high proliferation rate of 139% for A549 cells. Although HaCaT cells showed toxicity at 67%, they showed a relatively high survival rate. In the case where light was not irradiated, A549 cells showed a survival rate of 70% upon treatment with one-fourth MIC of SO and 98% upon treatment with one-fourth MIC of UG, indicating no toxicity. HaCaT cells showed a survival rate of 29% upon treatment with one-fourth MIC of SO. However, they showed a survival rate of 71% upon treatment with one-fourth MIC of UG (Figure 4a).

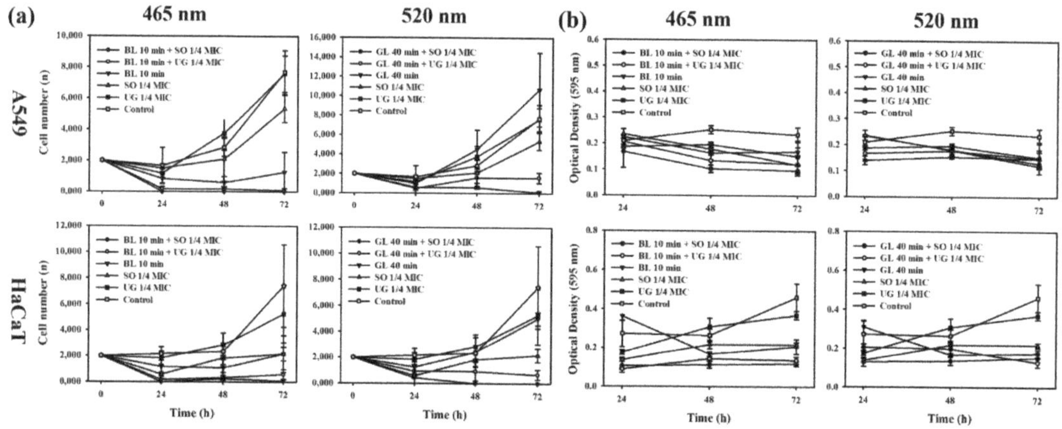

Figure 4. Cell physiological activities when simultaneously treated with 1/4 MIC of natural phytochemical extract and irradiated at 465 nm for 10 min against A549 and HaCaT cell lines. (**a**) Cell proliferation. (**b**) Cellular metabolic activity.

For cellular metabolic activity, A549 cells showed a decrease in absorbance compared to controls under all conditions. The metabolic activity decreased over time at 465 nm. Metabolic activity of HaCaT cells increased over time in control or single treatment group with UG one-fourth MIC, but decreased for the remaining conditions at 465 nm. Both A549 cells and HaCaT cells at 520 nm showed results similar to those at 465 nm (Figure 4b).

These results indicate that the combination therapy of the natural phytochemicals contained in the natural phytochemical extract used in this study with visible light showing synergistic effect on antibacterial activity was not specifically toxic to bacteria. Therefore, it is expected to be a mechanism that caused non-specific damage by increasing ROS production. Through this, the possibility of photodynamic utilization in the visible light region with a long wavelength was confirmed, as using 520 nm compared to 465 nm could reduce damage to areas other than the affected area when using combination therapy of natural phytochemicals and visible light.

4. Conclusions

In this study, we confirmed the synergy of antibacterial activity of four natural phytochemical extracts and visible light against MRSA. As a result, SO and UG showed synergistic effect on antibacterial activity at 465 nm and 520 nm. Antibacterial activity was confirmed when both SO and UG were irradiated for 10 min at 465 nm and when SO was irradiated for 40 min and UG was irradiated for 60 min at 520 nm. Antibacterial activity correlation between the absorption peak of the crude extract and the visible light wavelength seemed to be small, and synergistic effect on antibacterial activity was confirmed to increase in proportion to the light irradiation time and inversely proportional to the length of the wavelength. Also, the antibacterial activity of SO and UG by visible light was confirmed to be active regardless of antibiotic resistance. It was confirmed that the antibacterial activity mechanism causes non-specific damage regardless of the cell and bacteria, and it was confirmed that 520 nm causes less damage to cells than 465 nm under conditions where the one-fourth MICs of SO and UG show antibacterial activity. These results confirmed that certain plant extracts can be used as a photosensitizer through visible light. Additionally, it was shown that more efficient antibacterial activity against MRSA was possible when using the fusion therapy compared to using the plant extract and photodynamic therapy alone.

Currently, blue light is mainly used in the case of antibacterial activity in the visible light area using natural phytochemicals. Blue light exhibits antibacterial activity by activating bacterial protoporphyrin IX (PpIX) to increase ROS. Various studies are being conducted on blue light because it is less cytotoxic than ultraviolet rays. Some studies show that it can be specifically toxic when used with natural phytochemicals such as carvacrol [7,18–20]. However, the low human tissue permeability due to the short wavelength of blue light is underutilized [22,25,36,37]. Blue light can damage not only bacteria but also host cells [21,38,39]. This study showed that certain natural phytochemicals could be active according to specific wavelengths or irradiation time, not because they were active at absorption peaks among the four wavelengths used in the experiment.

Therefore, if the light of a longer wavelength than blue light is used in treatment in combination with a specific natural phytochemical, it will solve the problem related to short human tissue permeability and damage to host cells, which are disadvantages of a conventional blue light therapy. In addition, red light and green light can affect cell proliferation and regeneration without significantly affecting cell metabolic activity when a single treatment is performed on cells [31]. It is thought that natural phytochemicals active at various wavelengths can have various advantages in treating human tissue lesions if used in photodynamic treatment. However, since the experiment time was limited to one hour in this study, whether there was antibacterial activity during a single treatment of a wavelength other than BL and whether the antibacterial activity was enhanced when sufficient time was given at wavelengths longer than GL was unclear. Therefore, in future studies, it will be necessary to prove that natural phytochemicals do not increase antibacterial activity at a specific wavelength. Also, because this study was conducted using only crude extract, there is a lack of analysis of ingredients that can be used as a photosensitizer. To solve this problem, in future research, it is necessary to confirm the antibacterial activity of each fraction according to the characteristics of the ingredients and analyze the ingredients using methods such as total phenol content and total flavonoid content and analysis of additional antibacterial activity mechanisms through methods such as total ROS detection is also necessary. In addition, if visible light, which is effective in cell physiological activity, and natural phytochemical extracts, which show antibacterial activity enhancement through photoactivation, can be combined to confirm that both antibacterial and cell physiological activities are enhanced, it will increase the utilization of photodynamic therapy in the treatment of human tissue lesions.

Author Contributions: Conceptualization, Y.-J.H. and J.-Y.J.; Formal analysis, J.-Y.J.; Investigation, J.-Y.J.; Methodology, Y.-J.H. and J.-Y.J.; Project administration, Y.-J.H.; Funding acquisition, Y.-J.H.; Resources, Y.-J.H.; Supervision, Y.-J.H.; Validation, J.-Y.J.; Writing—original draft preparation, J.-Y.J.; Writing—review and editing, Y.-J.H. and J.-Y.J. All authors have read and agreed to the published version of the manuscript.

Funding: This study was supported by a grant from the RIS (NO. 202305530001) funded by Gachon University.

Institutional Review Board Statement: Not applicable.

Informed Consent Statement: Not applicable.

Data Availability Statement: Data are contained within the article.

Conflicts of Interest: The authors declare no conflicts of interest.

References

1. Del Giudice, P. Skin infections caused by *Staphylococcus aureus*. *Acta Derm. Venereol.* **2020**, *100*, adv00110. [CrossRef] [PubMed]
2. Hatlen, T.J.; Miller, L.G. Staphylococcal skin and soft tissue infections. *Infect. Dis. Clin. N. Am.* **2021**, *35*, 81–105. [CrossRef] [PubMed]
3. Nowicka, D.; Grywalska, E. *Staphylococcus aureus* and host immunity in recurrent furunculosis. *Dermatology* **2019**, *235*, 295–305. [CrossRef] [PubMed]
4. van Duin, D.; Paterson, D.L. Multidrug-resistant bacteria in the community: An update. *Infect. Dis. Clin. N. Am.* **2020**, *34*, 709–722. [CrossRef] [PubMed]

5. Song, K.H.; Kim, C.J.; Choi, N.K.; Ahn, J.; Choe, P.G.; Park, W.B.; Kim, N.J.; Choi, H.J.; Bae, J.Y.; Kim, E.S.; et al. Clinical and economic burden of bacteremia due to multidrug-resistant organisms in Korea: A prospective case control study. *J. Glob. Antimicrob. Resist.* **2022**, *31*, 379–385. [CrossRef] [PubMed]
6. Lu, M.; Dai, T.; Murray, C.K.; Wu, M.X. Bactericidal property of oregano oil against multidrug-resistant clinical isolates. *Front. Microbiol.* **2018**, *9*, 2329. [CrossRef]
7. Lu, M.; Wong, K.I.; Li, X.; Wang, F.; Wei, L.; Wang, S.; Wu, M.X. Oregano oil and harmless blue light to synergistically inactivate multidrug-resistant *Pseudomonas aeruginosa*. *Front. Microbiol.* **2022**, *13*, 810746. [CrossRef] [PubMed]
8. Song, M.; Liu, Y.; Li, T.; Liu, X.; Hao, Z.; Ding, S.; Panichayupakaranant, P.; Zhu, K.; Shen, J. Plant natural flavonoids against multidrug resistant pathogens. *Adv. Sci.* **2021**, *8*, e2100749. [CrossRef] [PubMed]
9. Wang, S.; Liu, X.Q.; Kang, O.H.; Kwon, D.Y. Combination of sanguisorbigenin and conventional antibiotic therapy for methicillin-resistant *Staphylococcus aureus*: Inhibition of biofilm formation and alteration of cell membrane permeability. *Int. J. Mol. Sci.* **2022**, *23*, 4232. [CrossRef]
10. Zhang, Y.; Zhu, Y.; Gupta, A.; Huang, Y.; Murray, C.K.; Vrahas, M.S.; Sherwood, M.E.; Baer, D.G.; Hamblin, M.R.; Dai, T. Antimicrobial blue light therapy for multidrug-resistant *Acinetobacter baumannii* infection in a mouse burn model: Implications for prophylaxis and treatment of combat-related wound infections. *J. Infect. Dis.* **2014**, *209*, 1963–1971. [CrossRef]
11. Correia, J.H.; Rodrigues, J.A.; Pimenta, S.; Dong, T.; Yang, Z. Photodynamic therapy review: Principles, photosensitizers, applications, and future directions. *Pharmaceutics* **2021**, *13*, 1332. [CrossRef] [PubMed]
12. do Prado-Silva, L.; Brancini, G.T.P.; Braga, G.Ú.L.; Liao, X.; Ding, T.; Sant'Ana, A.S. Antimicrobial photodynamic treatment (aPDT) as an innovative technology to control spoilage and pathogenic microorganisms in agri-food products: An updated review. *Food Control* **2022**, *132*, 108527. [CrossRef]
13. Le, T.D.; Phasupan, P.; Nguyen, L.T. Antimicrobial photodynamic efficacy of selected natural photosensitizers against food pathogens: Impacts and interrelationship of process parameters. *Photodiagnosis Photodyn. Ther.* **2020**, *32*, 102024. [CrossRef] [PubMed]
14. Leelanarathiwat, K.; Katsuta, Y.; Katsuragi, H.; Watanabe, F. Antibacterial activity of blue high-power light-emitting diode activated flavin mononucleotide against *Staphylococcus aureus* biofilm on a sandblasted and etched surface. *Photodiagnosis Photodyn. Ther.* **2020**, *31*, 101855. [CrossRef] [PubMed]
15. Paolillo, F.R.; Rodrigues, P.G.S.; Bagnato, V.S.; Alves, F.; Pires, L.; Corazza, A.V. The effect of combined curcumin-mediated photodynamic therapy and artificial skin on *Staphylococcus aureus*-infected wounds in rats. *Lasers Med. Sci.* **2021**, *36*, 1219–1226. [CrossRef]
16. Narita, K.; Asano, K.; Morimoto, Y.; Igarashi, T.; Hamblin, M.R.; Dai, T.; Nakane, A. Disinfection and healing effects of 222-nm UVC light on methicillin-resistant *Staphylococcus aureus* infection in mouse wounds. *J. Photochem. Photobiol. B* **2018**, *178*, 10–18. [CrossRef] [PubMed]
17. Senapathy, G.J.; George, B.P.; Abrahamse, H. Exploring the role of phytochemicals as potent natural photosensitizers in photodynamic therapy. *Anticancer Agents Med. Chem.* **2020**, *20*, 1831–1844. [CrossRef] [PubMed]
18. Wang, Y.; Wu, X.; Chen, J.; Amin, R.; Lu, M.; Bhayana, B.; Zhao, J.; Murray, C.K.; Hamblin, M.R.; Hooper, D.C.; et al. Antimicrobial blue light inactivation of gram-negative pathogens in biofilms: In vitro and in vivo studies. *J. Infect. Dis.* **2016**, *213*, 1380–1387. [CrossRef] [PubMed]
19. Wang, Y.; Ferrer-Espada, R.; Baglo, Y.; Goh, X.S.; Held, K.D.; Grad, Y.H.; Gu, Y.; Gelfand, J.A.; Dai, T. Photoinactivation of *Neisseria gonorrhoeae*: A paradigm-changing approach for combating antibiotic-resistant gonococcal infection. *J. Infect. Dis.* **2019**, *220*, 873–881. [CrossRef]
20. Lu, M.; Wang, S.; Wang, T.; Hu, S.; Bhayana, B.; Ishii, M.; Kong, Y.; Cai, Y.; Dai, T.; Cui, W.; et al. Bacteria-specific phototoxic reactions triggered by blue light and phytochemical carvacrol. *Sci. Transl. Med.* **2021**, *13*, eaba3571. [CrossRef]
21. Bauer, R.; Hoenes, K.; Meurle, T.; Hessling, M.; Spellerberg, B. The effects of violet and blue light irradiation on ESKAPE pathogens and human cells in presence of cell culture media. *Sci. Rep.* **2021**, *11*, 24473. [CrossRef]
22. Rkein, A.M.; Ozog, D.M. Photodynamic therapy. *Dermatol. Clin.* **2014**, *32*, 415–425. [CrossRef]
23. Gao, J.; Chen, Z.; Li, X.; Yang, M.; Lv, J.; Li, H.; Yuan, Z. Chemiluminescence in combination with organic photosensitizers: Beyond the light penetration depth limit of photodynamic therapy. *Int. J. Mol. Sci.* **2022**, *23*, 12556. [CrossRef]
24. Finlayson, L.; Barnard, I.R.M.; McMillan, L.; Ibbotson, S.H.; Brown, C.T.A.; Eadie, E.; Wood, K. Depth penetration of light into skin as a function of wavelength from 200 to 1000 nm. *Photochem. Photobiol.* **2022**, *98*, 974–981. [CrossRef] [PubMed]
25. Stolik, S.; Delgado, J.A.; Perez, A.; Anasagasti, L. Measurement of the penetration depths of red and near infrared light in human "ex vivo" tissues. *J. Photochem. Photobiol. B* **2000**, *57*, 90–93. [CrossRef] [PubMed]
26. Jung, I.G.; Jeong, J.Y.; Yum, S.H.; Hwang, Y.J. Inhibitory effects of selected medicinal plants on bacterial growth of methicillin-resistant *Staphylococcus aureus*. *Molecules* **2022**, *27*, 7780. [CrossRef] [PubMed]
27. Motelica, L.; Vasile, B.S.; Ficai, A.; Surdu, A.V.; Ficai, D.; Oprea, O.C.; Andronescu, E.; Mustatea, G.; Ungureanu, E.L.; Dobre, A.A. Antibacterial activity of zinc oxide nanoparticles loaded with essential oils. *Pharmaceutics* **2023**, *15*, 2470. [CrossRef] [PubMed]
28. Mun, Y.S.; Hwang, Y.J. Novel spa and multi-locus sequence types (mlst) of *Staphylococcus aureus* samples isolated from clinical specimens in Korean. *Antibiotics* **2019**, *8*, 202. [CrossRef] [PubMed]
29. Jeong, J.Y.; Jung, I.G.; Yum, S.H.; Hwang, Y.J. In vitro synergistic inhibitory effects of plant extract combinations on bacterial growth of methicillin-resistant *Staphylococcus aureus*. *Pharmaceuticals* **2023**, *16*, 1491. [CrossRef]

30. Chraibi, M.; Farah, A.; Elamin, O.; Iraqui, H.M.; Fikri-Benbrahim, K. Characterization, antioxidant, antimycobacterial, antimicrobial effcts of moroccan rosemary essential oil, and its synergistic antimicrobial potential with carvacrol. *J. Adv. Pharm. Technol. Res.* **2020**, *11*, 25–29. [CrossRef]
31. Rohringer, S.; Holnthoner, W.; Chaudary, S.; Slezak, P.; Priglinger, E.; Strassl, M.; Pill, K.; Mühleder, S.; Redl, H.; Dungel, P. The impact of wavelengths of LED light-therapy on endothelial cells. *Sci. Rep.* **2017**, *7*, 10700. [CrossRef] [PubMed]
32. Mueller, M.; Weinmann, D.; Toegel, S.; Holzer, W.; Unger, F.M.; Viernstein, H. Compounds from Caesalpinia sappan with anti-inflammatory properties in macrophages and chondrocytes. *Food Funct.* **2016**, *7*, 1671–1679. [CrossRef] [PubMed]
33. Assar, D.H.; Elhabashi, N.; Mokhbatly, A.A.; Ragab, A.E.; Elbialy, Z.I.; Rizk, S.A.; Albalawi, A.E.; Althobaiti, N.A.; Al Jaouni, S.; Atiba, A. Wound healing potential of licorice extract in rat model: Antioxidants, histopathological, immunohistochemical and gene expression evidences. *Biomed. Pharmacother.* **2021**, *143*, 112151. [CrossRef] [PubMed]
34. Lachowicz, S.; Oszmianski, J.; Rapak, A.; Ochmian, I. Profile and content of phenolic compounds in leaves, flowers, roots, and stalks of Sanguisorba officinalis L. Determined with the lc-dad-esi-qtof-ms/ms analysis and their in vitro antioxidant, antidiabetic, antiproliferative potency. *Pharmaceuticals* **2020**, *13*, 191. [CrossRef] [PubMed]
35. Ibrahim, N.; Mohd Yusoff, N.Z.; Ahmad, R. Quantification of catechin in leaves and stems of malaysian uncaria gambir (hunter) roxb. By hplc-dad. *Malays. J. Anal. Sci.* **2016**, *20*, 567–572. [CrossRef]
36. Ash, C.; Dubec, M.; Donne, K.; Bashford, T. Effect of wavelength and beam width on penetration in light-tissue interaction using computational methods. *Lasers Med. Sci.* **2017**, *32*, 1909–1918. [CrossRef] [PubMed]
37. Austin, E.; Geisler, A.N.; Nguyen, J.; Kohli, I.; Hamzavi, I.; Lim, H.W.; Jagdeo, J. Visible light. Part i: Properties and cutaneous effects of visible light. *J. Am. Acad. Dermatol.* **2021**, *84*, 1219–1231. [CrossRef] [PubMed]
38. Kleinpenning, M.M.; Smits, T.; Frunt, M.H.; van Erp, P.E.; van de Kerkhof, P.C.; Gerritsen, R.M. Clinical and histological effects of blue light on normal skin. *Photodermatol. Photoimmunol. Photomed.* **2010**, *26*, 16–21. [CrossRef]
39. Yin, R.; Dai, T.; Avci, P.; Jorge, A.E.; de Melo, W.C.; Vecchio, D.; Huang, Y.Y.; Gupta, A.; Hamblin, M.R. Light based anti-infectives: Ultraviolet c irradiation, photodynamic therapy, blue light, and beyond. *Curr. Opin. Pharmacol.* **2013**, *13*, 731–762. [CrossRef]

pharmaceutics

MDPI

Article

Cytotoxic and Immunomodulatory Effects of Hypericin as a Photosensitizer in Photodynamic Therapy Used on Skin Cell Cultures

Magdalena Krupka-Olek [1,2,*], Andrzej Bożek [2], Zenon P. Czuba [3], Małgorzata Kłósek [3], Grzegorz Cieślar [4] and Aleksandra Kawczyk-Krupka [4,*]

1 Doctoral School of the Medical University of Silesia, 40-055 Katowice, Poland
2 Clinical Department of Internal Diseases and Geriatrics, Chair of Internal Diseases, Dermatology and Allergology in Zabrze, Medical University of Silesia, 40-055 Katowice, Poland; andrzej.bozek@sum.edu.pl
3 Department of Microbiology and Immunology, Faculty of Medical Sciences in Zabrze, Medical University of Silesia, 40-055 Katowice, Poland; zczuba@sum.edu.pl (Z.P.C.); mklosek@sum.edu.pl (M.K.)
4 Department of Internal Diseases, Angiology and Physical Medicine, Center for Laser Diagnostics and Therapy, Faculty of Medical Sciences in Zabrze, Medical University of Silesia, 40-055 Katowice, Poland; cieslar1@tlen.pl
* Correspondence: magda.krupka94@gmail.com or d201054@365.sum.edu.pl (M.K.-O.); akawczyk@gmail.com (A.K.-K.)

Abstract: Determination of the hypericin–photodynamic (HY–PDT) effect on the secretion of cytokines secreted by the skin cells, may be the basis for using the immunomodulatory effect of photodynamic action in the treatment of inflammatory skin diseases. The study aimed to evaluate the cytotoxic and immunomodulatory effects of hypericin (HY) in photodynamic therapy (PDT) performed in vitro on cultures of selected skin cell lines. The study used two human cell lines, primary dermal fibroblast (HDFa) and primary epidermal keratinocytes (HEKa). The MTT test was used to define the metabolic activity of treated cells. Cell supernatants subjected to sublethal PDT were assessed to determine the interleukins: IL-2, IL-8, IL-10, IL-11, IL-19, IL-22, and metalloproteinase 1 (MMP-1). The results confirm the destructive effect of HY–PDT and the immunomodulatory effects of sublethal doses on the selected skin cells, depending on the concentration of HY and the light doses. No statistically significant differences were noted in IL-2 and IL-10 concentration after HY–PDT for HEKa and HDFa lines. After using HY–PDT, the concentration of IL-8, MMP-1, IL-22, and IL-11 significantly decreased in the HEKa line. Moreover, the concentration of IL-19 and MMP-1 significantly decreased in the HDFa line. The concentration of IL-11 in the HDFa line after using only the HY, without the light, increased but decreased after HY–PDT. Our experiment confirmed that HY–PDT has not only a cytotoxic effect but, used in sublethal doses, also presents immunomodulatory properties. These may be an advantage of HY–PDT when used in the treatment of persistent skin inflammation, connected with the release of pro-inflammatory cytokines resistant to conventional treatment methods.

Keywords: photodynamic therapy; hypericin; skin cell cultures; immunomodulatory effect

1. Introduction

Hypericin (HY) (4,5,7,4′,5′,7′-hexahydroxy-2,2′-dimethylnaphthodianthrone) is a natural dye with hydrophobic properties found in some species of the genus Hypericum, especially *Hypericum perforatum* L. (St. John's wort), basidiomycetes (*Dermocybe* spp.) and endophytic fungi (*Thielavia subthermophila*). As a natural substance with unexpectedly diverse and beneficial medical effects, it has been explored in recent decades for its wide pharmacological spectrum [1–6]. HY has antibacterial and antiviral, anticancer, antioxidant and neuroprotective properties, and has therefore been used in the treatment of many diseases, either as an independent substance or, using its photosensitizing properties, in photodynamic therapy [7,8]. *Hypericum perforatum* extracts have been used for thousands of years to treat abrasions, cuts and wounds [7] (Figure 1).

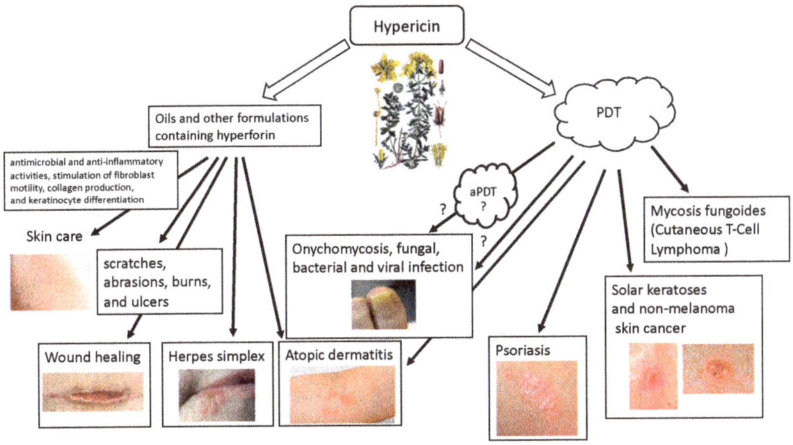

Figure 1. Use of hypericin in skin diseases (HY).

Oils containing hyperforin and hypericin or their derivatives are appropriate for application on scratches, abrasions, burns, and ulcers. The effectiveness of oil containing HY in the treatment is thanks to its antimicrobial and anti-inflammatory properties, which also follow from the stimulation of fibroblast motility, collagen production, and keratinocyte differentiation. The inflammation-reducing effects of HY are partly related to its antibacterial (e.g., directed against methicillin-resistant Staphylococcus aureus (MRSA) and penicillin-resistant (PRSA)) and antiviral (targeted against murine cytomegalovirus (MCMV), Sindbis virus, Friend's virus, herpes virus and Ranscher virus). The advantage of HY is that it is highly photoreactive. Due to the relatively short distance between oxygen atoms (about 2.5 Å), hydroxyl hydrogen can transfer between hydroxyl oxygen and carbonyl oxygen in the presence of fluorescent light. The fluorescence spectrum of hypericin and its analogues shows a "protonated" carbonyl group, which supports hydrogen transfer and acidification of the surrounding environment. Therefore, hydrogen flows constantly between two oxygen atoms under the influence of fluorescent light. Having as many as two negative charges in its structure, it can diffuse through the plasma membrane and move in intracellular membranes. HY interacts with hydrophobic structures through non-covalent bonds such as hydrogen bonds, van der Waals forces, hydrophobic effects, and π-π stacking. Due to the balance between the anionic and hydrophobic nature in the compound structure, HY can localize to various parts of the cell, such as lysosomes and the Golgi apparatus, cytoplasm and endoplasmic reticulum.

Hypericin is known as a natural photosensitizing agent used in photodynamic therapy. In addition to its anticancer effect, it is characterized by fungicidal, bactericidal and antiviral properties [9–21]. HY's optical properties configure its absorption of the visible light spectrum from 500 to 620 nm, with a maximum absorption at 595 nm, showing light emission of the order of 603 nm and is characterized by an intense red fluorescence [22]. The use of HY is made difficult by its phototoxicity, high temperature and pH, poor water solubility and high light sensitivity. The molar extinction coefficients of HY at approximately 590 nm range from 27,000 to 52,000 depending on the solvent, raw material, manufacturing process, aggregation, storage conditions, moisture, etc. The absorbance of the peak at 595 nm decreases upon increasing the pH, with the concomitant formation of a new, broad absorption band near 620–640 nm [23]. The quantum yield of singlet oxygen photosensitized by HY in air-saturated DMSO is $\Phi_\Delta = 0.4 \pm 0.03$. The rate constant for HY triplet state depopulation in reaction with ground state molecular oxygen is $k_q = 1.6 \pm 0.3 \times 10^9\ M^{-1}\ s^{-1}$. HY may act as a sensitizer in photodynamic reactions (mainly by type II mechanism). After activation with light, HY is effective primarily in the production of singlet oxygen (type II mechanism) but also superoxide anion (type I mechanism), which ultimately leads to necrosis, apoptosis, and autophagy, while, as an ICD type II inducer, HY–PDT can activate the immune system. There are two types of PDT reactions. Reactions that fall within the type I mechanism lead to the formation of radicals and radical ions that react with molecular oxygen, leading to the production of reactive oxygen species (ROS), such as superoxide anion, hydrogen peroxide (H_2O_2) and hydroxyl radical. In a second mechanism, the photosensitizer can transfer its energy to molecular oxygen via a triplet–triplet annihilation reaction, producing singlet oxygen ($^1O_2$). The production of ROS leads to lipid peroxidation and membrane damage, which is why hypericin and similar substances that sensitize to $^1O_2$ are highly phototoxic. This type II reaction mechanism has been shown to predominate during PDT. However, it has been proven that the photosensitization reaction carried out by HY can be transferred from type II to type I and vice versa, using different concentrations of antioxidants [24]. Regardless of the initial reaction, both type I and type II mechanisms lead to oxidative damage and tumor destruction. The photocytotoxicity of hypericin is highly oxygen-dependent, resulting in the activation of various forms of cell death (Figure 2). Probably the main mechanism of action of HY–PDT is the release of mitochondrial cytochrome c and secondary impairment of mitochondrial respiratory functions. Nevertheless, the final effect of HY–PDT depends on many factors. It has been proven that the phototoxicity of hypericin depends on the light dose and its concentration, and it has also been shown that the location of the photosensitizer in the cell and the mechanisms of cell death (apoptosis and necrosis) depend on the cell type.

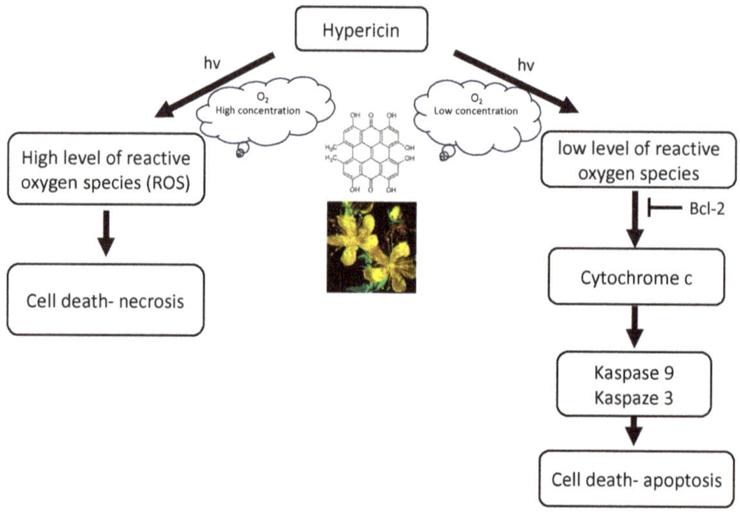

Figure 2. The mechanism of action of hypericin (HY).

The anticancer effect of HY involves the induction of apoptosis by activating caspases, which are cysteine proteases that trigger a cascade of proteolytic cleavages in cells. In addition, HY also causes the release of cytochrome c from mitochondria, inhibiting the growth of cancerous tissues, including glioma, neuroblastoma, adenoma, mesothelioma, melanoma, carcinoma, sarcoma, and leukemia. Additionally, in the presence of light and oxygen, hypericin, acting as a natural photosensitizer, leads to the production of superoxide radicals, which in turn create superoxide or hydroxyl radicals, i.e., singlet oxygen molecules, with cytotoxic properties towards cancer cells. Furthermore, death signals other than the mitochondria-mediated caspase activation cascade contribute to the enhancement of hypericin-induced photokilling in some cell types. When using necrotic concentrations of HY, no activation of caspases is observed, despite the rapid release of mitochondrial cytochrome c into the cytosol, which is probably the result of direct inactivation of caspases as a result of oxidation of the cysteinyl residue, which in turn may block the apoptotic pathway and shift the balance towards necrosis. High levels of oxidative stress induced by necrotic PDT states can cause rapid and irreversible impairment of mitochondrial function, causing a decrease in ATP levels and inhibiting the possibility of cell death through apoptosis. Thus, HY–PDT is a potent inducer of the mitochondrial caspase activation pathway; however, the "extrinsic" caspase activation pathway may also contribute to cell photokilling. HY interferes with the release of anti-apoptotic Bcl-2 family members, including Bcl-2 and Bcl-XL, and inhibit cytochrome c efflux, while pro-apoptotic members such as Bid, Bax, and Bad promote its release. At the same time, immediately after irradiation, JNK1 and p38 MAPK are activated, while ERK are inhibited [1]. Clinical trials have shown that the use of HY–PDT has potential in the treatment of different neoplasmatic diseases, including recurrent mesothelioma and basal cell, and squamous cell carcinoma as well as psoriasis, warts and skin cancer malignant glioma, pituitary adenoma and cutaneous T-cell lymphoma [20,25–28].

There are various possibilities for using HY in skin diseases. Both in the form of traditionally used oils and in external application for the treatment of burns, including sunburns, wounds, blunt injuries, hemorrhoids, ulcers, bedsores, and colloidal scars [7]. In these skin diseases, the antibacterial, antifungal, antiviral, anti-inflammatory and antioxidant properties of hypericin are used. Hypericin also shows potential in the treatment of inflammatory skin diseases with autoimmune deficiencies, such as atopic dermatitis or psoriasis. Moreover, hypericin's second form of use in the treatment of dermatological diseases is as a photodynamic therapy in the treatment of basal cell carcinoma of the skin, mycosis fungoides, and even as a potential treatment for melanoma. In a clinical trial, 8 patients with squamous cell carcinoma (SCC (40–100 μg) 2–4 weeks) and 11 patients with basal cell carcinoma (BCC (40–200 μg) 2–6 weeks) were treated with local application of intralesional hypericin and visible light irradiation 3–5 times a week [26]. Clinical remissions were observed after 6–8 weeks [26]. A clinical trial using HY–PDT in actinic keratosis (8 with AK), basal cell carcinoma (21 with BCC) and Bowen's disease (5 with carcinoma in situ) (0.15–0.25% HY, 2 h, 75 J/cm^2 red light) has also been described [29]. After this HY–PDT, authors described complete remission in 50% for AK, 28% in patients with superficial BCC, and 40% in patients with Bowen's disease and partial remission in patients with nodular BCC.

Recently, the results of a multicenter, placebo-controlled, double-blind, randomized phase III clinical trial (FLASH study) conducted from December 2015 to November 2020 in medical centers in the USA using local application of 0.25% HY ointment in photodynamic therapy of patients were published in the early stage of mycosis fungoides (MF, chronic T cutaneous lymphoma (CTCL)). The study confirmed the effectiveness of such treatment, emphasizing its good safety profile and lack of mutagenic effect. The study population included 169 patients, and, after 6 weeks of treatment, HY–PDT was 49% more effective than placebo after 3 cycles. There were no serious drug-related side effects [30,31]. Additionally, Rook et al. confirmed, in a phase II placebo-controlled study, the effectiveness of photodynamic therapy with topical hypericin and visible light irradiation in the treatment of cutaneous T-cell lymphoma and psoriasis [32]. A new, undeniably interesting direction may be the use of antimicrobial PDT (aPDT) with HY, which is confirmed by research and the associated published results using HY–PDT f.e. in onychomycosis [33,34]. It has been observed that HY inhibits the proliferation of various tumor cells, including lung cancers, bladder, colon, glioma, breast, cervical, leukemia, hepatic, melanoma and lymphoma [20,21]. Its use in inflammatory skin diseases, with its immunomodulating effect, may allow this form of therapy in chronic inflammatory skin diseases that cannot be treated conventionally, such as psoriasis, atopic dermatitis, or skin infection [7,28,32,35].

Inflammatory skin diseases, such as atopic dermatitis or psoriasis, are always difficult medical problems. They are usually chronic and require various forms of therapy, and, unfortunately, some patients require lifelong treatment. Cytokines are involved in initiating and maintaining inflammation and are responsible for the chronic and recurrent nature of the disease [36,37]. When cytokines induce inflammation, macrophages activate their production. The newest group of drugs used to treat psoriasis and atopic dermatitis are substances that affect the immune system [38,39]. Anti-interleukin (IL) therapies are the primary treatment for patients with moderate-to-severe psoriasis, therefore an important topic would be the impact of photodynamic therapy on the release of interleukins that play a major role in the etiopathogenesis of psoriasis [40].

Inflammatory skin diseases, including atopic dermatitis and psoriasis, constitute an important clinical problem. The primary physical effective dermatology method for treating inflammatory skin diseases is phototherapy, including laser therapy, photodynamic therapy (PDT), bath-PUVA, and extracorporeal photochemotherapy [41,42]. It has been confirmed that photodynamic therapy has cytotoxic and immunomodulatory effects [43]. PDT targets inflammatory cells, interferes with the production of cytokines and has a significant antibacterial effect on atopic skin [44]. Therefore, it is important to determine the PDT effect on skin cells and their secretion of cytokines.

In recent years, the significant role of the immune system, including cytokines, in the etiopathogenesis and course of autoimmune inflammatory skin diseases has been demonstrated [45,46]. Determination of the immunological profile of patients with severe inflammatory skin diseases that are resistant to conventional treatment methods, such as atopic dermatitis and psoriasis, supported by in vitro studies of the effect of PDT on the cytokine production by cells of the skin, may be the basis for the possible qualification of this group of patients for photodynamic therapy. This would act through an immunomodulatory mechanism and would be minimally invasive, thus avoiding severe side effects. To test the hypothesis that HY–PDT has an immunoregulatory effect by influencing the secretion of cytokines from the keratinocytes and fibroblasts responsible for the inflammatory process, we examined the effect of HY–PDT on the immunological activity of keratinocytes and fibroblasts in culture, measuring the secretion of IL-2, IL-8, IL-10, IL-11, IL-19, IL-22, and MMP-1.

2. Materials and Methods

2.1. Chemicals

Dimethyl sulfoxide (DMSO), hydrocortisone, HY (Hypericin Calbiochem), and MTT (3-[4,5-dimethylthiazol-2-yl]-2,5-diphenyltetrazolium bromide) were acquired from Sigma–Aldrich (St. Louis, MO, USA). From ATCC (Manassas, VA, USA) provided DMEM: F-12, Dulbecc's Modified Eagle's Medium (DMEM), trypsin (0.23%)-ethylenediaminetetraacetic acid (EDTA) (0.53 mM), and inactivated fetal bovine serum (FBS). PAA Laboratories (Cölbe, Germany) supplied Dulbecc's phosphate-buffered saline (DPBS) free of calcium and magnesium ions. The supplier of Bio-Plex Pro Assays was BIO-RAD Laboratories, Inc. (Hercules, CA, USA). All additional substances were pure or of analytical grade.

2.2. Cell Cultures

The scheme of the HY–PDT experiment is presented on the Figure 3.

The experiments were conducted on HEKa (Figure 4) primary epidermal keratinocytes (PCS-200-011) and HDFa (Figure 4) primary dermal fibroblasts (PCS-201-012). The supplier of cell lines was ATCC (Manassas, VA, USA). The cells HEKa were grown in monolayer cultures in dermal cell basal medium with 0.4% bovine pituitary extract (BPE), supplemented with rh TGF-α, L-glutamine, hydrocortisone hemisuccinate, rh insulin, epinephrine, apotransferrin, 100 U/mL penicillin, 10 µg/mL streptomycin, and 25 ng/mL amphotericin B solution. The HDFa cells were grown in monolayer cultures in fibroblast basal medium supplemented with rh FGF-β, L-glutamine, ascorbic acid, hydrocortisone hemisuccinate, rh insulin, 2% bovine fetal serum, penicillin 100 U/mL, streptomycin 10 µg/mL, and amphotericin B solution 25 ng/mL. The cells were incubated in a humidified atmosphere at 37 °C with 5% CO_2. The passages were conducted twice a week. The adhered HEKa and HDFa cells were treated with EDTA 0.02%, trypsin 0.05%, and trypsin neutralizing solution. The suspensions of 1.5×10^5/mL HEKa cells and 1×10^5/mL HDFa cells were used for the experiments. The next step of the study was to seed the skin cells in equivalent amounts of 200 μL per well into a 96-well plate. Incubation was then performed for 24 h to obtain adhesion.

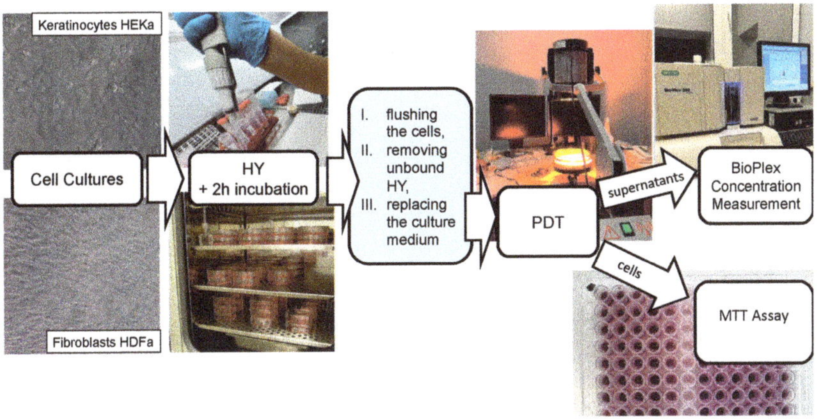

Figure 3. The scheme of the experiment HY–PDT.

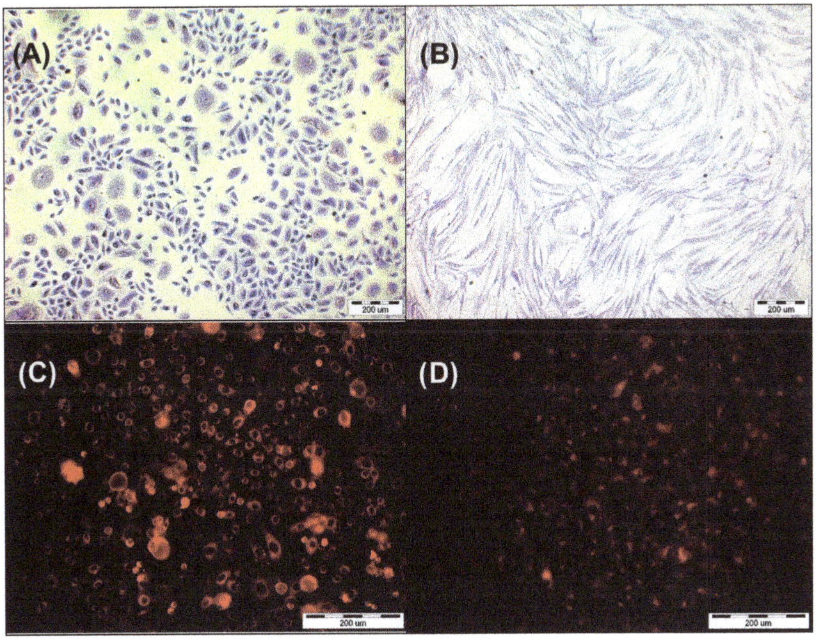

Figure 4. (**A**) Primary epidermal keratinocytes; normal, human, adult (HEKa) stained by Giemsa's solution. (**B**) Primary dermal fibroblast (HDFa) stained by Giemsa's solution. (**C**) HEKa line cells after incubation with HY in concentration 1 μM. (**D**) HDFa line cells after incubation with HY in concentration 1 μM.

2.3. Fluorescence Microscopy

The HEKa primary epidermal keratinocytes and HDFa primary dermal fibroblast adhered for 24 h in 96-well plates. The next day, the growth medium was removed, and the cells were washed with DPBS without calcium and magnesium ions. For two hours, HY was given to cells at the following final concentrations: 0.125 μM, 0.25 μM, 0.5 μM, and

1 μM. Dissolving HY in DMSO to a final concentration of ≤0.01% obtained the solution of 1 mM stock. After two hours, cells were rinsed with DPBS without calcium and magnesium ions, and the culture fresh medium was added. Using an Olympus IX51 inverted research microscope equipped with a color view camera (Tokyo, Japan, Olympus Inc.) and version 2.6 of Cell F software (Soft Imaging System GmbH, Münster, Germany) for capturing and analyzing images from microscope, the presence of HY in the cells was verified (Figure 4).

2.4. Photodynamic Therapy

In the next step of the research, following a 24 h period of adhesion, HEKa and HDFa cells were incubated for a 2 h period with HY at levels of 0 μM, 0.125 μM, 0.25 μM, 0.5 μM, and 1 μM. Since HY was added, the experiment was carried out without direct access to light. Following incubation of the cells with the PS, PBS without magnesium and calcium was flushed and replaced with the culture medium. Then, using an incoherent light source TO-1 (Cosmedico Medizintechnik Gm-bH, Schwenningen, Germany), the cells were exposed to visible light (VIS; 450–720 nm) as PDT (Figure 3). The infrared and orange light filters permitted the passage of wavelengths between 580–720 nm. For the experiment used the light doses of 1 J/cm^2, 2 J/cm^2, and 5 J/cm^2 were used and the fluence rate was 35 mW/cm^2. The distance between the light source and the plate containing the cells was 30 cm. To avoid the heating effect in the experiment a double water filter was used. Later, the cells were incubated for 24 h in the dark. The controls were cells without light exposure.

2.5. MTT Assay

The colorimetric MTT examination was performed to measure cell metabolic activity. MTT was used according to the typical protocol. Supernatants were gathered after 24 h of incubation and frozen at −80 °C, to preserve them for further experiment. The fresh medium with MTT was inserted into the cells at a concentration of 0.5 mg/mL and lasted four hours for incubation time. Subsequently, after incubation, the medium was injected with unreduced MTT, and DMSO was added in order to dissolve the formazan. The crystals were liquefied for ten minutes by shaking the plates after adding DMSO. After the transfer of the solution to a polypropylene plate, the absorbance was determined spectrophotometrically at a wavelength of 550 nm using a microplate reader (Bio-Tek Instruments Inc., eLx 800, Winooski, VT, USA). In the study, reduction of MTT was calculated as a percentage of the dark group control for each cell line.

2.6. Cytokines Measurements

In the next step of the experiment, IL-2, IL-8, IL-10, IL-11, IL-19, IL-22, and MMP-1 markings were undertaken with Bio-Plex Pro™ Assay kit and with Bio-Plex Suspension Array System (BIO-RAD Laboratories Inc., Hercules, CA, USA) (Figure 3). Assays were performed for control samples and samples treated with sublethal doses of HY–PDT at concentrations 0 μM, 0.25 μM, and 0.5 μM of HY. When we used the irradiation at a dose of 5 J/cm^2, a decrease in the metabolic activity of cells measured by the MTT test was observed, which indicates the cytotoxic effect of HY PDT. Therefore, irradiation doses of 1 J/cm^2 and 2 J/cm^2 were considered sublethal and subsequent experiments aimed at measuring cytokines secreted by living cells were carried out only for doses of 1 J/cm^2 and 2 J/cm^2. After centrifugation, the supernatants were transferred to 96-well microplates and diluted with buffer to a volume of 50 μL. Standards of the analyses to be determined were also placed in the plate wells. Then, a suspension of magnetic beads coated with specific antibodies was added to the analyses. Further proceedings followed the manufacture's instructions. The Bio-Plex Pro™ Assay kit consisted of 5.6 μm diameter fluorescent-dyed polystyrene beads that varied in color depending on the bound detection substance, a flow cytometer, and compatible software that automatically analyzed fluorescence results. After pre-wetting the well filter plate with wash buffer, the solution in each well was aspirated using a vacuum manifold. In the next step, the culture supernatants of the tested cells were incubated with antibody-conjugated beads for 30 min. Cytokines are determined using an antibody covalently bound to an appropriately colored polystyrene bead. After incubation, the test suspension was washed to remove unbound cytokine antibodies. In the next step, biotinylated specific detection antibodies that bind to the epitopes of the tested cytokines were added.

After another incubation and a series of washes, detection antibodies and streptavidin–phycoerythrin were added to the tested material for 30 min. Streptavidin has an affinity for the biotinylated detection antibody, and phycoerythrin is used as a fluorescent marker. After incubation, unbound streptavidin–PE was again removed from the solution by a series of buffer washes. The finally obtained beads covered with complexes labelled with phycoerythrin were analyzed in the Bio-Plex 3D Suspension Array System (Bio-Rad Laboratories Inc., USA). Beads associated with each cytokine were analyzed in a Bioplex Array Reader (Bio-Plex® 200 system). The fluorescence intensity was assessed using the Bio-Plex Manager™ program and the concentrations of the tested cytokines corresponding to the fluorescence intensity were automatically calculated using this program. The concentrations of the determined cytokines were obtained based on standard curves using the manufacture's software. The experiments were repeated four times ($n = 4$).

2.7. Statistical Analysis

The Shapiro–Wilk test was performed to check the normality of distribution. Regularity of distribution was gained in the case of the MTT test, and the proportion of MTT reduction of the examined unit concerning the control group was compared using the Student's *t*-test. To calculate cytokine denseness, Kruskal–Wallis analysis of variance (ANOVA) with post hoc examination using the multiple comparison test was used to define cytokine concentrations. The statistical examination was used in Statistica version 13 (TIBCO Software Inc., Palo Alto, CA, USA, 2017), and the diagrams were arranged using Excel® (Microsoft 365, 2303 version). Statistical significance was achieved for values of $p < 0.05$ (**) or $p < 0.01$ (***). The experiments were repeated four times ($n = 4$).

3. Results

3.1. Fluorescence Microscopy

HY uptake by both cell lines was observed by using a fluorescent microscope. The control groups that were not administered HY were shown to have no fluorescence. When HY concentrations in the culture medium increased, fluorescence in the HY-incubated cells increased as well (Figure 4).

3.2. MTT Cytotoxicity Assay

In the dark, HY showed a cytotoxic effect on both lines in the MTT assay. The cytotoxic effect is more visible in the case of the HDFa cell line, with a significant reduction in MTT reduction noticeable at a dose of 0.25 µM HY (MTT reduction = 79.62% ± 1.77, $p > 0.01$), while in the case of the HEKa line, a statistically significant cytotoxic effect occurred for the highest dose of HY 1 µM (MTT reduction = 87.90% ± 1.80, $p > 0.05$) (Figures 5 and 6).

For a light dose of 1 J/cm^2, light-only therapy and also in combination with a low HY dose of 0.125 µM had a stimulating effect on HEKa line cells (MTT reduction = 127.18% ± 1.71, *** $p < 0.01$; MTT reduction = 125.63% ± 1.06, *** $p < 0.01$, respectively). In the case of HY concentration of 1 µM on this cell line, it already had a cytotoxic effect (MTT reduction = 55.77% ± 0.74, *** $p < 0.01$) (Figures 5 and 6).

For a light dose of 2 J/cm^2, a similarly light-only therapy, without HY and in combination with small doses of HY 0.125 µM, 0.25 µM had a stimulating effect on HEKa line cells (respectively, MTT reduction = 130.58% ± 1.03, *** $p < 0.01$; MTT 114.85% ± 0.84, *** $p < 0.01$; MTT reduction = 122.29 ± 1.94, *** $p < 0.01$). The cytotoxic effect in HEKa is noticeable at a 1 µM dose (MTT reduction = 33.71 ± 1.41, *** $p < 0.01$). In the HDFa line, a stimulating effect also appears in the concentration of HY 0.125 µM and light-only exposure (MTT reduction = 106.29 ± 1.68, *** $p < 0.01$, MTT reduction = 108.49 ± 1.22, *** $p < 0.01$). The cytotoxic effect in HDFa is visible in doses of HY 1µM (Figures 5 and 6).

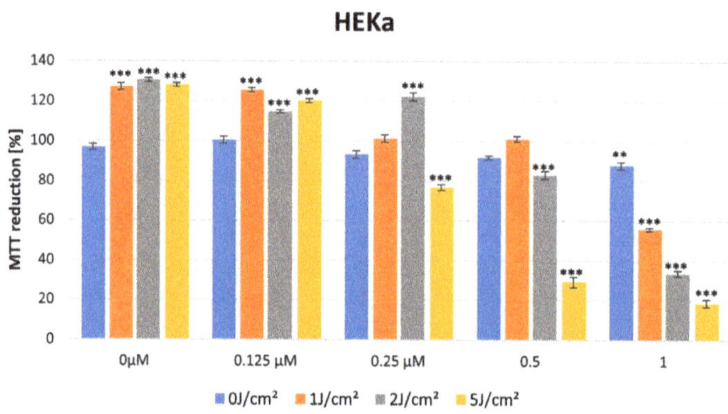

Figure 5. MTT reduction in the HEKa cell lines for different HY concentrations: 0 μM, 0.125 μM, 0.25 μM, 0.5 μM, and 1 μM and different light doses: 0 J/cm^2, 1 J/cm^2, 2 J/cm^2, 5 J/cm^2. The values represent the means ± SE. ** $p < 0.05$, *** $p < 0.01$.

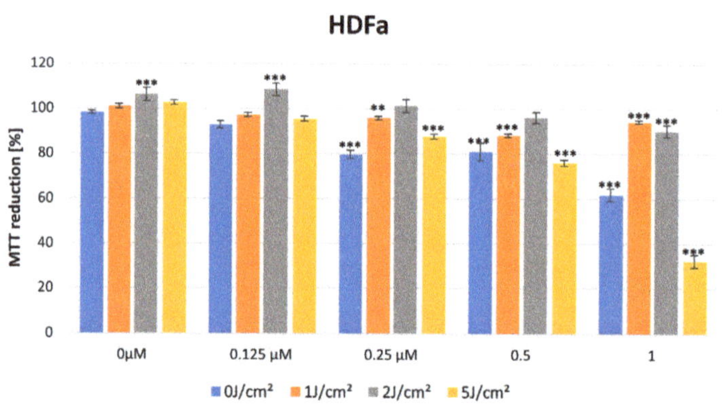

Figure 6. MTT reduction in the HDFa cell lines for different HY concentrations: 0 μM, 0.125 μM, 0.25 μM, 0.5 μM, and 1 μM and different light doses: 0 J/cm^2, 1 J/cm^2, 2 J/cm^2, 5 J/cm^2. The values represent the means ± SE. ** $p < 0.05$, *** $p < 0.01$.

When a higher light dose of 5 J/cm^2 was used, cytotoxicity significantly increased in both cell lines with increasing HY concentration (HEKa: MTT reduction = 18.55 ± 0.79, *** $p < 0.01$; HDFa: MTT reduction = 32.48 ± 2.42, *** $p < 0.01$) (Figures 5 and 6).

3.3. *Effect of HY–PDT on the Secretory Activity of IL-2, IL-10, MMP-1, IL-19, IL-22, IL-11, and IL-8*

3.3.1. IL-2

No statistically significant differences were noted in IL-2 concentration after HY–PDT for both HEKa and HDFa lines. For the dark control without PS, in the case of HEKa cells, the IL-2 level was 9.01 pg/mL ± 0.70 pg/mL and in HDFa cells the level was 8.63 pg/mL ± 5.07 pg/mL (Figures 7 and 8).

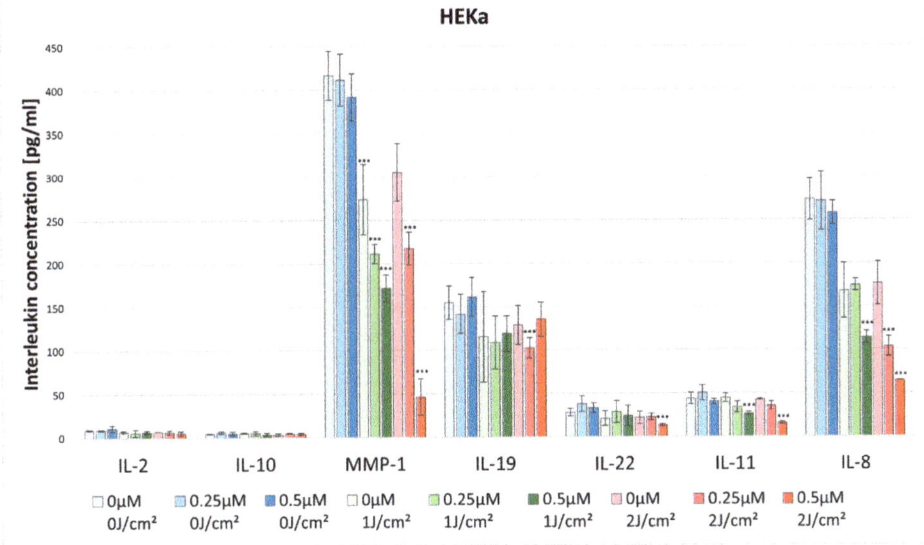

Figure 7. The concentration of IL-2, IL-10, MMP-1, IL-19, IL-22, IL-11, and IL-8 in the supernatants from cell culture HEKa line in different light doses (0 J/cm^2, 1 J/cm^2, 2 J/cm^2) and HY concentrations (0 μM, 0.25 μM, 0.5 μM). Statistical differences were marked concerning the dark control group within a given cytokine. The values represent the means ± SD. *** $p < 0.01$.

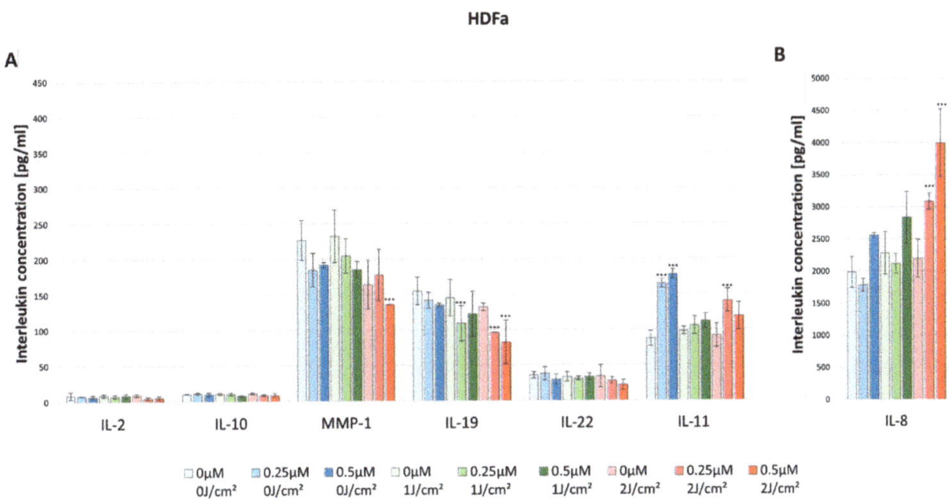

Figure 8. (**A**) The concentration of IL-2, IL-10, MMP-1, IL-19, IL-22, and IL-11 in the supernatants from cell culture HDFa line in different light doses (0 J/cm^2, 1 J/cm^2, 2 J/cm^2) and HY concentrations (0 μM, 0.25 μM, 0.5 μM). Statistical differences were marked concerning the dark control group within a given cytokine. The values represent the means ± SD. *** $p < 0.01$. (**B**) The concentration of IL-8 in the supernatants from cell culture HDFa line in different light doses (0 J/cm^2, 1 J/cm^2, 2 J/cm^2) and HY concentrations (0 μM, 0.25 μM, 0.5 μM). The values represent the means ± SD. *** $p < 0.01$.

3.3.2. IL-8

The concentration of IL-8 after using HY–PDT significantly decreased in the HEKa line. For the dark control the cytokine concentration was 272.96 pg/mL ± 23.91 pg/mL, and for the 0.5 μM at the light dose 1 J/cm^2 the concentration significantly decreased to 113.64 pg/mL ± 7.30 pg/mL. Additionally, for the light dose of 2 J/cm^2 the concentration dropped significantly at a dose of 0.25 μM HY to 103.19 pg/mL ± 11.29 pg/mL, and for the dose of 0.5 μM HY it decreased to 64.38 pg/mL (Figure 7).

In the case of the HDFa line, the concentration significantly increased after irradiation with a light dose of 2 J/cm^2 in the concentrations of HY 0.25 μM (3084.52 pg/mL ± 123.60 pg/mL) and 0.5 μM (3991.77 pg/mL ± 530.95 pg/mL) compared with the dark control (1986.98 pg/mL ± 238.72 pg/mL). As one can see, the HDFa line produced much higher IL-8 concentrations than the HEKa line (Figure 8).

3.3.3. IL-10

There were higher observed levels of IL-10 produced by HDFa than by HEKa cell line. For the dark control in the case of HDFa, the cytokine level was 10.60 pg/mL ± 0.39 pg/mL, while in the HEKa line it was 4.53 pg/mL ± 0.26 pg/mL. However, HY–PDT did not affect the levels of IL-10 secretion (Figures 7 and 8).

3.3.4. MMP-1

The concentration of MMP-1 after the use of HY–PDT significantly decreased in the HEKa line using the light dose of 1 J/cm^2 with 0.25 μM (211.16 pg/mL ± 11.06 pg/mL) and 0.5 μM HY (171.50 pg/mL ± 15.67 pg/mL), and at the dose of 2 J/cm^2 with 0.5 μM HY (46.41 pg/mL ± 20.89 pg/mL) compared with the control group (416.66 pg/mL ± 28.07 pg/mL). It is observable that, after using only the light dose of 1 J/cm^2 with no HY, the concentration has decreased from 416.66 pg/mL ± 28.07 pg/mL to 273.70 pg/mL ± 40.55 pg/mL (Figure 7). Furthermore, the HEKa line produced significantly higher concentrations of MMP-1 than the HDFa line. In the case of the HDFa line, the statistically significant reduction of MMP-1 concentration was observed in the light dose of 2 J/cm^2 with 0.5 μM HY (135.84 pg/mL ± 00.0 pg/mL) when compared with the control group (241.90 pg/mL ± 21.10 pg/mL) (Figure 8).

3.3.5. IL-19

The concentration of IL-19 in HEKa line cells after HY–PDT significantly decreased in the light dose of 2 J/cm^2 with a concentration of 0.5 μM HY (135.29 pg/mL ± 19.62 pg/mL) in comparison with the control group (154.82 pg/mL ± 19.45 pg/mL) (Figure 7).

In HDFa line cells, one can notice a decrease in the concentration of IL-19 at a light dose of 1 J/cm^2 and a concentration of 0.25 μM HY (108.89 pg/mL ± 25.01 pg/mL) related to the dark control (154.82 pg/mL ± 19.45 pg/mL). In the case of a light dose of 2 J/cm^2 a decrease in the concentration was also observed at the concentrations of 0.25 μM HY (95.70 pg/mL) and 0.5 μM HY (81.98 pg/mL ± 30.92 pg/mL) (Figure 8).

3.3.6. IL-22

The concentration of IL-22 after the use of HY–PDT significantly decreased in the HEKa line during light irradiation of 2 J/cm^2 and with a concentration of 0.5 μM HY (13.34 pg/mL ± 1.40 pg/mL) in comparison with the control group (28.09 pg/mL ± 4.55 pg/mL) (Figure 7). No statistically significant differences were noted in IL-22 concentration after HY–PDT for the HDFa line. For the dark control without PS, the level of IL-22 was 35.60 pg/mL ± 4.65 pg/mL (Figure 8).

3.3.7. IL-11

The concentration of IL-11 significantly decreased in the HEKa line after using HY–PDT compared to the control group (43.82 pg/mL ± 6.70 pg/mL). After light irradiation of 1 J/cm^2 and 2 J/cm^2 in the concentration of 0.5 μM HY the level of IL-11 reduced respectively by 26.34 pg/mL ± 1.88 pg/mL; 15.88 pg/mL ± 1.33 pg/mL (Figure 7).

In contrast, in the HDFa line, the usage of only HY in doses of 0.25 μM (164.87 pg/mL ± 6.44 pg/mL) and 0.5 μM (177.67 pg/mL ± 2.52 pg/mL) increased the secretion of IL-11 compared to the control group of HDFa (87.07 pg/mL ± 10.47 pg/mL). However, after HY–PDT, the concentration decreased to the baseline. Additionally, at a light dose of 2 J/cm^2 and 0.25 μM HY, the concentration of IL-11 increased again to 140.54 pg/mL ± 16.39 pg/mL (Figure 8).

4. Discussion

The idea of our study was to assess the impact of the PDT on skin cells, fibroblasts, and keratinocytes, to assess its immunomodulatory effect and possible possibilities of its use in inflammatory skin diseases such as atopic dermatitis (AD) and psoriasis. In our experiment, hypericin was chosen as the photosensitizer (PS), whose properties have previously attracted the attention of many researchers [31–37].

No such studies have examined the effects of HY–PDT on human skin cell types in an in vitro system; however, both in vitro experiments and clinical studies conducted with this natural photosensitizer indicate its effective and multidirectional effect.

Woźniak and Nowak-Perlak have confirmed that HY–PDT may be an effective method of treating patients with skin cancer, with the reservation that the use of hypericin is not easy due to disadvantages such as its poor solubility in water and sensitivity to heat and pH [47]. Nevertheless, we decided to choose this photosensitizer, taking into account its properties, natural origin, effectiveness and the possibility of safe use in inflammatory skin diseases not due to its cytotoxic effect but its immunomodulatory effect, which we wanted to demonstrate and prove in the experiment. In our experiment we used different doses of HY at 0.125 μM, 0.25 μM, 0.5 μM, and 1 μM for two hours as well. Then, after assessing the metabolic activity of cells using the MTT assay, doses of HY and light were selected, at which the cells showed viability comparable to the control. That was to examine the effect of the photodynamic reaction on the secretion of cytokines responsible for the inflammatory process in the skin by keratinocytes and fibroblasts. In this study, we reveal that small doses of HY, 0.125 μM and 0.25 μM, and light, 1 J/cm^2 and 2 J/cm^2, stimulate the metabolic activity of cells measured by the MTT test. In contrast, higher concentrations of HY and light doses (0.5 μM HY and 5 J/cm^2) have an inhibitory effect, both in the study on fibroblast (HDFa) and keratinocyte (HEKa) lines, confirming the cytotoxic effect, dependent on the photosensitizer dose and light, previously demonstrated in the work by Woźniak.

Popovic et al. also experimented to assess HY–PDT effects in vitro on the skin cell types. In a similar manner to our experiment, normal primary human keratinocytes, melanocytes, and fibroblasts were chosen in the study, which represented both the epidermal and dermal cellular compartments of human skin. The authors prepared an HY extract in dimethyl sulfoxide to obtain a 2 mM stock solution. Cells were incubated for four hours in different solutions in the range of 0.25–4 μM, and then HY was triggered with a diode-pumped laser at 561 nm light in the power density of 20 mW and a fluence rate of 5 J/cm^2. The use of 3 μM HY–PDT (four hours incubation period, tunable laser 561 nm, 5 J/cm^2, 20 mW) was cytotoxic to Fb and Mc, but not to Kc, and showed that lower doses of HY (0.25 μM, 0.5 μM, 0.75 μM, 1 μM, 2 μM) result in changes in cell morphology and thus affect various cellular functions. However, the authors discovered differences in the in vitro model between the susceptibility of primary cultured human skin cells to HY–PDT. They found that 3 μM HY–PDT is cytotoxic to fibroblasts to a minor extent in melanocytes but completely obstinate to keratinocytes. Additionally, the authors reveal that significant differences exist in cell viability and morphology between the cells [48]. Therefore, in our experiment, we examined not only the effect of cytotoxic doses of HY–PDT on fibroblasts and keratinocytes but, furthermore, the immunomodulatory activity of photodynamic action using hypericin for its possible use in skin inflammations that are characterized by the high production of cytokines involved in psoriasis and atopic dermatitis. One of the main cytokines involved in atopic dermatitis (AD) and psoriasis is interleukin-2 (IL-2). This cytokine has essential roles in key functions of the immune system, tolerance, and immunity, primarily via its direct effects on T cells [49]. IL-2, depending on its concentration, may exert both immunostimulatory and immuno-suppressive effects in autoimmune diseases, because, at high doses, IL-2 activates the differentiation and expansion of effector and memory T cells, while, at low doses, IL-2 activates the differentiation, survival and function of regulatory T cells (Tregs), a subset of CD4+ T cells [50]. In our experiment, we noted no statistically significant differences in IL-2, which may be related to the dose of photosensitizer, and energy dose, and may also have some beneficial clinical implications in terms of not triggering a possible controversial or unfavorable effect of HY–PDT on the release of this cytokine.

Another important cytokine for AD and psoriasis is interleukin 8. IL-8 levels are increased in psoriatic scale extracts and suction blister fluids in psoriatic skin lesions [51]. In our experiment, although we did not note the effect of HY–PDT on IL-2 secretion, the concentration of IL-8 significantly decreased in the HEKa line, which, considering the role of this cytokine in AD and psoriasis, seems to be an extremely beneficial effect. In our study we noted no statistically significant differences in IL-10 concentration after HY–PDT for HEKa and HDFa lines, which would mean no effect on anti-inflammatory cytokines; however, the lack of inhibition of the secretion of this interleukin, obtained in our experiment, can be taken into account as a beneficial factor.

In a study conducted by Larisch et al., the authors showed that a low dose of HY–PDT affects the secretion of cytokines tested on three human cell lines: HaCat cells, immortalized dermal keratinocytes, A431 cells epidermoid carcinoma cell line (keratinocytes from squamous cell carcinoma), and a primary dermal fibroblast cell line. The authors demonstrated that HY–PDT reduces IL-6 levels in all cell lines. Depending on the conditions, HY–PDT can cause an increase in IL-6 in malignant cells, which induces a specific anti-tumor immune response. The authors showed that, after treatment with HY–PDT, the level of IL-6 in A431 cells in both inflammatory conditions becomes significantly reduced when using a wavelength of 435 nm, while irradiation using a red wavelength of 610 nm had an IL-6-stimulating effect. Moreover, research has confirmed that hypericin itself can increase the level of anti-inflammatory cytokines IL-4, -5 and -10, which is extremely important in terms of its anti-inflammatory effect, alleviating inflammation in skin diseases or accelerating wound healing [52,53]. The effect of HY on its own, without photodynamic action, on the secretory activity of cells observed by these authors was also confirmed in our experiment.

In our study, we used an incoherent light source that enabled 580–720 nm wavelengths to flow through orange and infrared light filters. The concentration of IL-8, MMP-1, IL-22, and IL-11 significantly decreased in the HEKa line. Moreover, the concentration of IL-19 and MMP-1 significantly decreased in the HDFa line. This may confirm the results of Larisch et al. that the wavelength has an impact on the reduction of pro-inflammatory cytokines tested in our experiment, such as IL-8, MMP-1, IL-22, L-11 in the HEKa line and IL-19 and MMP-1 in the HDFa line. Moreover, we observed that the concentration of IL-19 and MMP-1 significantly decreased in the HDFa line. The concentration of IL-11 in the HDFa line after using only the HY, without the light, increased; however, after HY–PDT, it decreased, which would indicate not only the photodynamic effect but also the strong properties of hypericin itself. Larisch et al. have also noted a similar situation, though in the case of IL-10 expression in A431 cells, where hypericin itself caused an increase in this interleukin, and where this effect was intensified after lipopolysaccharide (LPS) induction and irradiation. This is an extremely desirable effect, given that IL-10 is one of the most important anti-inflammatory cytokines, and is involved in infections, acute and chronic inflammation and autoimmune disorders, particularly psoriasis and atopic dermatitis [52].

IL-22 plays an important role in psoriasis, atopic dermatitis, scleroderma and contact dermatitis. Furthermore, the PASI score, which measures the severity of the disease, is significantly linked with IL-22 plasma levels, suggesting that this interleukin may have a role in the etiology of psoriasis [54,55]. In our research, we showed that IL-22 significantly decreased in the HEKa line. Considering the important role of this cytokine in the skin's defense process, this is, unfortunately, not a very beneficial or expected effect. Nevertheless, considering the dependence of the photodynamic effect on the type of photosensitizer, energy dose and research model, it can be hoped that this effect will not be confirmed in clinical trials. In our experiment we reveal that, after HY–PDT, the concentration of IL-11 significantly decreased in the HEKa line, which seems to be a favourable result from the point of view of the unfavorable and excessive effect of fibrosis, often occurring after photodynamic therapy during the healing phase. IL-11 has also been shown to stimulate the release of the alarm cytokine IL-33 in fibroblasts, triggering an inflammatory response in the local microenvironment. Unfortunately, such long-term stimulation ultimately leads to fibrosis, playing an important role in diseases such as systemic sclerosis (SSc) [56,57]. Extensive clinical trials remain necessary to confirm the efficacy of rhIL-11 as an anti-inflammatory agent in psoriasis patients [46].

In our study, we reveal that MMP-1 significantly decreased in the HDFa line, in terms of its antifibrogenic effect, the effect we obtained in terms of the benefits of the healing process after photodynamic therapy may be questionable. Metalloproteinases play a very important role in both physiological and pathological conditions of the body. They take part in the process of wound healing, and scar formation, they also participate in the processes of angiogenesis and apoptosis, autoimmune and inflammatory diseases such as psoriasis, atopic dermatitis and scleroderma. MMP-1 may be a potentially effective antifibrogenic agent for the prevention or treatment of hypertrophic scars [58]. In our study, the concentration of IL-19 significantly decreased in the HDFa line and, considering the role of this cytokine in atopic dermatitis, this seems to be an extremely beneficial phenomenon. The concentration of IL-19 in HEKa line cells, after using HY–PDT, significantly decreased in the light dose of 2 J/cm^2 with a concentration of 0.5 μM HY, in comparison with the control group. In HDFa line cells one can notice a decrease in the concentration of IL-19 at a light dose of 1 J/cm^2 and a concentration of 0.25 μM HY related to the dark control. This anti-inflammatory effect of photodynamic therapy is extremely desirable in inflammatory skin diseases. It has been shown that, in atopic dermatitis, IL-19 is highly expressed in skin lesions [59]. IL-19 shows the most robust differential expression between psoriatic lesions and healthy skin. Cutaneous IL-19 overproduction is reflected by elevated IL-19 blood levels that correlate with psoriasis severity [60].

We simultaneously conducted a clinical trial in our center, which included 139 people suffering from AD, 115 with PS and a control group of 142. Of all of these people, cytokine profiles were determined in the blood serum for IFN-γ, IL-4, IL-2, IL-6, IL-5, IL-12, IL-8, IL-17, TNF-α, IL-22, IL-18, and IL-24 in ELISA. The examination of the above cytokines showed their high similarity in the examined individuals and validated the fact that AD and PS are active inflammatory diseases. Therefore, the next step in our investigations was to determine the effect of HY–PDT on cytokine secretion in vitro studies, in order to use HY–PDT in AD and PS patients [61]. Of course, the complex nature of the mechanism of action of cytokines and their mutual relations are extremely complicated; however, it seems that HY–PDT, which is a natural substance with multidirectional action, may find its place in the treatment of persistent inflammatory skin diseases, such as atopic dermatitis or psoriasis, that cannot be treated with conventional methods.

HY itself also has very interesting effects. This substance inhibits the breakdown of serotonin, a neurotransmitter also called the "happiness hormone", and is also an inhibitor of the reuptake of serotonin, norepinephrine, and dopamine. Classic antidepressants work similarly. Studies have shown that, for patients with mild-to-moderate depression, which has also been shown in AD and PS patients, St. John's wort has comparable effectiveness and safety to SSRIs. All of these reports are extremely interesting and indicate the great potential of HY–PDT in inflammatory skin diseases, not only due to the immunomodulatory effect of HY–PDT, but also the interesting properties of HY itself, which confirms the sense of our research and the possibility of using it in a clinical trial.

5. Conclusions

Hypericin is an effective and natural photosensitizer that can be used in the PDT of inflammatory skin diseases that do not respond to conventional therapy. There are still many cases of patients that require additional forms of therapy to alleviate the course of this disease. HY–PDT may be such an option, as a minimally invasive method based on a natural photosensitizer. Determining the cytokine profile in patients suffering from atopic dermatitis and psoriasis and assessing the effect of HY–PDT on these proteins seems advisable to determine the effectiveness and sense of using this form of therapy and its safety. Additional fundamental and clinical research remains necessary to fully elucidate the roles of various interleukin proteins in the pathogenesis of inflammatory dermatologic diseases and HY–PDT outcomes in patients.

Author Contributions: Conceptualization: M.K.-O., A.K.-K. and A.B.; methodology, Z.P.C., M.K. and A.K.-K.; validation: A.B.; formal analysis: Z.P.C., G.C. and A.B.; data curation: M.K.-O.; writing—original draft preparation: M.K.-O., A.B. and A.K.-K.; writing—review and editing: M.K.-O., A.B. and A.K.-K.; investigation: M.K.; resources: M.K.; funding acquisition: G.C.; visualization: M.K.-O.; supervision: A.B., A.K.-K., Z.P.C. and G.C. All authors have read and agreed to the published version of the manuscript.

Funding: This research was funded by the Medical University of Silesia, Katowice, grant number PCN-2-061/N/2/K.

Institutional Review Board Statement: Not applicable.

Informed Consent Statement: Not applicable.

Data Availability Statement: Data are available on request.

Conflicts of Interest: The authors declare no conflicts of interest.

References

1. Agostinis, P.; Vantieghem, A.; Merlevede, W.; de Witte, P.A. Hypericin in cancer treatment: More light on the way. *Int. J. Biochem. Cell Biol.* **2002**, *34*, 221–241. [CrossRef] [PubMed]
2. Theodossiou, T.A.; Hothersall, J.S.; De Witte, P.A.; Pantos, A.; Agostinis, P. The multifaceted photocytotoxic profile of hypericin. *Mol. Pharm.* **2009**, *6*, 1775–1789. [CrossRef] [PubMed]
3. Zhang, J.; Gao, L.; Hu, J.; Wang, C.; Hagedoorn, P.L.; Li, N.; Zhou, X. Hypericin: Source, determination, separation, and properties. *Sep. Purif. Rev.* **2020**, *51*, 1–10. [CrossRef]
4. Doroshenko, A.; Tomkova, S.; Kozar, T.; Stroffekova, K. Hypericin, a potential new BH3 mimetic. *Front. Pharmacol.* **2022**, *13*, 991554. [CrossRef] [PubMed]
5. Kiesslich, T.; Krammer, B.; Plaetzer, K. Cellular mechanisms and prospective applications of hypericin in photodynamic therapy. *Curr. Med. Chem.* **2006**, *13*, 2189–2204. [CrossRef] [PubMed]
6. Sanovic, R.; Verwanger, T.; Hartl, A.; Krammer, B. Low dose hypericin-PDT induces complete tumor regression in BALB/c mice bearing CT26 colon carcinoma. *Photodiagn. Photodyn. Ther.* **2011**, *8*, 291–296. [CrossRef] [PubMed]
7. Wölfle, U.; Seelinger, G.; Schempp, C.M. Topical application of St. John's wort (*Hypericum perforatum*). *Planta Med.* **2014**, *80*, 109–120. [CrossRef] [PubMed]
8. Ng, Q.X.; Venkatanarayanan, N.; Ho, C.Y. Clinical use of *Hypericum perforatum* (St John's wort) in depression: A meta-analysis. *J. Affect. Disord.* **2017**, *210*, 211–221. [CrossRef]
9. Allison, R.R.; Moghissi, K. Photodynamic therapy (PDT): PDT mechanisms. *Clin. Endosc.* **2013**, *46*, 24–29. [CrossRef]
10. Plaetzer, K.; Krammer, B.; Berlanda, J.; Berr, F.; Kiesslich, T. Photophysics and photochemistry of photodynamic therapy: Fundamental aspects. *Lasers Med. Sci.* **2009**, *24*, 259–268. [CrossRef]
11. Kwiatkowski, S.; Knap, B.; Przystupski, D.; Saczko, J.; Kędzierska, E.; Knap-Czop, K.; Kotlińska, J.; Michel, O.; Kotowski, K.; Kulbacka, J. Photodynamic therapy—Mechanisms, photosensitizers and combinations. *Biomed. Pharmacother.* **2018**, *106*, 1098–1107. [CrossRef] [PubMed]
12. Agostinis, P.; Berg, K.; Cengel, K.A.; Foster, T.H.; Girotti, A.W.; Gollnick, S.O.; Hahn, S.M.; Hamblin, M.R.; Juzeniene, A.; Kessel, D.; et al. Photodynamic therapy of cancer: An update. *CA Cancer J. Clin.* **2011**, *61*, 250–281. [CrossRef] [PubMed]
13. Wachowska, M.; Muchowicz, A.; Demkow, U. Immunological aspects of antitumor photodynamic therapy outcome. *Cent. Eur. J. Immunol.* **2015**, *40*, 481–485. [CrossRef] [PubMed]
14. Oniszczuk, A.; Wojtunik-Kulesza, K.A.; Oniszczuk, T.; Kasprzak, K. The potential of photodynamic therapy (PDT)-Experimental investigations and clinical use. *Biomed. Pharmacother.* **2016**, *83*, 912–929. [CrossRef]

15. Reginato, E.; Wolf, P.; Hamblin, M.R. Immune response after photodynamic therapy increases anti-cancer and anti-bacterial effects. *World J. Immunol.* **2014**, *4*, 1–11. [CrossRef]
16. Dougherty, T.J.; Gomer, C.J.; Henderson, B.W.; Jori, G.; Kessel, D.; Korbelik, M.; Moan, J.; Peng, Q. Photodynamic therapy. *J. Natl. Cancer Inst.* **1998**, *90*, 889–905. [CrossRef]
17. Allison, R.R.; Moghissi, K. Oncologic photodynamic therapy: Clinical strategies that modulate mechanisms of action. *Photodiagn. Photodyn. Ther.* **2013**, *10*, 331–341. [CrossRef] [PubMed]
18. Yang, D.; Lei, S.; Pan, K.; Chen, T.; Lin, J.; Ni, G.; Liu, J.; Zeng, X.; Chen, Q.; Dan, H. Application of photodynamic therapy in immune-related diseases. *Photodiagn. Photodyn. Ther.* **2021**, *34*, 102318. [CrossRef]
19. Sitnik, T.M.; Hampton, J.A.; Henderson, B.W. Reduction of tumour oxygenation during and after photodynamic therapy in vivo: Effects of fluence rate. *Br. J. Cancer* **1998**, *77*, 1386–1394. [CrossRef]
20. Dong, X.; Zeng, Y.; Zhang, Z.; Fu, J.; You, L.; He, Y.; Hao, Y.; Gu, Z.; Yu, Z.; Qu, C.; et al. Hypericin-mediated photodynamic therapy for the treatment of cancer: A review. *J. Pharm. Pharmacol.* **2021**, *73*, 425–436. [CrossRef]
21. Saw, C.L.; Heng, P.W.; Olivo, M. Potentiation of the photodynamic action of hypericin. *J. Environ. Pathol. Toxicol. Oncol.* **2008**, *27*, 23–33. [CrossRef] [PubMed]
22. Yamazaki, T.; Ohta, N.; Yamazaki, I.; Song, P.S. Excited-state properties of hypericin: Electronic spectra and fluorescence decay kinetics. *J. Phys. Chem.* **1993**, *97*, 7870–7875. [CrossRef]
23. Kubin, A.; Wierrani, F.; Burner, U.; Alth, G.; Grünberger, W. Hypericin--the facts about a controversial agent. *Curr. Pharm. Des.* **2005**, *11*, 233–253. [CrossRef] [PubMed]
24. Ehrenberg, B.; Anderson, J.L.; Foote, C.S. Kinetics and yield of singlet oxygen photosensitized by hypericin in organic and biological media. *Photochem. Photobiol.* **1998**, *68*, 135–140. [CrossRef]
25. Koren, H.; Schenk, G.M.; Iindra, R.H.; Alth, G.; Ebermann, R.; Kubin, A.; Koderhold, G.; Kreitner, M. Hypericin in phototherapy. *J. Photochem. Photobiol. B Biol.* **1996**, *36*, 113–119. [CrossRef] [PubMed]
26. Alecu, M.; Ursaciuc, C.; Hălălău, F.; Coman, G.; Merlevede, W.; Waelkens, E.; de Witte, P. Photodynamic treatment of basal cell carcinoma and squamous cell carcinoma with hypericin. *Anticancer Res.* **1998**, *18*, 4651–4654.
27. Sharman, W.M.; Allen, C.M.; van Lier, J.E. Photodynamic therapeutics: Basic principles and clinical applications. *Drug Discov. Today* **1999**, *4*, 507–517. [CrossRef]
28. Lavie, G.; Meruelo, D.; Aroyo, K.; Mandel, M. Inhibition of the CD8+ T cell-mediated cytotoxicity reaction by hypericin: Potential for treatment of T cell-mediated diseases. *Int. Immunol.* **2000**, *12*, 479–486. [CrossRef]
29. Dirschka, T.; Radny, P.; Dominicus, R.; Mensing, H.; Brüning, H.; Jenne, L.; Karl, L.; Sebastian, M.; Oster-Schmidt, C.; Klövekorn, W.; et al. Photodynamic therapy with BF-200 ALA for the treatment of actinic keratosis: Results of a multicentre, randomized, observer-blind phase III study in comparison with a registered methyl-5-aminolaevulinate cream and placebo. *Br. J. Dermatol.* **2012**, *166*, 137–146. [CrossRef]
30. Kim, E.J.; Mangold, A.R.; DeSimone, J.A.; Wong, H.K.; Seminario-Vidal, L.; Guitart, J.; Appel, J.; Geskin, L.; Lain, E.; Korman, N.J.; et al. Efficacy and safety of topical hypericin photodynamic therapy for early-stage cutaneous T-cell Llymphoma (*Mycosis fungoides*): The FLASH phase 3 randomized clinical trial. *JAMA Dermatol.* **2022**, *158*, 1031–1039. [CrossRef]
31. Liu, W.T.; Wang, H.T.; Yeh, Y.H.; Wong, T.W. An update on recent advances of photodynamic therapy for primary cutaneous lymphomas. *Pharmaceutics* **2023**, *15*, 1328. [CrossRef]
32. Rook, A.H.; Wood, G.S.; Duvic, M.; Vonderheid, E.C.; Tobia, A.; Cabana, B. A phase II placebo-controlled study of photodynamic therapy with topical hypericin and visible light irradiation in the treatment of cutaneous T-cell lymphoma and psoriasis. *J. Am. Acad. Dermatol.* **2010**, *63*, 984–990. [CrossRef]
33. Conrado, P.C.V.; Vaine, A.A.; Arita, G.S.; Sakita, K.M.; Gonçalves, R.S.; Caetano, W.; de Souza, M.; Baesso, M.L.; Malacarne, L.C.; Razzolini, E.; et al. Promising onychomycosis treatment with hypericin-mediated photodynamic therapy: Case reports. *Photodiagn. Photodyn. Ther.* **2023**, *42*, 103498. [CrossRef]
34. Galinari, C.B.; Biachi, T.P.; Gonçalves, R.S.; Cesar, G.B.; Bergmann, E.V.; Malacarne, L.C.; Kioshima Cotica, É.; Bonfim-Mendonça, P.S.; Svidzinski, T.I.E. Photoactivity of hypericin: From natural product to antifungal application. *Crit. Rev. Microbiol.* **2023**, *49*, 38–56. [CrossRef]
35. Choi, Y.M.; Adelzadeh, L.; Wu, J.J. Photodynamic therapy for psoriasis. *J. Dermatol. Treat.* **2015**, *26*, 202–207. [CrossRef]
36. Marek-Jozefowicz, L.; Nedoszytko, B.; Grochocka, M.; Żmijewski, M.A.; Czajkowski, R.; Cubała, W.J.; Slominski, A.T. Molecular mechanisms of neurogenic inflammation of the skin. *Int. J. Mol. Sci.* **2023**, *24*, 5001. [CrossRef]
37. Morgner, B.; Tittelbach, J.; Wiegand, C. Induction of psoriasis- and atopic dermatitis-like phenotypes in 3D skin equivalents with a fibroblast-derived matrix. *Sci. Rep.* **2023**, *13*, 1807. [CrossRef]
38. Su, Z.; Zeng, Y.P. Dupilumab-associated psoriasis and psoriasiform manifestations: A scoping review. *Dermatology* **2023**, *239*, 646–657. [CrossRef]
39. Navarro-Triviño, F.; Alcantara-Luna, S.; Domínguez-Cruz, J.; Galán-Gutiérrez, M.; Ruiz-Villaverde, R.; Pereyra-Rodriguez, J.J.; Armario-Hita, J.C. Upadacitinib for moderate to severe atopic dermatitis. *Immunotherapy* **2023**, *15*, 799–808. [CrossRef]
40. Turchin, I.; Bourcier, M. The role of interleukins in the pathogenesis of dermatological immune-mediated diseases. *Adv. Ther.* **2022**, *39*, 4474–4508. [CrossRef]
41. Rathod, D.G.; Muneer, H.; Masood, S. Phototherapy. In *StatPearls*; StatPearls Publishing LLC.: Treasure Island, FL, USA, 2024.

42. Kurz, B.; Berneburg, M.; Bäumler, W.; Karrer, S. Phototherapy: Theory and practice. *J. Dtsch. Dermatol. Ges.* **2023**, *21*, 882–897. [CrossRef]
43. Ding, Y.N.; Ding, H.Y.; Li, H.; Yang, R.; Huang, J.Y.; Chen, H.; Wang, L.H.; Wang, Y.J.; Hu, C.M.; An, Y.L.; et al. Photosensitive small extracellular vesicles regulate the immune microenvironment of triple negative breast cancer. *Acta Biomater.* **2023**, *167*, 534–550. [CrossRef]
44. Grundmann, S.A.; Beissert, S. Modern aspects of phototherapy for atopic dermatitis. *J. Allergy* **2012**, *2012*, 121797. [CrossRef]
45. Ruscitti, P.; Esposito, M.; Di Cola, I.; Pellegrini, C.; De Berardinis, A.; Mastrangelo, M.; Gianneramo, C.; Barile, A.; Fargnoli, M.C.; Cipriani, P. Cytokine profile characterization of naïve patients with psoriasis and psoriatic arthritis: Implications for a pathogenic disease continuum. *Front. Immunol.* **2023**, *14*, 1229516. [CrossRef]
46. Numerof, R.P.; Asadullah, K. Cytokine and anti-cytokine therapies for psoriasis and atopic dermatitis. *BioDrugs* **2006**, *20*, 93–103. [CrossRef]
47. Woźniak, M.; Nowak-Perlak, M. Hypericin-based photodynamic therapy displays higher selectivity and phototoxicity towards melanoma and squamous cell cancer compared to normal keratinocytes in vitro. *Int. J. Mol. Sci.* **2023**, *24*, 16897. [CrossRef]
48. Popovic, A.; Wiggins, T.; Davids, L.M. Differential susceptibility of primary cultured human skin cells to hypericin PDT in an in vitro model. *J. Photochem. Photobiol. B* **2015**, *149*, 249–256. [CrossRef]
49. Zhang, Y.; Su, J. Interleukin-2 family cytokines: An overview of genes, expression, signaling and functional roles in teleost. *Dev. Comp. Immunol.* **2023**, *141*, 104645. [CrossRef]
50. Yuan, Y.; Kolios, A.G.A.; Liu, Y.; Zhang, B.; Li, H.; Tsokos, G.C.; Zhang, X. Therapeutic potential of interleukin-2 in autoimmune diseases. *Trends Mol. Med.* **2022**, *28*, 596–612. [CrossRef]
51. Matsushima, K.; Shichino, S.; Ueha, S. Thirty-five years since the discovery of chemotactic cytokines, interleukin-8 and MCAF: A historical overview. *Proc. Jpn. Acad. Ser. B Phys. Biol. Sci.* **2023**, *99*, 213–226. [CrossRef]
52. Larisch, P.; Verwanger, T.; Linecker, M.; Krammer, B. The interrelation between a pro-inflammatory milieu and fluorescence diagnosis or photodynamic therapy of human skin cell lines. *Photodiagn. Photodyn. Ther.* **2014**, *11*, 91–103. [CrossRef] [PubMed]
53. Safarini, O.A.; Keshavamurthy, C.; Patel, P. Calcineurin inhibitors. In *StatPearls*; StatPearls Publishing: Treasure Island, FL, USA, 2024.
54. Ke, Y.; Li, B.Z.; Nguyen, K.; Wang, D.; Wang, S.; Young, C.D.; Wang, X.J. IL-22RA2 Is a SMAD7 target mediating the alleviation of dermatitis and psoriatic phenotypes in mice. *J. Investig. Dermatol.* **2023**, *143*, 2243–2254.e2210. [CrossRef] [PubMed]
55. Wölfle, U.; Haarhaus, B.; Schempp, C.M. Amarogentin displays immunomodulatory Effects in Human Mast Cells and Keratinocytes. *Mediat. Inflamm.* **2015**, *2015*, 630128. [CrossRef] [PubMed]
56. Steadman, T.; O'Reilly, S. Elevated interleukin-11 in systemic sclerosis and role in disease pathogenesis. *J. Dermatol.* **2023**, *50*, 1255–1261. [CrossRef] [PubMed]
57. O'Reilly, S. Interleukin-11 and its eminent role in tissue fibrosis: A possible therapeutic target. *Clin. Exp. Immunol.* **2023**, *214*, 154–161. [CrossRef] [PubMed]
58. Keskin, E.S.; Keskin, E.R.; Öztürk, M.B.; Çakan, D. The effect of MMP-1 on wound healing and scar formation. *Aesthetic Plast. Surg.* **2021**, *45*, 2973–2979. [CrossRef] [PubMed]
59. Oka, T.; Sugaya, M.; Takahashi, N.; Nakajima, R.; Otobe, S.; Kabasawa, M.; Suga, H.; Miyagaki, T.; Asano, Y.; Sato, S. Increased interleukin-19 expression in cutaneous T-cell lymphoma and atopic dermatitis. *Acta Derm.-Venereol.* **2017**, *97*, 1172–1177. [CrossRef] [PubMed]
60. Ge, G.; Shang, J.; Gan, T.; Chen, Z.; Pan, C.; Mei, Y.; Long, S.; Wu, A.; Wang, H. Psoriasis and leprosy: An arcane relationship. *J. Inflamm. Res.* **2023**, *16*, 2521–2533. [CrossRef]
61. Krupka-Olek, M.; Bożek, A.; Kawczyk-Krupka, A. The immunological and allergen profiles of patients with atopic dermatitis or psoriasis. *Medicina* **2022**, *58*, 367. [CrossRef]

pharmaceutics

Systematic Review

Riboflavin- and Hypericin-Mediated Antimicrobial Photodynamic Therapy as Alternative Treatments for Oral Candidiasis: A Systematic Review

Maciej Łopaciński [1], Jakub Fiegler-Rudol [2,*], Wojciech Niemczyk [1], Dariusz Skaba [1] and Rafał Wiench [1]

1 Department of Periodontal Diseases and Oral Mucosa Diseases, Faculty of Medical Sciences in Zabrze, Medical University of Silesia, 40-055 Katowice, Poland; mlopacinski@sum.edu.pl (M.Ł.); niemczykwojciech00@gmail.com (W.N.); dskaba@sum.edu.pl (D.S.); rwiench@sum.edu.pl (R.W.)
2 Faculty of Medical Sciences in Zabrze, Medical University of Silesia, 40-055 Katowice, Poland
* Correspondence: jakub.fieglerrudol@gmail.com

Abstract: Background: Oral candidiasis, predominantly caused by *Candida albicans*, presents significant challenges in treatment due to increasing antifungal resistance and biofilm formation. Antimicrobial photodynamic therapy (aPDT) using natural photosensitizers like riboflavin and hypericin offers a potential alternative to conventional antifungal therapies. **Material and Methods**: A systematic review was conducted to evaluate the efficacy of riboflavin- and hypericin-mediated aPDT in reducing Candida infections. The PRISMA framework guided the selection and analysis of 16 eligible studies published between 2014 and 2024. Data on light parameters, photosensitizer concentrations, and outcomes were extracted to assess antifungal effects. **Results**: Both riboflavin- and hypericin-mediated aPDT demonstrated significant antifungal activity, achieving substantial reductions in Candida biofilm and planktonic cell viability. Riboflavin activated by blue light and hypericin activated by yellow or orange light effectively targeted fluconazole-resistant Candida strains with minimal cytotoxicity to host tissues. However, complete biofilm eradication remained challenging, and variations in protocols highlighted the need for standardization. **Conclusions**: Riboflavin- and hypericin-mediated aPDT present promising, biocompatible alternatives for managing antifungal resistance in Candida infections. Further clinical trials and standardized protocols are essential to optimize outcomes and confirm efficacy in broader clinical settings.

Keywords: aPDT; biofilm; Candida; denture stomatitis; diode laser; planktonic cells

1. Introduction

The oral cavity of humans is colonized by a diverse microbial community, predominantly composed of bacteria, with fungi constituting a smaller fraction [1]. Among these, *Candida* species are a natural part of the oral flora in healthy individuals, with *Candida albicans* being the most prevalent, accounting for 60–70% of cases, followed by *Candida tropicalis* and *Candida glabrata* [2]. While typically commensal, these yeasts can become pathogenic under specific conditions, leading to oral candidiasis [3]. *C. albicans* is the primary causative agent of oral candidiasis, responsible for up to 95% of cases [4]. Host factors such as xerostomia, smoking, oral prostheses, dental caries, diabetes, and cancer treatments can accelerate the disease process [5]. The immune response of the host mucosa plays a critical role in controlling *C. albicans*. Adaptive immune mechanisms, especially those mediated by Th1 and Th17 cellular responses, are essential for maintaining tissue homeostasis and combating fungal proliferation. Dendritic cells are pivotal in initiating these defenses by presenting antigens and producing cytokines [6,7]. However, systemic diseases or periods of immunosuppression may compromise these defenses, allowing *Candida* to exploit its virulence factors to establish and propagate infections [8]. The management of oral candidiasis typically involves topical or systemic antifungal agents, such as azoles and polyenes. However, the extensive use of these agents has led to the emergence of fluconazole-resistant *Candida* species [9]. Additionally, the formation of microbial biofilms provides a protective barrier, enhancing resistance to antifungal treatments and complicating disease management [10]. Given the rising prevalence of antifungal-resistant pathogens and the associated toxicity of conventional therapies, there is a pressing need for alternative strategies to control yeast infections [11]. Antimicrobial photodynamic therapy (aPDT) is emerging as a promising alternative. This technique involves the administration of a photosensitizing agent, which is activated by visible light at an appropriate wavelength to generate Reactive Oxygen Species (ROS) with antimicrobial effects [12]. The underlying mechanism of aPDT lies in its ability to induce oxidative stress, leading to microbial cell damage without significantly affecting host tissues. Importantly, aPDT has demonstrated efficacy against biofilm-associated infections and resistant strains, highlighting its clinical potential in managing recalcitrant fungal infections [13]. A critical aspect of aPDT is the selection of photosensitizers (PSs). In recent years, natural polyphenolic compounds have garnered interest due to their unique chemical structures, inherent antimicrobial properties, and favorable safety profiles. Curcumin, methylene blue, hypericin, and riboflavin have demonstrated strong antifungal activity in various studies [12–14]. Hypericin, derived from *Hypericum perforatum* (commonly known as St. John's Wort), and riboflavin (vitamin B2) have shown promise against fluconazole-resistant strains of *Candida* [15–19]. Riboflavin, activated by blue light, produces ROS that induce oxidative damage to microbial cells, offering a natural and effective solution [20,21]. Given the increasing challenge of antifungal resistance and the need for innovative solutions, this review aims to systematically summarize the evidence supporting the use of polyphenolic natural products as photosensitizers in aPDT. By exploring their potential to counteract biofilm-related infections and resistant pathogens, this study seeks to establish a foundation for future clinical applications of aPDT in antifungal therapy.

2. Materials and Methods

2.1. Focused Question and Null Hypothesis

A systematic review was conducted following the PICO framework [22], as follows: In patients with *Candida* infections (Population), does treatment with riboflavin- or hypericin-mediated antimicrobial photodynamic therapy (Intervention), compared to blue light irradiation alone, the use of riboflavin or hypericin as photosensitizers alone, or other pharmacological treatments (Comparison), result in more effective eradication or reduction of *Candida* infections (Outcome)? The null hypothesis for our article stated that there is no significant difference in the eradication or elimination effectiveness of *Candida* strains when subjected to riboflavin- or hypericin-mediated antimicrobial photodynamic therapy compared to blue light irradiation alone, riboflavin or hypericin as photosensitizers alone, or other pharmacological treatments.

2.2. Search Strategy

This review has been registered with PROSPERO under the ID CRD42024617727. The review was conducted following the Preferred Reporting Items for Systematic Reviews and Meta-Analyses (PRISMA) 2020 guidelines [23]. An electronic search was performed through PubMed/Medline, Embase, Scopus, and Cochrane Library databases (search phrases detailed in Figure 1). The databases were searched by three authors independently (M.Ł., J.F.-R. and R.W.) using the same search terms. Additional electronic filters were applied to include only articles published between 1 January 2014 and 3 December 2024 and restricted to publications in English. After initial screening, potential studies were selected based on titles and abstracts to determine if they met all inclusion criteria (Table 1). Two authors (J.F.-R. and R.W.) then conducted a full-text review of the selected studies to collate the desired data. Additionally, a snowball search was performed by examining the reference lists of articles deemed eligible for full-text review to identify further relevant studies. This research proposed that hypericin and riboflavin-mediated antimicrobial photodynamic therapy could serve as an effective approach for reducing Candida strains, potentially functioning as a complementary or alternative treatment for oral candidiasis compared to conventional pharmacological methods. Articles included in this review were selected based on specific inclusion and exclusion criteria.

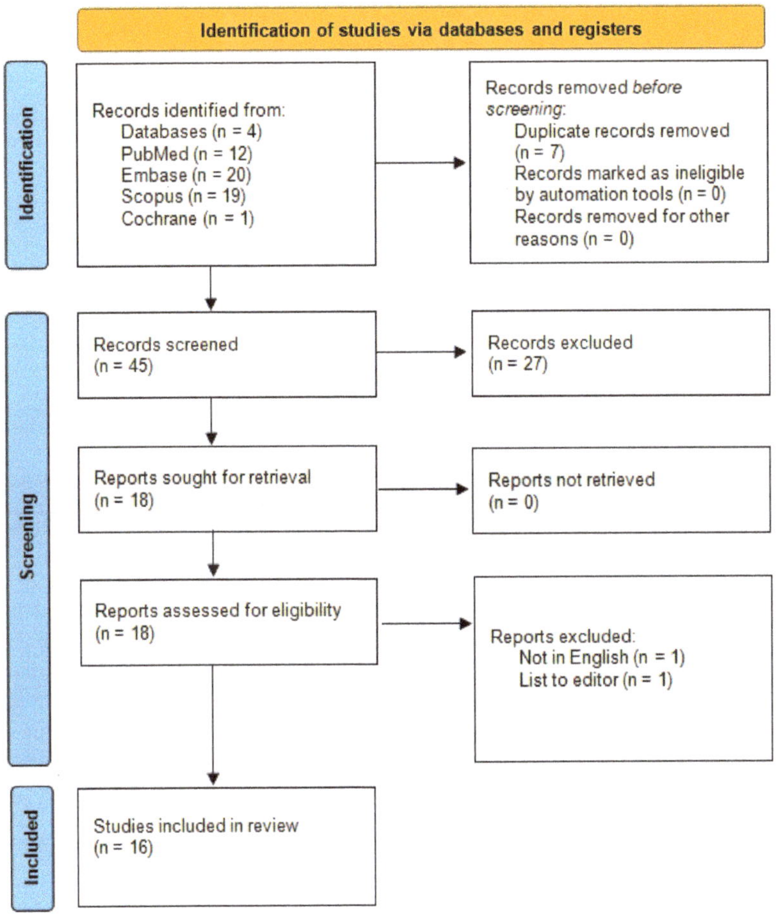

Figure 1. PRISMA 2020 flow diagram.

Table 1. Search syntax used in the study.

Source	Search Term	Filters	Number of Results
PubMed/MEDLINE	(Candida [Title/Abstract] OR candidiasis oral [Title/Abstract] OR denture stomatitis [Title/Abstract]) AND (photodynamic therapy [Title/Abstract] OR aPDT [Title/Abstract] OR antimicrobial photodynamic therapy [Title/Abstract] OR photodynamic antimicrobial chemotherapy [Title/Abstract] OR PACT [Title/Abstract] OR photodynamic inactivation [Title/Abstract] OR PDI [Title/Abstract]) AND (riboflavin [Title/Abstract] OR hypericin [Title/Abstract])	English language Publicationyears: 2014–2024 Full text	12
Embase	('candida':ti,ab OR 'candidiasis oral':ti,ab OR 'denture stomatitis':ti,ab) AND ('photodynamic therapy':ti,ab OR 'aPDT':ti,ab OR 'antimicrobial photodynamic therapy':ti,ab OR 'photodynamic antimicrobial chemotherapy':ti,ab OR 'PACT':ti,ab OR 'photodynamic inactivation':ti,ab OR 'PDI':ti,ab) AND ('riboflavin':ti,ab OR 'hypericin':ti,ab)	Publication years: 2014–2024 Controlled Clinical Trial Randomized Controlled Trial	20
Scopus	(TITLE-ABS ("Candida") OR TITLE-ABS ("candidiasis oral") OR TITLE-ABS ("denture stomatitis")) AND (TITLE-ABS ("photodynamic therapy") OR TITLE-ABS ("aPDT") OR TITLE-ABS ("antimicrobial photodynamic therapy") OR TITLE-ABS ("photodynamic antimicrobial chemotherapy") OR TITLE-ABS ("PACT") OR TITLE-ABS ("photodynamic inactivation") OR TITLE-ABS ("PDI")) AND (TITLE-ABS ("riboflavin") OR TITLE-ABS ("hypericin"))	Article Publication years: 2014–2024	19
Cochrane	((mh "Candida" OR "candidiasis" OR "denture stomatitis") AND ("Photodynamic Therapy" OR "antimicrobial photodynamic therapy" OR "PDI" OR "aPDT") AND ("Riboflavin" OR "Hypericin"))	Publication years: 2014–2024	1

2.3. Selection of Studies

During the study selection process for this systematic review, reviewers independently evaluated the titles and abstracts of the identified articles to minimize bias. Any disagreements regarding the eligibility of studies were resolved through collaborative discussions until a unanimous decision was achieved. This rigorous methodology, adhering to PRISMA guidelines, helped ensure that only the most relevant and high-quality studies were included in the analysis, thereby strengthening the review's reliability and reproducibility [23].

2.4. Risk of Bias in Individual Studies

During the preliminary stage of study selection, reviewers independently examined titles and abstracts to minimize potential bias in the evaluation. Inter-reviewer agreement was measured using Cohen's kappa statistic to ensure consistency in decision-making [24]. Disagreements concerning the inclusion or exclusion of studies were resolved through thorough discussions among the authors until a unanimous decision was achieved.

2.5. Quality Assessment

The quality of the included studies was independently assessed by two reviewers (J.F-R. and R.W.). The evaluation centered on critical elements of aPDT design, execution, and data analysis, with an emphasis on ensuring objectivity and result validation. The risk of bias was determined by assigning a score of 1 toeach "yes" response and 0 to each "no" response to a predefined set of evaluation criteria, as outlined below:

1. Was a specific concentration of riboflavin or hypericin as the photosensitizer indicated?
2. Was the origin or source of the photosensitizer (riboflavin or hypericin) provided?
3. Was the incubation time for the photosensitizer clearly stated?
4. Were detailed parameters of the light source (such as type, wavelength, output power, fluence, and power density) provided?
5. Was a power meter used in the study?
6. Was a negative control group included in the experimental design?
7. Were numerical results reported, including relevant statistics?
8. Was there no missing outcome data?
9. Was the study independent from its source of funding?

The data extracted from each study were analysed and categorized based on the total count of affirmative ("yes") responses to the specified criteria. The level of bias was determined using the following scoring thresholds: high risk: 0–3; moderate risk: 4–6; and low risk: 7–9. Each study's scores were compiled, and a corresponding level of bias risk—classified as low, moderate, or high—was determined in accordance with the guidelines specified in the Cochrane Handbook for Systematic Reviews of Interventions [25].

2.6. Risk of Bias Across Studies

The results of the quality assessment and risk of bias across the studies are presented in Section 3.3.

2.7. Data Extraction

After reaching a consensus on the selection of included articles, the two reviewers (J.F.-R. and R.W.) extracted data on various aspects, including the citation details (first author and publication year), type of study, Candida strains used, test and control groups, follow-up period, outcomes, type and parameters of the light source, concentration of riboflavin or hypericin, and the use of nanocarriers, additional substances, as well as incubation and irradiation times.

3. Results

3.1. Study Selection

Figure 1 illustrates the detailed research methodology per PRISMA guidelines [23]. The initial search yielded 52 articles, which were narrowed down to 45 after duplicate removal. Following the screening of titles and abstracts, 18 studies qualified for full-text evaluation. Of these, two were excluded. One study was excluded for not including *C. albicans*. One study was omitted as it was primarily written in a non-English language, with only the title and abstract available in English, and another was excluded for being a letter to the editor. Ultimately, 16 studies were included in the final review, all published within the last 10 years.

3.2. Quality Assessment Presentation

The risk of bias assessment for the 16 studies included after a full-text review is detailed in Table 2. Studies were required to score at least six points to be included in the analysis. Among these, all studies were identified as having a low risk of bias, with three achieving the maximum score of 9. None of the studies were rated as high or moderate risk.

Table 2. Selection criteria for papers included in the systematic review.

Inclusion Criteria	Exclusion Criteria
Studies that assess Candida elimination through riboflavin-mediated aPDT or hypericin-mediated aPDT in both in vitro and animal models. In vitro animal studies involving strains from the Candida genus of yeasts. RCTs where riboflavin or hypericin was used as the primary photosensitizer in aPDT for Candida treatment. Studies evaluating synergistic effects of riboflavin or hypericin aPDT combined with other antifungal agents. Research with control groups that assess the effects of aPDT with riboflavin or hypericin against untreated controls or alternative therapies. Comparative studies that directly compare the efficacy of riboflavin- and hypericin-mediated aPDT with other antifungal treatments. Longitudinal studies or studies with follow-up periods to monitor the antifungal effects of riboflavin or hypericin aPDT.	"Gray literature" sources Study types: case reports or case series, letters to the editor, historical overviews, narrative or systematic reviews, books, documents, and other non-journal sources. Non-peer-reviewed sources Studies published in languages other than English. Duplicate publications or studies sharing the same ethical approval number. General medical applications unrelated to oral candidiasis. Studies lacking a control group or comparison group Use of aPDT not intended as a therapeutic method for Candida. Other photosensitizers than riboflavin or hypericin. Studies on non-Candida infections or studies that do not evaluate Candida strains. In vitro studies that do not simulate oral conditions relevant to Candida infections

aPDT: antimicrobial photodynamic therapy; RCT: randomized controlled trial.

3.3. Data Presentation

The extracted data from the 16 studies that met the eligibility criteria and were included in the review are summarized in Tables 3–5. These include an overview of the general study characteristics, the specifications of the light sources used, and the attributes of hypericin or riboflavin as a photosensitizer in aPDT protocols. The results of the quality assessment and risk of bias across the studies are presented in Table 3.

Table 3. The results of the quality assessment and risk of bias across the studies.

Reference Number	Author and Year	1	2	3	4	5	6	7	8	9	Sum	Risk
[26]	Agut et al. (2011)	1	1	1	1	0	1	1	1	1	8	Low
[27]	Alam et al. (2019)	1	1	1	1	1	1	1	1	1	9	Low
[28]	Alshehri et al. (2021)	1	1	1	1	1	1	1	1	1	9	Low
[29]	Arboleda et al. (2014)	1	1	1	1	0	1	1	1	1	8	Low
[30]	Ardakani et al. (2024)	1	1	1	1	1	1	1	1	1	8	Low
[31]	Bernala et al. (2011)	1	1	1	1	0	1	1	1	1	8	Low
[32]	Troichenko et al. (2021)	1	1	1	1	0	1	1	1	1	8	Low
[33]	Sakita et al. (2019)	1	1	1	1	0	1	1	1	1	8	Low
[34]	Sato et al. (2022)	1	1	1	1	0	1	1	1	1	8	Low
[35]	Tunccan et al. (2018)	1	1	1	1	0	1	1	1	1	8	Low
[36]	Rezusta et al. (2012)	1	1	1	1	0	1	1	1	1	8	Low
[37]	Morelato et al. (2022)	1	1	1	1	0	1	1	1	1	8	Low
[38]	Paz-Cristobal et al. (2014)	1	1	1	1	0	1	1	1	1	8	Low
[39]	Sato et al. (2023)	1	1	1	1	0	1	1	1	1	8	Low
[40]	Kashiwabuchi et al. (2013)	1	1	1	1	0	1	1	1	1	8	Low
[41]	Sousa et al. (2019)	1	1	1	1	1	1	1	1	1	9	Low

A comprehensive overview of the included studies is presented in Table 4.

Table 4. A general overview of the studies.

Reference Number	Author and Year	Country	Study Design
[26]	Agut et al. (2011)	Spain	In vitro study
[27]	Alam et al. (2019)	South Korea	In vitro and in vivo study
[28]	Alshehri et al. (2021)	Saudi Arabia	In vitro study
[29]	Arboleda et al. (2014)	USA	In vitro study
[30]	Ardakani et al. (2024)	Iran	In vitro study
[31]	Bernala et al. (2011)	Brazil	In vitro study
[32]	Troichenko et al. (2021)	Ukraine	In vitro study
[33]	Sakita et al. (2019)	Brazil	In vitro study
[34]	Sato et al. (2022)	Brazil	In vitro and in vivo study
[35]	Tunccan et al. (2018)	Turkey	In vitro study
[36]	Rezusta et al. (2012)	Spain	In vitro study
[37]	Morelato et al. (2022)	Croatia	In vitro study
[38]	Paz-Cristobal et al. (2014)	Spain	In vitro study
[39]	Sato et al. (2023)	Brazil and UK	In vitro and in vivo study
[40]	Kashiwabuchi et al. (2013)	Brazil and USA	In vitro study
[41]	Sousa et al. (2019)	Portugal	In vitro study

Main outcomes and details from each study are presented in Table 5.

Table 5. Main outcomes and details from each study.

Reference Number	Author and Year	Study Design	Species Evaluated	Study Groups	Outcomes
[26]	Agut et al. (2011)	In vitro study	*C. albicans*, *C. parapsilopsis*, *C. krusei*, *S. cerevisiae*	Hyp concentrations ranged from 0.625 μM to 320 μM +602 nm LED lamp at fluence levels of 0, 18, and 37 J/cm^2.	Hyp was effective in aPDT for inactivating various yeast strains, including *C. albicans*, *Candida parapsilopsis*, *Saccharomyces cerevisiae*, and *C. krusei*. A 3-log reduction in fungal survival was achieved with lower concentrations of Hyp (0.625–40 μM), using a fluence of 37 J/cm^2. For a 6-log reduction, higher concentrations of Hyp were required. The most sensitive strain was *C. albicans*. The aPDT treatment did not result in significant cytotoxicity in keratinocytes and dermal fibroblasts at the tested concentrations, suggesting the potential for therapeutic use with minimal side effects.
[27]	Alam et al. (2019)	In vitro and in vivo study	*C. albicans*, *S. aureus*, *MRSA*, *P. aeruginosa*	1. Control Group (no treatment) 2. Hyp only 3. Orange light only 4. Ampicillin only 5. Hyp + orange light (aPDT) 6. Hyp + Ampicillin + orange light 7. Positive Control Group (gentamicin or nystatin) 8. Gram-positive bacteria (*Staphylococcus aureus*, *MRSA*) 9. Gram-negative bacteria (*Pseudomonas aeruginosa*) 10. Fungal strains (*C. albicans*) 11. *C. elegans* in vivo model (treated vs. untreated pathogens)	aPDT using Hyp combined with orange light effectively inhibited *C. albicans*. A 4.8-log reduction in fungal growth was observed after treating *C. albicans* with 10 μM Hyp followed by orange light exposure for 1 h. This result demonstrated significant efficacy, comparable to the antifungal agent nystatin (20 μg/mL), confirming the potential of HY-PDT as an effective antifungal treatment.

Table 5. *Cont.*

Reference Number	Author and Year	Study Design	Species Evaluated	Study Groups	Outcomes
[28]	Alshehri et al. (2021)	In vitro study	*C. albicans*	1. No decontamination 2. Nystatin suspension 3. RF 0.1% in darkness 4. Blue LED light only 5. RF-PDT with RF 0.1% + blue LED light	RF-PDT is highly effective in reducing *C. albicans* viability on acrylic denture surfaces. RF-PDT achieved the lowest *C. albicans* viability (41.1%) compared to nystatin (56.3%), riboflavin alone (81.7%), and no treatment (95.6%). SEM and CLSM analyses confirmed that RF-PDT-treated surfaces were almost completely free of *C. albicans*. Furthermore, RF-PDT caused no significant surface degradation or changes in mechanical properties of the acrylic resin, maintaining flexural strength and modulus. These results suggest that RF-PDT is a safe and effective antifungal method for denture disinfection.
[29]	Arboleda et al. (2014)	In vitro study	*C. albicans*, *F. solani*, *A. fumigatus*	1. Control—no treatment 2. 0.1% RB alone 3. 518 nm irradiation alone 4. RF-PDT (375 nm UV-A LED + riboflavin) 5. RB-PDT (518 nm green LED + rose bengal)	RB-PDT with 518 nm green light achieved the highest inhibition (95.6% ± 3%) of *C. albicans* growth compared to other treatment groups, including riboflavin-mediated aPDT with 375 nm UV-A light (35.3% ± 10%) and controls. RB alone and green light alone showed less inhibition (42.2% ± 3.7% and 35.6% ± 6.7%, respectively), while the untreated control exhibited 24.2% ± 2.6% inhibition. These findings indicate that RB-PDT is significantly more effective against *C. albicans* than riboflavin-mediated aPDT or individual components alone.
[30]	Ardakani et al. (2024)	In vitro study	*C. albicans*, *C. glabrata* (with *S. mutans* *S. sanguinis*)	1. Control 2. 0.2% chlorhexidine 3. 5.25% sodium hypochlorite 4. Curcumin 5. Riboflavin 6. Phycocyanin (each with and without LED)	aPDT using natural photosensitizers—curcumin, riboflavin, and phycocyanin—activated by LED light, was effective in reducing *C. albicans* in a multispecies biofilm model. aPDT with curcumin and LED light achieved the highest reduction in *C. albicans* biofilm, followed by riboflavin and phycocyanin. Significant decreases in biofilm mass and fungal cell viability were observed compared to untreated controls and groups treated with photosensitizers alone. The treatment showed promise for safe and effective antifungal disinfection of denture materials while maintaining their structural integrity.
[31]	Bernala et al. (2011)	In vitro study	*C. albicans*, *C. krusei*, *C. tropicalis*	1. Control group (*Candida* spp. without treatment) 2. PS group (Hyp only) 3. Light-only group (590 nm yellow LED light without Hyp) 4. aPDT group (Hyp + 590 nm yellow LED light) 5. Host cell control group (HEp-2 epithelial cells and McCoy fibroblasts treated with Hyp and light)	HY-PDT inactivation effectively reduced *C. albicans* viability under selective conditions. The optimal parameters included Hyp concentrations of 0.1–0.4 μg/mL, a short incubation time of 10 min, and irradiation with 590 nm yellow LED light at a dose of 6 J/cm^2. These conditions resulted in significant photoinactivation of *C. albicans* without affecting mammalian fibroblast and epithelial cell viability, indicating high selectivity. The results suggest the potential of HY-PDT for treating oral candidiasis, particularly in immunocompromised patients, while minimizing damage to host tissues.

Table 5. *Cont.*

Reference Number	Author and Year	Study Design	Species Evaluated	Study Groups	Outcomes
[32]	Troichenko et al. (2021)	In vitro study	*C. albicans* biofilm in ophthalmic model	1. Control group—no treatment 2. aPDT group—methylene blue + 630–670 nm laser 3. CXL group—riboflavin + 365 nm UV light 4. aPDT + CXL group—riboflavin, methylene blue, 365 nm UV light, and 630–670 nm laser 5. aPDT + CXL + antifungal group (fluconazole)	The study demonstrated that *C. albicans* is susceptible to aPDT with methylene blue (0.1%) and low-energy laser irradiation (630–670 nm), as well as CXL with RF (0.1%) and 365-nm ultraviolet light. Growth inhibition zones for aPDT alone ranged from 15 to 28 mm (mean 21.9 ± 4.7 mm), and for CXL alone, they ranged from 0 to 19 mm (mean 9.1 ± 9.6 mm). When combined (aPDT + CXL), inhibition zones ranged from 14 to 30 mm (mean 22.4 ± 7.27 mm). The most effective treatment was aPDT + CXL combined with fluconazole, producing the largest inhibition zones (36–38 mm, mean 36.9 ± 0.87 mm), 6.3 mm larger than the fluconazole control alone. These findings highlight the potential of combination treatments for enhanced antifungal effects against *C. albicans*.
[33]	Sakita et al. (2019)	In vitro study	*C. albicans*, *C. tropicalis*, *C. parapsilosis*, *C. glabrata*	1. Positive control 2. Light-only control 3. Photosensitizer-only control 4. aPDT + P123-Hyp at varying concentrations (0.25–32 μM) with specific light fluences (10.8–16.2 J/cm^2) 5. Combination therapy with fluconazole (varied concentration) + P123-HY-PDT	P123-Hyp effectively inactivated *Candida albicans* through PDI. Using low Hyp concentrations (0.25–1.0 μmol/L) and light fluences of 10.8–16.2 J/cm^2, the treatment achieved a significant reduction in *C. albicans* planktonic cells, with complete fungicidal effects at certain conditions. Additionally, P123-HY-PDT significantly inhibited biofilm formation, reducing *C. albicans* cell viability, metabolic activity, and total biomass by up to 87%. The therapy was synergistic with fluconazole, effectively overcoming fluconazole-resistant *C. albicans* strains by reducing the required drug concentrations up to eightfold. These findings support P123-Hyp-PDI as a promising strategy for treating *C. albicans* infections and preventing biofilm formation.
[34]	Sato et al. (2022)	In vitro and in vivo study	*C. albicans*	1. Negative control group: no treatment. 2. Infected positive control group: *C. albicans* inoculum without intervention. 3. Solvent control group—treated with 20% DMSO only. 4. Antifungal control group: Bio-vagin® vaginal antifungal cream (contains benzoylmetronidazole, nystatin, and benzalkonium chloride). 5. Empty NLC-group. 6. Free Hyp-group: analyzed in the dark. 7. NLC-HYP-group: analyzed in the dark. 8. Free Hyp+ group: exposed to white LED light (113 J/cm^2, 5 min). 9. NLC-HYP+ group: exposed to white LED light (113 J/cm^2, 5 min).	NLC-HYP combined with aPDT effectively inhibited *Candida albicans* both in vitro and in vivo. In vitro, aPDT with NLC-HYP achieved a significant reduction in *C. albicans* planktonic viability, with a 90% reduction in fungal growth observed after a 5 min LED light irradiation. In vivo, using a murine vulvovaginal candidiasis model, NLC-HYP combined with aPDT significantly reduced fungal burden in vaginal lavages compared to untreated controls. Additionally, the treatment prevented the formation of pathogenic hyphae, promoting a predominance of yeast forms, which are less virulent. These results highlight the potential of NLC-HYP and aPDT as a promising therapeutic approach for treating *C. albicans* infections.

Table 5. *Cont.*

Reference Number	Author and Year	Study Design	Species Evaluated	Study Groups	Outcomes
[35]	Tunccan et al. (2018)	In vitro study	*C. albicans*, *C. parapsilosis*	1. Red LED + MB group: biofilms treated with MB (25 μg/mL) and exposed to 660 nm red LED light. 2. Green LED + RB group: biofilms treated with RB (0.1%) and exposed to 518 nm green LED light. 3. RF + UV group: biofilms treated with RBF (0.1%) and exposed to 370 nm UV light. 4. Biofilm control: untreated biofilms grown on microplates and glass slides. 5. Negative control: biofilms treated with amphotericin B.	aPDT effectively reduced biofilm formation of *C. albicans* using a combination of red LED light (660 nm) and methylene blue as a photosensitizer. This treatment achieved a 45.4% reduction in biofilm formation, significantly outperforming other tested combinations such as riboflavin with UV-A and rose bengal with green LED light. In addition to biofilm reduction, aPDT markedly reduced the viability of *C. albicans* planktonic cells, with red LED + methylene blue treatment showing a 3-log10 reduction in fungal cell counts. These results highlight the potential of aPDT as a promising strategy to combat *C. albicans* biofilms, particularly in clinical settings involving catheter-associated infections.
[36]	Rezusta et al. (2012)	In vitro study	*C. albicans* strains resistant to azole	1. *Candida albicans* (ATCC and CECT strains): Hyp (0.625–640 μM), light fluences (18–37 J/cm^2), suspensions (0.5, 4.0 McFarland). 2. *Candida parapsilosis* (ATCC 22019): Hyp (1.25–320 μM), light fluences (18–37 J/cm^2), suspensions (0.5, 4.0 McFarland). 3. *Candida krusei* (ATCC 6258): Hyp (40–320 μM), light fluences (18–37 J/cm^2), suspensions (0.5, 4.0 McFarland). 4. Dark controls. 5. Light-only controls. 6. Untreated controls.	HY-PDT effectively inactivated C. *albicans* under controlled conditions. A 3-log10 reduction in *C. albicans* viability was achieved at Hyp concentrations as low as 0.625 μM and light fluences of 18 J/cm^2, while a 6-log10 reduction required higher Hyp concentrations (5 μM) and light fluences of 37 J/cm^2. The treatment preserved the viability of human keratinocytes and fibroblasts when Hyp concentration and light fluence were maintained below these thresholds. These findings indicate that *C. albicans* is particularly susceptible to HY-PDT, making it a promising candidate for antifungal therapies with minimal damage to host cells.
[37]	Morelato et al. (2022)	In vitro study	*C. albicans*, *S. aureus*	1. Negative control 2. Positive control: Surface treated with a sterile cotton pellet soaked in 0.2% chlorhexidine-based solution for 60 s. 3. PDT1: Surface treated with 0.1% methylene blue dye as the photosensitizer, followed by 660 nm diode laser irradiation (124.34 W/cm^2 power density, 1240 J/cm^2 energy density) for 60 s. 4. PDT2: Surface treated with 0.1% riboflavin dye as the photosensitizer, followed by 445 nm diode laser irradiation (124.34 W/cm^2 power density, 1.24 J/cm^2 energy density) for 60 s.	RF combined with 445 nm diode laser light effectively reduced *Candida albicans* biofilm on titanium dental implants. Both aPDT with riboflavin and 445 nm blue light (PDT2) and aPDT with methylene blue and 660 nm red light (PDT1) achieved significant reductions in *C. albicans* CFUs compared to the untreated control group, with no statistically significant difference between the two aPDT protocols. These findings suggest that riboflavin and blue light offer an effective, aesthetically favorable alternative to methylene blue for managing fungal biofilms on dental implant surfaces.

Table 5. *Cont.*

Reference Number	Author and Year	Study Design	Species Evaluated	Study Groups	Outcomes
[38]	Paz-Cristobal et al. (2014)	In vitro study	*C. albicans* (azole-resistant and azole-susceptible strains)	1. Negative control group 2. Hyp-group: different concentrations of Hyp (0.32–40 μmol/L), with light fluences of 18 or 37 J/cm^2. 3. DMMB group: different concentrations of DMMB (0.32–40 μmol/L), with light fluences of 18 or 37 J/cm^2. 4. ROS quencher groups: Sodium Azide: quenches singlet oxygen ($^1O_2$); Mannitol: quenches hydroxyl radicals (·OH); Catalase: quenches hydrogen peroxide (H_2O_2); Superoxide Dismutase: quenches superoxide anion radicals (O_2^-).	aPDT using Hyp and DMMB effectively inactivated *Candida albicans* strains, including azole-resistant variants, in a light-dose and photosensitizer concentration-dependent manner. Hyp achieved a ≥3-log10 reduction at concentrations as low as 0.62 μmol/L for most strains, while DMMB required slightly higher concentrations (0.62–2.5 μmol/L). At higher fungal densities, Hyp required increased concentrations to achieve a 6-log10 reduction, while DMMB maintained efficacy with smaller concentration adjustments. ROS analysis revealed that Hyp primarily relied on hydrogen peroxide for its phototoxic effect, whereas DMMB depended on singlet oxygen. These results highlight aPDT as a promising strategy against azole-resistant *C. albicans*, with Hyp performing better at low fungal densities and DMMB offering advantages in high-density infections.
[39]	Sato et al. (2023)	In vitro and in vivo study	*C. albicans* with Gram-negative bacteria	1. PBS/Non-PDT (negative control) 2. Pure NLC/Non-PDT 3. Pure HG/Non-PDT 4. Free Hyp/Non-PDT 5. Free RB/Non-PDT (positive control) 6. PBS/PDT 7. Free Hyp/PDT 8. Free RB/PDT 9. Hy.NLC/PDT 10. Hy.NLC-HG/PDT	Hy.NLC-HG, combined with PDT, effectively reduced *Candida albicans* biofilm viability both in vitro and in vivo. In vitro, the Hy.NLC-HG/PDT treatment achieved a 1.2 log reduction in *C. albicans* viability, while other formulations, including free Hyp and rose bengal under PDT, showed reductions up to 1.9 log. In vivo, mice treated with Hy.NLC-HG/PDT displayed significantly lower fungal colony counts and a reduction in hyphae formation in vaginal fluids compared to controls. This treatment promoted a predominance of less virulent yeast forms of *C. albicans*, highlighting its potential as a non-invasive and effective approach for managing vulvovaginal candidiasis.
[40]	Kashiwabuchi et al. (2013)	In vitro study	*C. albicans* *F. solani*	1. Negative control group 2. UV-A light-only group: exposed to 365 nm UV-A light for 30 min without riboflavin. 3. Riboflavin-only group: fungal cells treated with 0.1% riboflavin solution without UV-A light exposure. 4. Dead cell control group 5. UV-A + riboflavin: fungal cells treated with riboflavin and exposed to 365 nm UV-A light for 30 min.	Combining RF with long-wave UV-A light (365 nm) had no significant antifungal effect on *C. albicans* in terms of cell viability reduction. While no notable cell death occurred, some phenotypic changes were observed, including a slight decrease in cell diameter and non-uniform biofilm growth in treated samples. These results suggest that the treatment may induce minor structural changes but is ineffective for directly inactivating *C. albicans*. Further optimization of dose and exposure time is needed to explore its potential as an antifungal treatment.

Table 5. *Cont.*

Reference Number	Author and Year	Study Design	Species Evaluated	Study Groups	Outcomes
[41]	Sousa et al. (2019)	In vitro study	*C. albicans*	1. Tri-Py(+)-Me as photosensitizer: blood plasma samples treated with this porphyrinic compound at varying concentrations and subjected to photodynamic inactivation. 2. FORM as photosensitizer: a formulation based on a mixture of cationic porphyrins used for inactivation of *Candida albicans* in plasma and whole blood. 3. MB as reference photosensitizer: used for comparison in plasma and whole blood photodynamic therapy. 4. Light control group. 5. Dark control group. 6. DMSO control group: samples treated with the solvent used to dissolve porphyrinic photosensitizers to evaluate theirindependent effects.	The study found that PDT using porphyrinic photosensitizers, FORM and Tri-Py(+)-Me, effectively inactivated *Candida albicans* in blood plasma, achieving reductions of 1.7 log10 and 2.5 log10 in fungal viability at 10 μM concentrations, respectively, after 270 min of irradiation. Both photosensitizers outperformed MB, which only achieved a 0.5 log10 reduction under the same conditions. However, in whole blood, the reduction in *C. albicans* viability was modest, reaching only 0.7 log10 for both photosensitizers. Importantly, neither FORM nor Tri-Py(+)-Me caused significant hemolysis under isotonic conditions, supporting their potential for safe plasma disinfection applications.

PDT—Photodynamic Therapy, aPDT—Antimicrobial Photodynamic Therapy, Hyp—Hypericin, HY-PDT—Hypericin-mediated aPDT, LED—Light-Emitting Diode, CFU—Colony-Forming Units, SEM—Scanning Electron Microscopy, CLSM—Confocal Laser Scanning Microscopy, RB—Rose Bengal, RF-PDT—Riboflavin-mediated photodynamic therapy RB-PDT—rose bengal-mediated photodynamic therapy, UV-A—Ultraviolet A Light, DMMB—1,9-Dimethyl Methylene Blue, NLC—Nanostructured Lipid Carriers, Hy.NLC-HG—Hypericin-Loaded Nanostructured Lipid Carrier Hydrogel, MB—Methylene Blue, ROS—Reactive Oxygen Species, CXL—Collagen Cross-Linking, Tri-Py(+)-Me—Tri-Pyridyl Methyl, PC—Positive Control, NC—Negative Control, FLU—Fluconazole, P123-Hyp—Hypericin Encapsulated in P123 Micelles, RBF—Riboflavin, *C. albicans*—*Candida albicans*, *C. parapsilosis*—*Candida parapsilosis*, *C. krusei*—*Candida krusei*, *C. tropicalis*—*Candida tropicalis*, *C. glabrata*—*Candida glabrata*, *S. cerevisiae*—*Saccharomy cescerevisiae*, *S. aureus*—*Staphylococcus aureus*, MRSA—Methicillin-Resistant *Staphylococcus aureus*, *P. aeruginosa*—*Pseudomonas aeruginosa*, *F. solani*—*Fusarium solani*, *A. fumigatus*—*Aspergillus fumigatus*, SA—Sodium Azide, MAN—Mannitol, CAT—Catalase, SOD—Superoxide Dismutase, LC—Light Control, DC—Dark Control, HEp-2—Human Epithelial Type 2 Cells, MCF—McFarland Standard.

3.4. General Characteristics of the Included Studies

The general characteristics of the 16 studies that were included are shown in Table 4.

3.5. Main Study Outcomes

The reviewed studies collectively highlight the potential of aPDT using natural photosensitizers like hypericin or riboflavin as effective alternatives for managing *Candida* infections, especially in the context of rising antifungal resistance. Agut et al. demonstrated the broad-spectrum antifungal efficacy of hypericin, achieving a 3-log reduction in *C. albicans* and other yeast strains at low hypericin concentrations (0.625–40 μM) with a 37 J/cm^2 fluence, with no cytotoxic effects on human keratinocytes or fibroblasts [26]. Alam et al. further validated hypericin's effectiveness, showing significant inhibition of *C. albicans* and Gram-positive bacteria when activated by orange light, with combination therapy also enhancing outcomes for resistant strains like *P. aeruginosa* [27]. Alshehri et al. explored riboflavin-mediated photodynamic therapy (RF-PDT) on acrylic denture materials and found it highly effective for reducing *C. albicans* biofilm viability, outperforming other treatments and maintaining the mechanical properties of the materials [28]. Arboleda et al. demonstrated that rose bengal aPDT was more effective than RF-PDT at inhibiting *C. albicans*, while Ardakani et al. found that aPDT using riboflavin and other natural photosensitizers significantly reduced biofilm mass and *C. albicans* CFU counts in a multi-species biofilm model, showing promise for biofilm-related infections [29,30]. Bernala et al. highlighted hypericin fungicidal efficacy even at low concentrations, achieving selective

Candida inactivation without harming host cells [31]. Sakita et al. enhanced hypericin's efficacy by encapsulating it in micelles, leading to complete biofilm inhibition for multiple Candida species, with synergy observed when combined with fluconazole against resistant strains [33]. Sato et al. advanced these findings in vivo, showing that hypericin-loaded nanostructured lipid carriers combined with aPDT significantly reduced *C. albicans* colonies in a mouse model with minimal host tissue damage [39]. Troichenko et al. demonstrated the potential of combined aPDT and collagen cross-linking for inhibiting *C. albicans* biofilms in ophthalmic applications, while Morelato et al. found that riboflavin–PDT with blue LED and methylene blue–PDT with red LED both significantly reduced biofilm formation in peri-implantitis models [37]. Rezusta et al. showed that hypericin-mediated aPDT was effective against azole-resistant *C. albicans*, achieving a 3-log reduction at low fungal concentrations. These studies collectively underscore PDT's potential as a minimally invasive, biocompatible, and effective treatment for fungal infections, particularly those associated with biofilms or resistant strains [36]. While many studies demonstrate the efficacy of aPDT, limitations such as incomplete biofilm eradication, variability in the reduction of fungal cell viability, and the potential for regrowth under suboptimal conditions must be acknowledged. Differences in light source parameters, such as wavelength and energy density, were observed to significantly influence outcomes, with some protocols achieving higher efficacy due to optimized settings. These findings highlight the importance of standardized methodologies to ensure reproducibility and to maximize the therapeutic potential of aPDT [28–40]. However, differences in experimental protocols, including photosensitizer concentrations, light parameters, and fungal strains, highlight the need for standardization. The lack of large-scale clinical trials is a limitation, as most evidence comes from in vitro or small animal studies. Future research should prioritize clinical validation and explore standardized aPDT protocols, innovative delivery systems like micelles or hydrogels, and combinations with antifungal drugs to optimize treatment outcomes and expand aPDT's applicability across clinical settings. These findings suggest that aPDT, particularly with natural photosensitizers like hypericin and riboflavin, could offer a safe, sustainable, and effective alternative to traditional antifungal therapies [26–42].

3.6. Characteristics of Light Sources Used in aPDT

Table 6 outlines the physical parameters of the light sources used in studies that satisfied the inclusion criteria.

Table 6. Light sources' physical parameters of studies that fulfilled the eligibility criteria.

Reference Number	Author and Year	Light Source	Wavelength	Energy Density (Fluence) (J/cm^2)	Power Output (Standardized) (mW/cm^2)	Irradiation Time (s)	Spot Size/Fiber Surface Area (cm^2)
[26]	Agut et al. (2011)	LED	602	0, 18, 37	Not specified	Not specified	Not specified
[27]	Alam et al. (2019)	Orange LED	590	Not specified	15 ± 2	3600–10,800	Not specified
[28]	Alshehri et al. (2021)	Blue LED	450	15	25	600	4.5
[29]	Arboleda et al. (2014)	Green and UV LED	375 and 518	5.4	2.2	Not stated	28.3
[30]	Ardakani et al. (2024)	Blue LED Red LED	410–490 630–640	60	1100 ± 200	60 20	0.5
[31]	Bernala et al. (2011)	Yellow LED diffusion table	590	6	2000 ± 400	600	Not specified
[32]	Troichenko et al. (2021)	UV and low-energy lasers	365	Not specified	10	600 (UV) 180 (laser)	Not specified
[33]	Sakita et al. (2019)	Nanocarriers with PDT	450 to 750	16.2	Not specified	Not specified	Not specified
[34]	Sato et al. (2022)	Hypericin-loaded LED system	532	Not specified	3.0	Not specified	Not specified

Table 6. *Cont.*

Reference Number	Author and Year	Light Source	Wavelength	Energy Density (Fluence) (J/cm^2)	Power Output (Standardized) (mW/cm^2)	Irradiation Time (s)	Spot Size/Fiber Surface Area (cm^2)
[35]	Tunccan et al. (2018)	LED and UV-A	LED (660 and 528) UV-A (370)	0.233	Not specified	300	Not specified
[36]	Rezusta et al. (2012)	LED	602 ± 10	18, 37	0.077 (assumed area: 10 cm^2)	Not specified	Not specified
[37]	Morelato et al. (2022)	Diode laser	445	1.24	Not specified	60	Not specified
[38]	Paz-Cristobal et al. (2014)	LED	602 ± 10	37	124,340	Not specified	Not specified
[39]	Sato et al. (2023)	LED	525	113	10.3	900	Not specified
[40]	Kashiwabuchi et al. (2013)	UV-A (365 nm) with riboflavin	365	5.4	Not specified	1800	Not specified
[41]	Sousa et al. (2019)	PAR radiation, OSRAM 21 lamps of 18 W	380–700	Not specified	3.0	16200	Not specified

LED: Light-Emitting Diode; UV: Ultraviolet.

Table 7 summarises the concentration and incubation time of the photosenistisors used i the studies.

Table 7. Characteristics of PS used in studies meeting eligibility criteria.

Reference Number	Author and Year	Incubation Time (Minutes)	Concentration/s of PS Used
[26]	Agut et al. (2011)	Not specified	0.625 M hypericin 1.25 M hypericin 2.5 M hypericin 40 M hypericin
[27]	Alam et al. (2019)	30	0.1% hypericin
[28]	Alshehri et al. (2021)	10	0.1% riboflavin
[29]	Arboleda et al. (2014)	Not specified	0.1% riboflavin 0.1% rose bengal
[30]	Ardakani et al. (2024)	Not specified	Curcumin Riboflavin Phycocyanin
[31]	Bernala et al. (2011)	10	0.1–0.4 μg/mL hypericin
[32]	Troichenko et al. (2021)	10 (UV) 3 (Laser)	0.1% riboflavin 0.1% methylene blue
[33]	Sakita et al. (2019)	120	0.25–32.0 μM P123-Hyp
[34]	Sato et al. (2022)	Not specified	Hypericin in lipid carriers (specific concentration unspecified)
[35]	Tunccan et al. (2018)	4320	0.1% riboflavin 25 μg/mL methylene blue 0.1% rose bengal
[36]	Rezusta et al. (2012)	Not specified	0.625–320 μM hypericin
[37]	Morelato et al. (2022)	Not specified	0.1% riboflavin 0.1% methylene blue
[38]	Paz-Cristobal et al. (2014)	1–60	0.625–40 μM hypericin 1.25–2.5 μM DMMB
[39]	Sato et al. (2023)		
[40]	Kashiwabuchi et al. (2013)	30	Riboflavin, UV-A (not quantified)
[41]	Sousa et al. (2019)	10 in PBS, 30 in plasma/whole blood	5.0 μM Tri-Py(+)-Me 10 μM FORM

DMMB—Dimethyl Methylene Blue, P123-Hyp—Hypericin Encapsulated in P123 Micelles, Tri-Py(+)-Me—Tri-Pyridyl Methyl, UV—Ultraviolet Radiotaion.

4. Discussion

4.1. Results in the Context of Other Evidence

This systematic review provides compelling evidence to reject our null hypothesis, which posited no significant difference in the efficacy of riboflavin- and hypericin-mediated aPDT compared to conventional antifungal treatments for managing *Candida* infections, demonstrating that aPDT is a promising alternative for reducing fungal load, particularly in cases where conventional antifungals face challenges due to resistance or biofilm formation. Both riboflavin and hypericin exhibited substantial antifungal activity against *Candida* spp. in vitro, with multiple studies achieving complete eradication of planktonic cells under optimized conditions [27,28,31,36], and were effective in reducing biofilm mass and viability, although biofilms remained more resistant than planktonic cells due to their structural complexity and extracellular matrix [32,33,35,36]. The versatility of riboflavin, activated by blue light, and hypericin, which responds to yellow or orange light, underscores their clinical potential, supported by safety profiles showing minimal cytotoxicity to human keratinocytes and fibroblasts, indicating their suitability for clinical applications without damaging host tissues [31,36,39]. Riboflavin- and hypericin-mediated aPDT effectively targeted fluconazole-resistant *Candida* strains, offering a promising strategy to address antifungal drug resistance, while their combination with conventional antifungal agents like fluconazole enhanced effects, particularly against biofilm-associated infections, suggesting a dual-action therapeutic approach [32,33,36]. Despite significant reductions in *Candida* spp. cell counts, complete biofilm eradication was not consistently achieved due to the biofilm's protective extracellular matrix emphasizing the difficulty of treating biofilm-associated infections, and the findings remain limited by the predominance of in vitro studies and the variability in study designs, including differences in light parameters, photosensitizer concentrations, and incubation times, complicating direct comparisons and underscoring the need for standardized protocols [35–37]. Nonetheless, in vivo studies confirmed the effectiveness of hypericin-loaded hydrogels in reducing *Candida albicans* vaginal colonies and riboflavin-mediated aPDT in decreasing fungal loads on dental surfaces and prosthetic materials, with both photosensitizers identified as promising natural alternatives due to their biocompatibility, low toxicity, and sustainable use in aPDT though the scarcity of in vivo or clinical trials limits the generalizability of results, requiring future research with large-scale studies to establish standardized protocols and optimize outcomes [26,36]. These findings align with prior evidence emphasizing the potential of photodynamic therapy in overcoming antimicrobial resistance and managing biofilm-associated infections, underscoring its promise for clinical application in drug-resistant *Candida* infections and biofilm-associated conditions. Numerous studies have highlighted the promising role of photodynamic therapy in managing oral candidiasis, strongly supporting its potential as an effective alternative or adjunct to traditional antifungal treatments. For instance, Hu et al. evaluated the efficacy of PDT in comparison to conventional antifungal drugs and found it to be superior to nystatin in reducing *Candida* colonies [42]. Their findings also suggested that PDT might offer greater effectiveness than other antifungals, such as fluconazole and miconazole. Rodríguez-Cerdeira et al. similarly reported that PDT is a promising treatment option due to its broad antimicrobial spectrum and the ability to target drug-resistant strains of Candida, making it a viable alternative where traditional antifungal treatments might fail [43]. Supporting this, D'Amico et al. demonstrated that PDT significantly reduces *Candida albicans* biofilm without exerting cytotoxic effects on gingival cells. Their study compared various photosensitizers and reinforced PDT's potential as both a primary and adjunctive therapy for oral candidiasis [44]. The mechanisms underlying PDT's effectiveness were further explored by Kashef and Hamblin, who noted its ability to alter Candida cell permeability, ultimately leading to fungal death [45]. They also highlighted PDT's wide antibacterial spectrum, short therapeutic course, and strong targeting capabilities, which make it particularly advantageous in antifungal treatment strategies. However, the application of PDT shows variability depending on the site of treatment. For example, Agut et al. observed that PDT was more effective in reducing *Candida* colonies on the palate compared to the denture area [26]. This difference is attributed to the porous and irregular surfaces of dentures, which facilitate microbial adhesion and recolonization. The limited action of PDT on denture surfaces compared to broader oral areas treated with systemic drugs further underscores this finding. Studies by Pérez-Laguna et al. and others have emphasized that mechanical cleaning of dentures is essential to achieve optimal outcomes, as PDT alone is insufficient to address fungal growth on such surfaces [46]. Comparative analyses have further clarified PDT's position relative to other antifungaltreatments. For example, while PDT showed similar efficacy to fluconazole, miconazole was found to be more effective [47]. However, PDT's ability to target drug-resistant Candida strains gives it a distinct advantage over azoles in specific cases. Furthermore, systemic antifungals like amphotericin B demonstrated less effectiveness in removing fungal colonies from denture surfaces, further reinforcing the critical role of regular denture cleaning in managing oral candidiasis [48]. Despite these advancements, recurrence rates of candidiasis remain a significant concern. Studies by Mima et al., Macial et al., and Schwingel et al. have reported high recurrence rates, primarily due to inadequate denture cleaning and Candida recolonization [49–51]. Nevertheless, the combination of PDT with traditional antifungal agents has shown promise in mitigating these challenges [42]. Notably, the synergistic effect of PDT and nystatin has been demonstrated to significantly reduce Candida colonies and lower recurrence rates. This is attributed to their complementary mechanisms of action, which enhance overall treatment efficacy [42]. Studies by Paz-Cristobal et al. and Agut et al. highlighted that combination therapy with PDT and nystatin is both effective and safe, with adverse reactions reported as mild and self-limiting [26,38]. Common side effects, such as nausea and burning tongue, were mostly observed in immunodeficient patients and did not pose significant risks [42,52,53]. Overall, PDT presents itself as a valuable adjunct to traditional antifungal therapies due to its broad spectrum, strong targeting capability, and short therapeutic course. Combining PDT with antifungal agents like nystatin is recommended for achieving improved clinical outcomes and reducing the recurrence of oral candidiasis [42]. These findings collectively underline the potential of PDT as an innovative and effective approach tothe management of this challenging condition [36–42].

4.2. Limitations of the Evidence

The primary limitation lies in the significant variability of protocols across studies. Light source parameters, including wavelength, energy density, and fluence, as well as photosensitizer concentrations and incubation times, differed widely, making it difficult to compare outcomes or establish standardized guidelines. Furthermore, while many studies reported efficacy against *Candida* spp., most were conducted in vitro, with limited in vivo evidence or clinical trials available to confirm these findings in human populations. Additionally, while aPDT was effective in reducing biofilm mass, complete eradication of biofilms was rarely achieved, highlighting a persistent challenge in biofilm-associated infections. Finally, the studies included in this review often relied on subjective outcome measures, such as CFU reduction and visual biofilm assessment, without integrating advanced diagnostic tools like imaging or molecular analyses to substantiate their results.

4.3. Limitations of the Review Process

The lack of homogeneity among the included studies led to a narrative synthesis of results. The variability in study designs, intervention protocols, and outcome measures may have introduced bias in evaluating the overall efficacy of riboflavin- and hypericin-mediated aPDT. Moreover, the significant differences in the parameters used across studies prevented the authors from applying the GRADE tool, and as such, heterogeneity makes it challenging to formulate clear recommendations. To address this, future research should focus on conducting well-designed randomized controlled trials to directly compare specific parameters and establish standardized protocols. Furthermore, the exclusion of non-English studies and gray literature may have restricted the scope of the review, potentially overlooking relevant data. These limitations highlight the need for more rigorous research in this field to enable systematic comparisons and quantitative analyses.

4.4. Implications for Practice, Policy, and Future Research

Riboflavin- and hypericin-mediated aPDT shows promise as a safe and effective alternative or adjunct to conventional antifungal therapies, particularly for managing drug-resistant or recurrent Candida infections. Clinicians should consider incorporating aPDT into treatment protocols for conditions such as denture stomatitis and other mucosal infections. However, for this to become routine practice, standardized treatment protocols—including consistent light parameters, photosensitizer concentrations, and application techniques—must be developed and validated. Policymakers and research funding agencies should prioritize support for large-scale, multicenter clinical trials to confirm the efficacy and safety of aPDT in diverse patient populations. Furthermore, future research should explore the synergistic potential of combining aPDT with existing antifungal drugs, particularly for biofilm-associated infections where monotherapies often fall short. Innovations such as nanocarrier systems and hydrogels could enhance the delivery and stability of photosensitizers, improving therapeutic efficacy. While the current evidence highlights the potential of aPDT in combating oral candidiasis and related infections, addressing the identified gaps is crucial for its integration into routine clinical practice.

Future research should prioritize the standardization of parameters to enable more reliable and meaningful comparisons across studies. Moreover, further investigation is needed to examine the variations in efficacy between different regions of the mouth, such as tooth versus palate applications, to deepen our understanding of site-specific outcomes.

5. Conclusions

This systematic review demonstrates the potential of riboflavin- and hypericin-mediated antimicrobial photodynamic therapy as promising, non-invasive alternatives for managing Candida infections, particularly in cases resistant to conventional antifungal therapies. Significant reductions in fungal viability and biofilm mass, coupled with minimal cytotoxic effects, highlight the clinical promise of these photosensitizers. Riboflavin and hypericin, activated by blue and yellow/orange light, respectively, offer versatility and efficacy, particularly against fluconazole-resistant strains. Additionally, the reviewed evidence indicates that aPDT can achieve outcomes comparable to traditional antifungal agents while reducing systemic side effects and potentially enhancing efficacy through synergistic combinations. However, the lack of standardization in study protocols, such as variations in light parameters and photosensitizer concentrations, alongside a scarcity of large-scale clinical trials, limits the applicability of these findings. To address these limitations, future research should prioritize large-scale, multicenter studies with consistent methodologies and explore optimal treatment parameters to enhance the reproducibility and effectiveness of aPDT. Furthermore, focusing on areas where aPDT could have the most immediate clinical impact, such as the treatment of antifungal-resistant Candida strains and biofilm-associated infections, would maximize its relevance and utility. These targeted applications address critical gaps in current antifungal therapies and could accelerate the integration of aPDT into clinical practice.

Author Contributions: Conceptualization, M.Ł., W.N. and R.W.; methodology, W.N. and R.W.; software, M.Ł. and J.F.-R.; formal analysis, J.F.-R., W.N. and M.Ł.; investigation, J.F.-R., W.N. and M.Ł.; writing—original draft preparation, J.F.-R., W.N., R.W. and M.Ł.; writing—review and editing, W.N., J.F.-R., M.Ł., R.W. and D.S.; supervision, R.W. and D.S.; funding acquisition, R.W. and D.S. All authors have read and agreed to the published version of the manuscript.

Funding: This research received no external funding.

Data Availability Statement: Data are contained within the article.

Conflicts of Interest: The authors declare no conflicts of interest.

References

1. Rapala-Kozik, M.; Surowiec, M.; Juszczak, M.; Wronowska, E.; Kulig, K.; Bednarek, A.; Gonzalez-Gonzalez, M.; Karkowska Kuleta, J.; Zawrotniak, M.; Satała, D.; et al. Living Together: The Role of *Candida albicans* in the Formation of Polymicrobial Biofilms in the Oral Cavity. *Yeast* **2023**, *40*, 303–317. [CrossRef] [PubMed]
2. Stenderup, A. Oral Mycology. *Acta Odontol. Scand.* **1990**, *48*, 3–10. [CrossRef] [PubMed]
3. Fumes, A.C.; Da Silva Telles, P.D.; Corona, S.A.M.; Borsatto, M.C. Effect of APDT on Streptococcus Mutans and *Candida albicans* Present in the Dental Biofilm: Systematic Review. *Photodiagnosis Photodyn. Ther.* **2018**, *21*, 363–366. [CrossRef] [PubMed]
4. Vila, T.; Sultan, A.S.; Montelongo-Jauregui, D.; Jabra-Rizk, M.A. Oral Candidiasis: A Disease of Opportunity. *J. Fungi* **2020**, *6*, 15. [CrossRef]
5. Patel, M. Oral Cavity and *Candida albicans:* Colonisation to the Development of Infection. *Pathogens* **2022**, *11*, 335. [CrossRef]
6. Zhou, Y.; Cheng, L.; Lei, Y.L.; Ren, B.; Zhou, X. The Interactions Between *Candida albicans* and Mucosal Immunity. *Front. Microbiol* **2021**, *12*, 652725. [CrossRef]
7. Talapko, J.; Juzbašić, M.; Matijević, T.; Pustijanac, E.; Bekić, S.; Kotris, I.; Škrlec, I. *Candida albicans*—The Virulence Factors and Clinical Manifestations of Infection. *J. Fungi* **2021**, *7*, 79. [CrossRef]
8. Sanglard, D.; Coste, A.; Ferrari, S. Antifungal Drug Resistance Mechanisms in Fungal Pathogens from the Perspective of Transcriptional Gene Regulation. *FEMS Yeast Res.* **2009**, *9*, 1029–1050. [CrossRef]
9. Seneviratne, C.J.; Silva, W.J.; Jin, L.J.; Samaranayake, Y.H.; Samaranayake, L.P. Architectural Analysis, Viability Assessment and Growth Kinetics of *Candida albicans* and *Candida glabrata* Biofilms. *Arch. Oral Biol.* **2009**, *54*, 1052–1060. [CrossRef]
10. Carmello, J.C.; Alves, F.G.; Basso, F.; De Souza Costa, C.A.; Bagnato, V.S.; Mima, E.G.D.O.; Pavarina, A.C. Treatment of Oral Candidiasis Using Photodithazine®—Mediated Photodynamic Therapy In Vivo. *PLoS ONE* **2016**, *11*, e0156947. [CrossRef]
11. Pereira Gonzales, F.; Maisch, T. Photodynamic Inactivation for Controlling *Candida albicans* Infections. *Fungal Biol.* **2012**, *116*, 1–10. [CrossRef] [PubMed]
12. Kubizna, M.; Dawiec, G.; Wiench, R. Efficacy of Curcumin-Mediated Antimicrobial Photodynamic Therapy on *Candida* spp.—A Systematic Review. *Int. J. Mol. Sci.* **2024**, *25*, 8136. [CrossRef] [PubMed]
13. Suwannasom, N.; Kao, I.; Pruß, A.; Georgieva, R.; Bäumler, H. Riboflavin: The Health Benefits of a Forgotten Natural Vitamin. *Int. J. Mol. Sci.* **2020**, *21*, 950. [CrossRef] [PubMed]
14. Barroso, R.A.; Navarro, R.; Tim, C.R.; De Paula Ramos, L.; De Oliveira, L.D.; Araki, Â.T.; Fernandes, K.G.C.; Macedo, D.; Assis, L. Antimicrobial Photodynamic Therapy Against *Propionibacterium acnes* Biofilms Using Hypericin (*Hypericum perforatum*) Photosensitizer: In Vitro Study. *Lasers Med. Sci.* **2021**, *36*, 1235–1240. [CrossRef]
15. Boen, M.; Brownell, J.; Patel, P.; Tsoukas, M.M. The Role of Photodynamic Therapy in Acne: An Evidence-Based Review. *Am. J. Clin. Dermatol.* **2017**, *18*, 311–321. [CrossRef]
16. Li, S.-S.; Zhang, L.-L.; Nie, S.; Lv, T.; Wang, H.-W. Severe Acne in Monozygotic Twins Treated with Photodynamic Therapy. *Photodiagnosis Photodyn. Ther.* **2018**, *23*, 235–236. [CrossRef]
17. Galeotti, N. Hypericum Perforatum (St John's Wort) beyond Depression: A Therapeutic Perspective for Pain Conditions. *J. Ethnopharmacol.* **2017**, *200*, 136–146. [CrossRef]
18. Napoli, E.; Siracusa, L.; Ruberto, G.; Carrubba, A.; Lazzara, S.; Speciale, A.; Cimino, F.; Saija, A.; Cristani, M. Phytochemical Profiles, Phototoxic and Antioxidant Properties of Eleven Hypericum Species—A Comparative Study. *Phytochemistry* **2018**, *152*, 162–173. [CrossRef]
19. Polat, E.; Kang, K. Natural Photosensitizers in Antimicrobial Photodynamic Therapy. *Biomedicines* **2021**, *9*, 584. [CrossRef]
20. Kubrak, T.P.; Kołodziej, P.; Sawicki, J.; Mazur, A.; Koziorowska, K.; Aebisher, D. Some natural photosensitizers and their Medicinal properties for Use in Photodynamic Therapy. *Molecules* **2022**, *27*, 1192. [CrossRef]

21. Wang, X.; Wang, L.; Fekrazad, R.; Zhang, L.; Jiang, X.; He, G.; Wen, X. Polyphenolic Natural Products as Photosensitizers for Antimicrobial Photodynamic Therapy: Recent Advances and Future Prospects. *Front. Immunol.* **2023**, *14*, 1275859. [CrossRef] [PubMed]
22. Schardt, C.; Adams, M.B.; Owens, T.; Keitz, S.; Fontelo, P. Utilization of the PICO Framework to Improve Searching PubMed for Clinical Questions. *BMC Med. Inform. Decis. Making.* **2007**, *7*, 16. [CrossRef]
23. Page, M.J.; McKenzie, J.E.; Bossuyt, P.M.; Boutron, I.; Hoffmann, T.C.; Mulrow, C.D.; Shamseer, L.; Tetzlaff, J.M.; Akl, E.A.; Brennan, S.E.; et al. The PRISMA 2020 Statement: An Updated Guideline for Reporting Systematic Reviews. *BMJ* **2021**, *372*, n71. [CrossRef] [PubMed]
24. Watson, P.F.; Petrie, A. Method Agreement Analysis: A Review of Correct Methodology. *Theriogenology* **2010**, *73*, 1167–1179. [CrossRef] [PubMed]
25. Higgins, J.; Thomas, J.; Chandler, J.; Cumpston, M.; Li, T.; Page, M. *Welch Cochrane Handbook for Systematic Reviews of Interventions Version 6.4*; Cochrane: London, UK, 2023. Available online: http://www.training.cochrane.org/handbook (accessed on 20 October 2024).
26. Agut, M.; Rezusta, A.; Paz-Cristobal, M.P.; Vicente, P.M.; Díez, D.R.; López-Chicón, P.; Alemany, M.; Semino, C.; Gilaberte, Y.; Nonell, S. Photodynamic effect in vitro of hypericin on yeasts and evaluation of its photocytotoxicity in keratinocytes and fibroblasts. *Photodiagnosis Photodyn. Ther.* **2011**, *8*, 224. [CrossRef]
27. Alam, S.T.; Le, T.A.N.; Park, J.-S.; Kwon, H.C.; Kang, K. Antimicrobial Biophotonic Treatment of Ampicillin-Resistant *Pseudomonas aeruginosa* with Hypericin and Ampicillin Cotreatment Followed by Orange Light. *Pharmaceutics* **2019**, *11*, 641. [CrossRef]
28. Alshehri, A.H. Mechanical and antimicrobial effects of riboflavin-mediated photosensitization of in vitro *C. albicans* formed on polymethyl methacrylate resin. *Photodiagnosis Photodyn. Ther.* **2021**, *36*, 102488. [CrossRef]
29. Arboleda, A.; Miller, D.; Cabot, F.; Taneja, M.; Aguilar, M.C.; Alawa, K.; Amescua, G.; Yoo, S.H.; Parel, J.M. Assessment of rose bengal versus riboflavin photodynamic therapy for inhibition of fungal keratitis isolates. *Am. J. Ophthalmol.* **2014**, *158*, 64–70.e2. [CrossRef]
30. Shahi Ardakani, A.; Benedicenti, S.; Solimei, L.; Shahabi, S.; Afrasiabi, S. Reduction of Multispecies Biofilms on an Acrylic Denture Base Model by Antimicrobial Photodynamic Therapy Mediated by Natural Photosensitizers. *Pharmaceuticals* **2024**, *17*, 1232. [CrossRef]
31. Bernal, C.; Rodrigues, J.A.O.; Guimarães, A.P.P.; Ribeiro, A.O.; de Oliveira, K.T.; Imasato, H.; Perussi, J.R. Selective photoinactivation of *C. albicans* and *C. dubliniensis* with hypericin. *Laser Phys.* **2011**, *21*, 245–249. [CrossRef]
32. Troichenko, L.F.; Drozhzhyna, G.I.; Moloda, A.L.; Dolenko, L.V. In vitro investigation of the effect of photosensitizer-mediated 365-nm UV light and 630–670-nm low-energy laser irradiation on the fungal flora, *Candida albicans* and *Fusarium* spp. *Oftalmol. Zhurnal* **2021**, *92*, 34–40. [CrossRef]
33. Sakita, K.M.; Conrado, P.C.; Faria, D.R.; Arita, G.S.; Capoci, I.R.; Rodrigues-Vendramini, F.A.; Pieralisi, N.; Cesar, G.B.; Gonçalves, R.S.; Caetano, W.; et al. Copolymeric micelles as efficient inert nanocarrier for hypericin in the photodynamic inactivation of Candida species. *Future Microbiol.* **2019**, *14*, 519–531. [CrossRef] [PubMed]
34. Sato, M.R.; Oshiro-Junior, J.A.; Rodero, C.F.; Boni, F.I.; Araújo, V.H.S.; Bauab, T.M.; Nicholas, D.; Callan, J.F.; Chorilli, M. Photodynamic therapy-mediated hypericin-loaded nanostructured lipid carriers against vulvovaginal candidiasis. *J. Med. Mycol.* **2022**, *32*, 101296. [CrossRef] [PubMed]
35. Güzel Tunçcan, Ö.; Kalkancı, A.; Unal, E.A.; Abdulmajed, O.; Erdoğan, M.; Dizbay, M.; Çağlar, K. The in vitro effect of antimicrobial photodynamic therapy on Candida and *Staphylococcus biofilms. Turk. J. Med. Sci.* **2018**, *48*, 873–879. [CrossRef]
36. Rezusta, A.; López-Chicón, P.; Paz-Cristobal, M.P.; Alemany-Ribes, M.; Royo-Díez, D.; Agut, M.; Semino, C.; Nonell, S.; Revillo, M.J.; Aspiroz, C.; et al. In vitro fungicidal photodynamic effect of hypericin on Candida species. *Photochem. Photobiol.* **2012**, *88*, 613–619. [CrossRef]
37. Morelato, L.; Budimir, A.; Smojver, I.; Katalinić, I.; Vuletić, M.; Ajanović, M.; Gabrić, D. A Novel Technique for Disinfection Treatment of Contaminated Dental Implant Surface Using 0.1% Riboflavin and 445 nm Diode Laser—An In Vitro Study. *Bioengineering* **2022**, *9*, 308. [CrossRef]
38. Paz-Cristobal, M.P.; Royo, D.; Rezusta, A.; Andrés-Ciriano, E.; Alejandre, M.C.; Meis, J.F.; Revillo, M.J.; Aspiroz, C.; Nonell, S.; Gilaberte, Y. Photodynamic fungicidal efficacy of hypericin and dimethyl methylene blue against azole-resistant *Candida albicans* strains. *Mycoses* **2014**, *57*, 35–42. [CrossRef]
39. Sato, M.R.; Oshiro-Junior, J.A.; Rodero, C.F.; Boni, F.I.; Araújo, V.H.S.; Bauab, T.M.; Nicholas, D.; Callan, J.F.; Chorilli, M. Enhancing Antifungal Treatment of *Candida albicans* with Hypericin-Loaded Nanostructured Lipid Carriers in Hydrogels: Characterization, In Vitro, and In Vivo Photodynamic Evaluation. *Pharmaceuticals* **2023**, *16*, 1094. [CrossRef] [PubMed] [PubMed Central]
40. Kashiwabuchi, R.T.; Carvalho, F.R.; Khan, Y.A.; Hirai, F.; Campos, M.S.; McDonnell, P.J. Assessment of fungal viability after long-wave ultraviolet light irradiation combined with riboflavin administration. *Graefes Arch. Clin. Exp. Ophthalmol.* **2013**, *251*, 521–527. [CrossRef]

41. Sousa, V.; Gomes, A.T.P.C.; Freitas, A.; Faustino, M.A.F.; Neves, M.G.P.M.S.; Almeida, A. Photodynamic Inactivation of *Candida albicans* in Blood Plasma and Whole Blood. *Antibiotics* **2019**, *8*, 221. [CrossRef]
42. Hu, Q.; Li, T.; Yang, J.; Peng, Y.; Liu, Q.; Liu, N. Efficacy of photodynamic therapy in the treatment of oral candidiasis: A systematic review and meta-analysis. *BMC Oral Health* **2023**, *23*, 802. [CrossRef] [PubMed]
43. Rodríguez-Cerdeira, C.; Martínez-Herrera, E.; Fabbrocini, G.; Sanchez-Blanco, B.; López-Barcenas, A.; El-Samahy, M.; Juárez-Durán, E.R.; González-Cespón, J.L. New Applications of Photodynamic Therapy in the Management of Candidiasis. *J. Fungi* **2021**, *7*, 1025. [CrossRef] [PubMed]
44. D'Amico, E.; Di Lodovico, S.; Pierfelice, T.V.; Tripodi, D.; Piattelli, A.; Iezzi, G.; Petrini, M.; D'Ercole, S. What Is the Impact of Antimicrobial Photodynamic Therapy on Oral Candidiasis? An In Vitro Study. *Gels* **2024**, *10*, 110. [CrossRef]
45. Kashef, N.; Hamblin, M.R. Can microbial cells develop resistance to oxidative stress in antimicrobial photodynamic inactivation? *Drug Resist. Updates* **2017**, *31*, 31–42. [CrossRef]
46. Pérez-Laguna, V.; Gilaberte, Y.; Millán-Lou, M.I.; Agut, M.; Nonell, S.; Rezusta, A.; Hamblin, M.R. A combination of photodynamic therapy and antimicrobial compounds to treat skin and mucosal infections: A systematic review. *Photochem. Photobiol. Sci.* **2019**, *18*, 1020–1029. [CrossRef]
47. Goldman, G.H.; da Silva Ferreira, M.E.; dos Reis Marques, E.; Savoldi, M.; Perlin, D.; Park, S.; Martinez, P.C.G.; Goldman, M.H.S.; Colombo, A.L. Evaluation of fluconazole resistance mechanisms in *Candida albicans* clinical isolates from HIV- infected patients in Brazil. *Diagn. Microbiol. Infect. Dis.* **2004**, *50*, 25–32. [CrossRef]
48. Yanxuan, X.; Yutong, S.; Yiming, X.; Xiaoting, D.; Xianwen, W.; Qianming, C.; Lu, J. Meta-analysis of the efficacy and safety of topical antifungal drugs in the treatment of oral candidiasis. In Proceedings of the 13th National Oral Mucosal Pathology and the 11th National Conference on Combination of Chinese and Western Medicine in Stomatology of the Chinese Society of Stomatology, Wuhan, China, 15 October 2021. [CrossRef]
49. Mima, E.G.; Vergani, C.E.; Machado, A.L.; Massucato, E.M.S.; Colombo, A.L.; Bagnato, V.S.; Pavarina, A.C. Comparison of Photodynamic Therapy versus conventional antifungal therapy for the treatment of denture stomatitis: A randomized clinical trial. *Clin. Microbiol. Infect.* **2012**, *18*, E380–E388. [CrossRef]
50. Maciel, C.M.; Piva, M.R.; Ribeiro, M.A.; de Santana Santos, T.; Ribeiro, C.F.; Martins-Filho, P.R. Methylene Blue-Mediated Photodynamic Inactivation Followed by Low-Laser Therapy versus Miconazole Gel in the Treatment of Denture Stomatitis. *J. Prosthodont.* **2016**, *25*, 28–32. [CrossRef]
51. Scwingel, A.R.; Barcessat, A.R.; Núñez, S.C.; Ribeiro, M.S. Antimicrobial photodynamic therapy in the treatment of oral candidiasis in HIV-infected patients. *Photomed. Laser Surg.* **2012**, *30*, 429–432. [CrossRef]
52. Zhao, Y. Efficacy of Photodynamic Antimicrobial Therapy on Oral Candidiasis in AIDS Patients with Combined Oral Cavity. Master's Thesis, Guangxi Medical University, Guangxi, China, 2018.
53. Qin, J.M. Study on the Antibacterial Effect of Photodynamic Therapy on Oral Candidiasis in Patients with AIDS. Master's Thesis, Guangxi Medical University, Guangxi, China, 2018.

pharmaceutics

MDPI

Systematic Review

Riboflavin-Mediated Photodynamic Therapy in Periodontology: A Systematic Review of Applications and Outcomes

Jakub Fiegler-Rudol *, Maciej Łopaciński, Artur Los, Dariusz Skaba and Rafał Wiench

Department of Periodontal Diseases and Oral Mucosa Diseases, Faculty of Medical Sciences in Zabrze, Medical University of Silesia, 40-055 Katowice, Poland; mlopacinski@sum.edu.pl (M.Ł.); s79893@365.sum.edu.pl (A.L.); dskaba@sum.edu.pl (D.S.); rwiench@sum.edu.pl (R.W.)

* Correspondence: jakub.fiegler@gmail.com

Abstract: Background: Riboflavin (vitamin B_2) has emerged as a promising photosensitizer in photodynamic therapy (PDT) due to its strong absorption of blue light and favourable safety profile. This systematic review aims to evaluate the efficacy of riboflavin-mediated PDT in periodontology, specifically examining its antimicrobial effects and potential to improve clinical outcomes compared to conventional or other PDT-based treatments. **Methods**: A systematic review was conducted following PRISMA guidelines. A comprehensive literature search was performed in PubMed/Medline, Embase, Scopus, and the Cochrane Library. Studies published in English within the last 10 years were considered, where riboflavin served as the primary photosensitizer for dental treatments. Data extraction focused on study design, photosensitizer concentration, light source parameters, and clinical or microbiological outcomes. The risk of bias was assessed independently by two reviewers using a predefined scoring system. **Results**: Ten studies met the inclusion criteria, all demonstrating a low risk of bias. Riboflavin-mediated PDT consistently reduced microbial biofilms and pathogen viability in periodontitis, peri-implantitis, and endodontic models. Although some studies reported slightly lower efficacy compared to chlorhexidine or toluidine blue–based PDT, riboflavin-mediated PDT exhibited advantages such as minimal staining, low cytotoxicity, and enhanced collagen crosslinking. However, most studies were in vitro or small-scale clinical trials, limiting conclusions on long-term effectiveness. **Conclusions**: Riboflavin-mediated PDT shows promise as a safe adjunctive therapy for periodontal infections. Larger, well-designed clinical trials with standardized parameters and extended follow-up are needed to further evaluate its efficacy and optimize treatment protocols for routine clinical application.

Keywords: riboflavin; photodynamic therapy; periodontics; periodontal infections; biofilms; antimicrobial therapy; blue light activation; dental treatments

1. Introduction

1.1. Rationale

Riboflavin, commonly known as vitamin B_2, is an essential water-soluble vitamin involved in numerous biochemical processes such as cellular metabolism, redox reactions, and the maintenance of tissue integrity [1–3]. In addition to its well-known nutritional benefits, riboflavin has gained prominence as a powerful photosensitizing agent in photodynamic therapy (PDT), a minimally invasive treatment modality that is increasingly used in various medical fields, including dentistry [4,5]. Photodynamic therapy integrates three core components: a photosensitizer, light of a specific wavelength, and molecular oxygen [6]. When these elements interact, they generate reactive oxygen species (ROS) that effectively mediate antimicrobial activity, induce cellular damage in pathogens, and modify target tissue structures [4,7]. The duration of action for riboflavin-mediated photodynamic therapy (PDT) depends on the specific treatment protocol, including factors such as the irradiation time, riboflavin concentration, light source used, and the clinical condition being treated [4,7–9]. A schematic representation of this is presented in Figure 1.

Riboflavin is ideally suited for PDT because it effectively absorbs blue light and exhibits excellent biocompatibility [8,9]. It shows absorption peaks around 225, 275, 380, and 450 nm. Although these wavelengths do not penetrate deeply into tissues, this limitation may not pose a major issue when bacterial contamination is largely superficial. Additionally, the limited tissue penetration of blue light (405–470 nm) can serve as a benefit by safeguarding patient tissues from extensive photodamage [10]. The gold standard treatment for periodontitis currently involves the combination of systemic and local antibiotic therapies with root planing, effectively targeting pathogenic bacteria and promoting the restoration of periodontal health [7,10,11].

The mechanism of riboflavin-mediated PDT is multifaceted. Upon exposure to light at an appropriate wavelength, riboflavin transitions from its ground state to an excited singlet state, enabling it to interact with molecular oxygen in its environment [11]. This interaction produces ROS, such as singlet oxygen and free radicals, that inflict oxidative damage on bacterial membranes, proteins, and DNA, thereby effectively inactivating pathogens [11,12]. Beyond its antimicrobial effects, photoactivated riboflavin also enhances collagen cross-linking within dentin. This process strengthens the organic matrix and improves the long-term stability of adhesive bonds, making riboflavin-mediated PDT a versatile tool for both microbial control and structural reinforcement in dental procedures [13].

Riboflavin-mediated PDT offers several advantages over traditional dental treatments. Conventional disinfectants such as sodium hypochlorite and chlorhexidine, while effective, carry risks of cytotoxicity and tissue irritation [14,15]. Likewise, techniques like phosphoric acid etching can be invasive and potentially weaken enamel or dentin [16]. In contrast, riboflavin-mediated PDT is minimally invasive, non-toxic, and preserves tissue integrity while delivering robust antimicrobial activity [17]. Moreover, its capacity to stabilize the dentin matrix through collagen cross-linking helps inhibit enzymatic degradation by matrix metalloproteinases (MMPs), which is crucial for maintaining the durability of adhesive bonds [18]. These beneficial properties position riboflavin-mediated PDT as an attractive alternative or adjunct to existing protocols, especially for applications such as disinfecting caries-affected dentin, reconditioning enamel, and enhancing bond strength in adhesive dentistry [15–19].

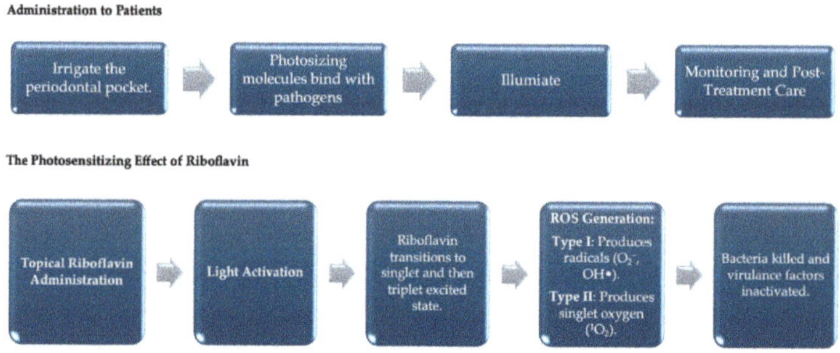

Figure 1. A Schematic representation of clinical and chemical aspects of riboflavin-mediated PDT [4].

1.2. Objectives

The primary objective of this systematic review is to assess the current evidence regarding the efficacy of riboflavin-mediated PDT in the treatment of various dental conditions. This includes evaluating its antimicrobial effects, its ability to reduce biofilm mass, and its potential to improve clinical outcomes when used alone or in combination with other treatments. Additionally, this review aims to identify the optimal parameters for riboflavin-mediated PDT, including light source specifications and photosensitizer concentrations, to provide evidence-based recommendations for its clinical application. By consolidating findings from in vitro, clinical, and animal studies, this review seeks to highlight the strengths and limitations of riboflavin-mediated PDT, inform future research directions, and potentially facilitate its integration into routine clinical practice.

2. Materials and Methods

2.1. Focused Question and Null Hypothesis

A systematic review was undertaken using the PICO framework and structured as follows [20]: For patients diagnosed with dental infections or conditions such as peri-implantitis, periodontitis, endodontic infections, or orthodontic biofilms (Population), does the implementation of riboflavin-mediated photodynamic therapy (Intervention), in comparison to conventional treatments such as mechanical debridement, curcumin-mediated PDT, or other non-surgical therapies (Comparison), lead to more effective management, reduced microbial load, or improved clinical outcomes (Outcome)? The null hypothesis for this study posits that there is no significant difference in the effectiveness of managing dental infections or improving clinical outcomes when using riboflavin-mediated photodynamic therapy compared to conventional mechanical debridement, curcumin-mediated PDT, or other non-surgical treatments.

2.2. Search Strategy

This systematic review was registered with PROSPERO CRD42025635828 and adhered to the PRISMA 2020 guidelines to ensure clarity and transparency in reporting [21]. A comprehensive search strategy was implemented across several databases, including PubMed/Medline, Embase, Scopus, and the Cochrane Library, using predefined keywords, which are listed in Table 1. Three researchers conducted the database searches independently, employing consistent methodologies. The review included studies published in English between 1 January 2015, and 3 January 2025, based on predefined inclusion criteria. Two authors (J.F-R. and R.W.) screened studies at the title, abstract, and full-text levels. Additionally, reference lists of eligible studies were examined to identify further relevant publications. The findings suggest that photodynamic therapy using riboflavin and curcumin may serve as a promising alternative or complementary approach to conventional peri-implantitis treatments, supported by a careful selection of high-quality studies.

Table 1. Search syntax used in the study.

Source	Search Term	Filters	Number of Results
Medline via PubMed	(riboflavin OR "vitamin B2") AND ("photodynamic therapy" OR photochemotherapy OR phototherapy OR PDT OR "light-activated disinfection" OR photosensitizer OR photosensitizing OR "light therapy") AND (periodontal OR periodontics OR periodontology OR periodontitis OR periodont* OR gingivitis OR "gum disease" OR "gum infection")	2015–2025	15

Table 1. *Cont.*

Source	Search Term	Filters	Number of Results
Web of Science Scopus	(TITLE-ABS-KEY (riboflavin OR "vitamin B2")) AND (TITLE-ABS-KEY("photodynamic therapy" OR photochemotherapy OR phototherapy OR PDT OR "light-activated disinfection" OR photosensitizer OR photosensitizing OR "light therapy")) AND (TITLE-ABS-KEY (periodontal OR periodontics OR periodontology OR periodontitis OR periodont* OR gingivitis OR "gum disease" OR "gum infection"))	2015–2025	14
Embase	(('riboflavin': ti, ab, kw OR 'vitamin B2': ti, ab, kw)) AND (('photodynamic therapy': ti, ab, kw OR photochemotherapy: ti, ab, kw OR phototherapy: ti, ab, kw OR pdt: ti, ab, kw OR 'light-activated disinfection': ti, ab, kw OR photosensitizer: ti, ab, kw OR photosensitizing: ti, ab, kw OR 'light therapy': ti, ab, kw)) AND ((periodontal: ti, ab, kw OR periodontics: ti, ab, kw OR periodontology: ti, ab, kw OR periodontitis: ti, ab, kw OR periodont*: ti, ab, kw OR gingivitis: ti, ab, kw OR 'gum disease': ti, ab, kw OR 'gum infection': ti, ab, kw))	2015–2025	7
Cochrane database	(MH "Riboflavin" OR "Riboflavin" OR "Vitamin B2") AND (MH "Photodynamic Therapy" OR "Photodynamic Therapy" OR "PDT" OR "Photochemotherapy" OR "Antimicrobial Photodynamic Therapy" OR "Light-Activated Disinfection" OR "Photosensitizer" OR "Photosensitizing" OR "Light Therapy") AND (MH "Dentistry" OR MH "Oral Health" OR "Periodontal" OR "Periodontics" OR "Periodontology" OR "Periodontitis" OR "Periodont*" OR "Gingivitis" OR "Gum Disease" OR "Gum Infection")	2015–2025	1

2.3. Selection of Studies

In the selection phase of this systematic review, each reviewer independently assessed the titles and abstracts of the retrieved studies to ensure objective inclusion. If disagreements about a study's eligibility arose, the reviewers collaborated and discussed the matter until a consensus was achieved. This rigorous process, adhering to PRISMA guidelines, ensured that only the most pertinent and methodologically sound studies were included, thereby improving the reliability and reproducibility of the review [21].

The inclusion criteria for this systematic review focused on studies that utilized riboflavin-based PDT for various dental conditions, including both in vitro and animal research. Additionally, research that explored the combined effects of riboflavin-mediated PDT with other antimicrobial or anti-inflammatory treatments was considered. Studies with control groups comparing riboflavin-based PDT to standard mechanical debridement, alternative non-surgical therapies, or no treatment were included, as well as investigations that directly compared the effectiveness of riboflavin-mediated PDT with other non-surgical treatments. Long-term studies assessing the sustained impact of riboflavin-mediated PDT on dental health outcomes, such as infection control, inflammation reduction, and tissue healing, were also included. Only publications that met predefined quality standards (Table 2) and specifically addressed the improvement or management of dental conditions using riboflavin-mediated PDT were considered.

Exclusion criteria included grey and unpublished literature, such as dissertations, conference abstracts, theses, and non-peer-reviewed materials, as well as articles published in languages other than English. Duplicate publications or those with identical ethical approval numbers were excluded. Studies focusing on dental or medical issues outside the scope of this review were also excluded, along with those using alternative photosensitizers other than riboflavin in PDT. Non-relevant in vitro studies that did not replicate clinical dental conditions or address pertinent microbial strains were not included. Furthermore, non-primary data formats such as case reports, case series, narrative reviews, systematic reviews, editorials, and books were excluded, as were studies lacking a control or comparison group. Lastly, studies involving non-therapeutic uses of PDT were not considered.

2.4. Risk of Bias in Individual Studies and Quality Assessment

At the start of the study selection process for this systematic review, each reviewer individually examined the titles and abstracts of the identified articles on riboflavin-mediated photodynamic therapy in dental treatments to reduce the risk of bias. The agreement between reviewers was measured using Cohen's kappa statistic, ensuring consistent and reliable decision-making [22]. In cases where disagreements about a study's eligibility occurred, the reviewers discussed the issues thoroughly until they reached a unanimous agreement.

The methodological quality of the included studies was independently assessed by two reviewers and focused on critical aspects of riboflavin-mediated photodynamic therapy (PDT) protocols, including study design, execution, and data analysis to maintain objectivity and reliable outcomes. Potential biases were identified by assigning a score of 1 for each "yes" and 0 for each "no" response, based on the following evaluation criteria: (1) Was a specific concentration of riboflavin clearly defined and utilized as the photosensitizer? (2) Was the origin or source of the riboflavin disclosed in the study? (3) Was the incubation period for the riboflavin photosensitizer explicitly stated? (4) Were detailed specifications of the light source provided, including type, wavelength, output power, fluence, and power density? (5) Was a power meter employed to accurately measure the light parameters used in the study? (6) Was a negative control group included in the experimental design to provide a baseline for comparison? (7) Were numerical results presented, accompanied by appropriate statistical analyses? (8) Was there complete reporting of outcome data without any missing information? (9) Funding Independence: Was the study conducted independently of its funding sources to prevent potential conflicts of interest? (10) Were participants and/or investigators blinded to the treatment allocations to minimize bias? Each study's risk of bias was then classified based on the total number of "yes" responses: High Risk of Bias (0–3 points), Moderate Risk of Bias (4–6 points), and Low Risk of Bias (7–10 points). The total score was calculated for each study, and the corresponding bias risk level (low, moderate, or high) was determined according to the guidelines outlined in the Cochrane Handbook for Systematic Reviews of Interventions [23]. This rigorous quality assessment process ensured that only studies with robust and reliable methodologies were included in the systematic review, thereby enhancing the overall validity and credibility of the review's findings.

Table 2 provides a detailed evaluation of the risk of bias for the 10 studies included in the final analysis. Inclusion criteria required each study to score at least six points according to the established evaluation framework. All selected studies demonstrated a low risk of bias, with one study achieving the highest possible score of 10 points [24]. Importantly, no studies were classified as having a moderate or high risk of bias, reinforcing the reliability and robustness of the systematic review's findings.

Table 2. The results of the quality assessment and risk of bias across the studies.

Author(s)	1	2	3	4	5	6	7	8	9	10	Total	Risk
Afrasiabi et al., 2023 [25]	1	1	1	1	1	0	1	1	1	0	8	Low
Bärenfaller et al., 2016 [26]	1	1	1	1	1	0	1	1	0	0	7	Low
Comeau et al., 2022 [27]	1	1	1	1	1	0	0	1	1	0	7	Low
Etemadi et al., 2023 [28]	1	1	1	1	1	1	1	1	1	0	9	Low
Kang et al., 2019 [29]	1	1	1	1	1	0	1	1	0	0	7	Low
Kunz et al., 2019 [30]	1	1	1	1	1	1	1	1	0	0	8	Low
Leelanarathiwata et al., 2020 [31]	1	1	1	1	1	1	1	1	0	0	8	Low
Morelato et al., 2022 [32]	1	1	1	1	1	1	1	1	1	0	9	Low
Nielsen et al., 2015 [33]	1	1	1	1	0	1	1	1	1	0	8	Low
Qamar et al., 2023 [24]	1	1	1	1	1	1	1	1	1	1	10	Low

2.5. Data Extraction

After finalizing the selection of pertinent studies, the two reviewers extracted detailed information from each included article. This extraction process encompassed bibliographic details such as the lead author's name and the year of publication, the study design, the specific dental conditions addressed, and the types of experimental and control groups utilized. Additionally, they documented the length of follow-up periods, the outcomes measured related to dental treatment effectiveness, and the technical specifications of the light sources used, including type, wavelength, and power parameters. Furthermore, the reviewers meticulously recorded the concentrations of riboflavin employed as the photosensitizer, the use of nanocarriers or other supplementary agents, as well as the incubation and irradiation durations during photodynamic therapy. They also captured information on any adjunctive treatments or methodologies integrated into the studies. This comprehensive data extraction ensured that all relevant variables were thoroughly captured, enabling a robust and exhaustive analysis of the efficacy and operational parameters of riboflavin-mediated photodynamic therapy in various dental treatments. This systematic approach to data extraction facilitated a nuanced understanding of how riboflavin-mediated PDT performs across different clinical scenarios, thereby strengthening the overall reliability and depth of the systematic review.

3. Results

3.1. Study Selection

Figure 2 presents an overview of the research workflow, meticulously designed to follow the PRISMA guidelines [23]. The process began with an initial literature search that identified 37 articles. After eliminating duplicates, 30 records remained. A thorough screening of titles and abstracts was conducted, resulting in 10 studies being chosen for a full-text review. Notably, no studies were excluded during this phase. In the end, 10 studies published within the last decade were included in the final analysis. Table 3 provides a detailed summary of these selected studies.

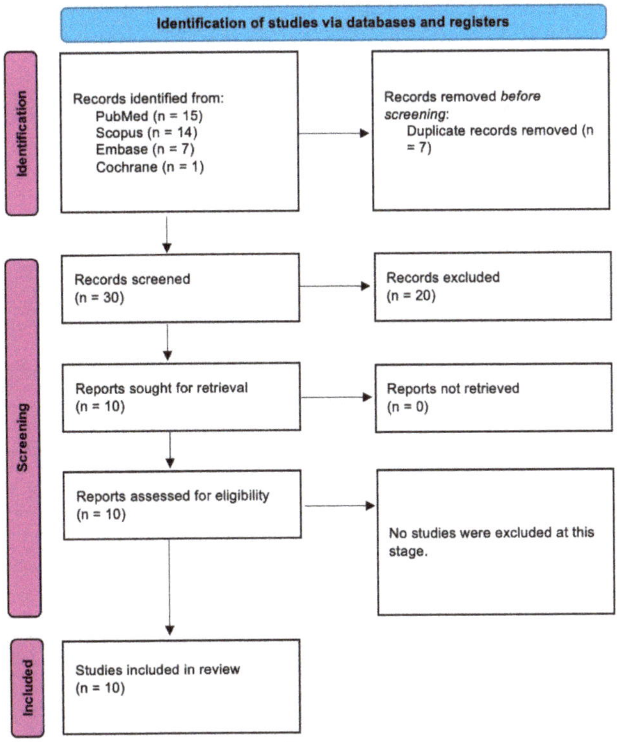

Figure 2. Prisma 2020 flow diagram.

Table 3. Summary of the studies.

Author and Year	Country	Study Design	Programs Used (Version, Specifications, Model, Brand, Company, City, State, Country)
Afrasiabi et al. 2023 [25]	Iran	in vitro study	Blue diode laser (0.4–1.0 W/cm^2), Curcumin and Riboflavin, Chlorhexidine, Laser Research Center of Dentistry, Tehran University of Medical Sciences, Tehran, Iran
Bärenfaller et al., 2016 [26]	Switzerland	in vitro study	Photoactivated disinfection using LED (Blue and Red), Riboflavin, University of Bern, Freiburgstrasse, Bern, Switzerland
Comeau et al., 2022 [27]	Canada	in vitro study	Blue LED (1.3 J/cm^2), Riboflavin-loaded dental resin, University of British Columbia, Vancouver, Canada
Etemadi et al., 2023 [28]	Iran	in vitro study	LED irradiation (390–480 nm), Curcumin and Riboflavin, Chlorhexidine 0.12%, Tehran Medical Sciences, Islamic Azad University, Tehran, Iran
Kang et al., 2019 [29]	South Korea	in vitro study	405 nm blue light (25.3 J), Curcumin, Protoporphyrin-IX, Resazurin, Riboflavin, Yonsei University College of Dentistry, Seoul, South Korea

Table 3. *Cont.*

Author and Year	Country	Study Design	Programs Used (Version, Specifications, Model, Brand, Company, City, State, Country)
Kunz et al., 2019 [30]	Switzerland	in vitro study	Blue LED (30 s, 60 s), Riboflavin, Hydrogen Peroxide, University of Bern, Switzerland
Leelanarathiwata et al., 2020 [31]	Thailand	in vitro study	Blue high-power LED, Flavin Mononucleotide, Mahidol University, Bangkok, Thailand
Morelato et al., 2022 [32]	Croatia	in vitro study	445 nm diode laser, Riboflavin, University of Rijeka, Croatia
Nielsen et al., 2015 [33]	Denmark	in vitro study	Blue LED, Riboflavin and Toluidine Blue O, Aarhus University, Denmark
Qamar et al., 2023 [24]	Saudi Arabia	Randomized controlled trial	Riboflavin-loaded Poly-L-glycolic acid nanoparticles, Aloe Vera gel, Riyadh Elm University, Riyadh, Saudi Arabia (Marked in Blue)

3.2. Data Presentation

Data from the 10 studies meeting the inclusion criteria were carefully extracted and are systematically summarized in Tables 3–6. These tables provide an extensive overview of each study's key features, including the characteristics of the light sources used and the specific properties of riboflavin employed as a photosensitiser in PDT protocols. This structured presentation enables detailed comparisons and comprehensive analysis of riboflavin-based PDT across the selected studies, supporting a robust assessment of its effectiveness and methodological aspects in addressing dental conditions.

Table 4. Main outcomes and study groups.

Author and Year	Study Groups	Main Outcomes
Afrasiabi et al., 2023 [25]	Negative Control: No treatment. Positive Control: Bacterial suspension exposed to CHX at 25 °C for 1 min. Curcumin Only: Bacterial suspension exposed to curcumin (40 μM) in the dark at 25 °C for 5 min. Riboflavin Only: Bacterial suspension exposed to riboflavin (100 μM) in the dark at 25 °C for 5 min. aPDT with Curcumin + Blue Diode Laser aPDT with Riboflavin + Blue Diode Laser	Riboflavin-mediated PDT demonstrates significant bactericidal effects against periodontal pathogens like *Streptococcus mutans*, particularly when combined with a blue diode laser at optimized power densities. The study found that riboflavin, activated by 445 nm blue light, induces oxidative stress, leading to microbial decontamination. The bactericidal efficacy improves with increased laser power density, with maximum effect observed at 1.0 W/cm^2. Compared to conventional antimicrobial agents such as chlorhexidine, riboflavin-mediated PDT offers a non-invasive alternative, reducing bacterial colonies without systemic side effects, thus enhancing its potential as a sustainable periodontal therapy.

Table 4. *Cont.*

Author and Year	Study Groups	Main Outcomes
Bärenfaller et al., 2016 [26]	Negative Control: No treatment. Light Control: light only. Photosensitizer Control: Without light. PAD30 (Blue LED): Photoactivated disinfection with blue LED for 30 s with riboflavin as photosensitizer. PAD60 (Blue LED): Photoactivated disinfection with blue LED for 60 s with riboflavin as photosensitizer. PADred: Photoactivated disinfection with red LED for 60 s with toluidine blue as photosensitizer.	Riboflavin-mediated PDT, often combined with blue spectrum LED, demonstrates notable antimicrobial effects against periodontopathogenic species. Studies highlight its efficacy in reducing planktonic bacterial counts, including pathogens such as *Porphyromonas gingivalis* and *Aggregatibacter actinomycetemcomitans*. However, the bactericidal impact is time and dose-dependent, with increased exposure enhancing outcomes. Riboflavin-mediated PDT shows diminished efficacy in complex multi-species biofilms and in the presence of serum, underlining the importance of mechanical biofilm removal as an adjunct. Despite its promising potential, riboflavin-mediated PDT's effectiveness is generally inferior to red-spectrum light systems using toluidine blue. Its clinical relevance lies in supplementing traditional periodontal therapies while minimizing antibiotic resistance risks
Comeau et al., 2022 [27]	Control Groups: Resin blend without riboflavin (0% B_2). Bacterial biofilm-only group (*Streptococcus mutans*) without resin disks. Experimental Resin Groups: Riboflavin-loaded resins with concentrations: 0.1%, 1.0%, and 1.5% B_2. Light Treatment Sub-Groups: Dark: No light exposure. Light: Exposure to blue LED light (440–460 nm) for 60 s at a fluence of 1.3 J/cm^2. Aging Conditions: Immediate: Resin specimens sterilized and tested immediately after fabrication. Aged: Resin specimens stored in 37 °C ultrapure water for 28 days before testing.	Riboflavin-mediated photodynamic therapy (PDT) in periodontology demonstrates significant antimicrobial and restorative potential. As a photosensitizer, riboflavin is activated by blue light to produce ROS that effectively reduce bacterial viability, particularly against pathogens like *Porphyromonas gingivalis*, *Aggregatibacter actinomycetemcomitans*, and *Streptococcus mutans*. Its efficacy is enhanced with optimized light parameters, such as higher fluence rates and appropriate exposure times, though it is less effective against complex biofilms and in the presence of serum. Studies show that riboflavin-mediated PDT can decrease biofilm formation on dental materials and integrate into resin-based restorations, providing mechanical stability and antimicrobial activity without compromising material properties. Further optimization of concentration, light parameters, and biofilm models is necessary to maximize its clinical applicability.

Table 4. *Cont.*

Author and Year	Study Groups	Main Outcomes
Etemadi et al., 2023 [28]	Negative Control: No treatment Positive Control: 0.12% chlorhexidine (5 s) Curcumin Group: 5 mg/mL curcumin in the dark for 5 min. Riboflavin Group: 0.5% riboflavin in the dark for 5 min. LED Group: Exposed to blue light (390–480 nm) for 60 s. Curcumin-mediated PDT: 5 mg/mL + LED. Riboflavin-mediated PDT: 0.5% + LED.	Riboflavin-mediated PDT in periodontology and peri-implantology exhibits promising antimicrobial effects, especially against *Aggregatibacter actinomycetemcomitans*. When activated by blue light or LEDs in the 390–480 nm range, riboflavin generates ROS that disrupt bacterial membranes, reducing biofilm viability on teeth and implant surfaces. Riboflavin mediated PDT effectively lowers bacterial CFU/mL in vitro, with better results under optimized conditions such as higher light intensity and adequate exposure time. Although generally less effective than curcumin-mediated PDT or chlorhexidine, riboflavin-mediated PDT offers a biocompatible, non-invasive alternative that avoids systemic side effects and minimizes antibiotic resistance risks. While its ability to kill biofilms is clear, clinical use may be limited by complex biofilm structures and low oxygen levels in deep periodontal pockets.
Kang et al., 2019 [29]	4 photosensitizers tested: Curcumin: 100 µg/mL, 10 µg/mL, 1 µg/mL, and 0.1 µg/mL. Protoporphyrin IX: Same concentrations as curcumin. Resazurin: Same concentrations as curcumin. Riboflavin: Same concentrations as curcumin. Light Exposure: 405 nm violet-blue LED irradiation (25.3 J). Dark Condition: No light exposure (PS only).	Riboflavin-mediated PDT demonstrated antimicrobial effects against *Veillonella parvula* but showed limited or no activity against *Lactobacillus gasseri* at lower concentrations. Its efficacy varied across bacterial strains, emphasizing its potential for selective bacterial inhibition in periodontal therapy while highlighting the need for optimization in biofilm models and clinical applications.
Kunz et al., 2019 [30]	Control Group: 0.9% NaCl. Riboflavin (0.1%) + 30 s of blue LED light. Riboflavin (0.1%) + 60 s of blue LED light. 0.25% H_2O_2 + Riboflavin + 30 s of blue LED light. 0.25% H_2O_2 + Riboflavin + 60 s of blue LED light. 3% H_2O_2 + Riboflavin + 30 s of blue LED light. 3% H_2O_2 + Riboflavin + 60 s of blue LED light. Mechanical biofilm removal only. Mechanical biofilm removal + 0.25% H_2O_2 + Riboflavin + 60 s of blue LED light. Mechanical biofilm removal + 3% H_2O_2 + Riboflavin + 60 s of blue LED light.	It demonstrates that while aPDT alone has limited activity against biofilms, its efficacy significantly increases when preceded by H_2O_2 pretreatment, particularly at a 3% concentration. This combined approach effectively eliminates planktonic bacteria and multi-species biofilms, with no detectable bacteria remaining when coupled with mechanical biofilm removal. This method could provide a potent alternative to traditional antimicrobial periodontal therapies, reducing the reliance on antibiotics and their associated resistance issues.

Table 4. *Cont.*

Author and Year	Study Groups	Main Outcomes
Leelanarathiwata et al., 2020 [31]	Control Group: No treatment. Light Irradiation Only Groups: Red diode laser (for 60 s). Blue high-power LED (for 10 s). Red Laser + Methylene Blue Blue LED + FMN	Riboflavin-mediated PDT, employing flavin mononucleotide activated by blue high-power LED light, demonstrates significant antibacterial efficacy against *Staphylococcus aureus* biofilms, a key contributor to peri-implantitis. This novel approach yields bacterial reductions comparable to established methylene blue–based PDT with red laser activation, achieving over 93% bacterial reduction. Riboflavin's natural presence and safer profile, combined with shorter treatment durations and effective biofilm penetration, position it as a promising alternative or adjunctive treatment to conventional scaling, root planing, and antibiotics, particularly amidst rising antibiotic resistance. While both PDT systems effectively reduce biofilm mass and bacterial viability, riboflavin's activation by blue light offers aesthetic and operational advantages, though further optimization and studies are needed for deeper tissue applications and enhanced biofilm eradication.
Morelato et al., 2022 [32]	Negative Control: Untreated implants. Positive Control: Implants treated with 0.2% CHX s for 60 s using brushing movements. PDT Groups: PDT1 (660 nm diode laser): Methylene blue (0.1%) as a photosensitizer, activated with a 660 nm diode laser for 60 s. PDT2 (445 nm diode laser): Riboflavin (0.1%) as a photosensitizer, activated with a 445 nm diode laser for 60 s.	Riboflavin-mediated PDT, specifically utilizing a 445 nm diode laser combined with 0.1% riboflavin as a photosensitizer, demonstrates significant efficacy in reducing biofilms of *Staphylococcus aureus* and *Candida albicans* on dental implant surfaces. This method shows comparable outcomes to conventional 660 nm diode laser PDT with methylene blue and 0.2% CHX treatments, without significant differences in microbial reduction among these methods. Advantages include minimal aesthetic disruption due to riboflavin's light-yellow colour, which contrasts with the staining caused by methylene blue. The technique proves to be a promising adjunct to mechanical debridement for peri-implantitis, particularly in aesthetic zones, although it does not completely eradicate all microorganisms or organic material.

Table 4. *Cont.*

Author and Year	Study Groups	Main Outcomes
Nielsen et al., 2015 [33]	Negative Control Group (P−L−): Microbial suspension treated with sterile saline without light or photosensitizer. Light Alone Group (P−L+): Microbial suspension irradiated with light (red or blue LED) without photosensitizer. Photosensitizer Alone Group (P+L−): Microbial suspension treated with photosensitizer without light. Photoactivated Disinfection (PAD) Groups (P+L+): Riboflavin + Blue Light: Treated with riboflavin and irradiated with 460 nm blue LED. Toluidine Blue O + Red Light: Treated with toluidine blue O and irradiated with 630 nm red LED.	Riboflavin-mediated PDT with blue light showed limited antimicrobial effects compared to TBO with red light for periodontal and endodontic pathogens. Although riboflavin effectively reduced *Porphyromonas gingivalis* and *Prevotella intermedia*, similar reductions occurred with blue light alone, indicating activation of bacterial endogenous chromophores. For other pathogens, riboflavin only caused minor to moderate bacterial reductions, and longer irradiation times did not enhance efficacy within clinical limits. In contrast, TBO-mediated PAD completely eradicated all tested pathogens even with short irradiation, demonstrating superior antimicrobial efficacy. Thus, riboflavin is unsuitable as a photosensitizer for periodontal or endodontic infections, while TBO shows significant promise.
Qamar et al., 2023 [24]	Group 1: PGA/RF/AV + MD Group 2: PDT + MD Group 3: MD Alone	While PDT alone significantly reduced BoP and microbial loads of Tf, the application of PGA/RF/AV demonstrated better outcomes. This compound significantly improved PD, PI, and MBL, with enhanced reductions in microbial counts of both *Porphyromonas gingivalis* and Tf. These findings highlight the potential of the PGA/RF/AV complex as a more effective treatment modality than PDT alone, leveraging the bactericidal and anti-inflammatory properties of riboflavin and aloe vera to achieve improved clinical and microbiological outcomes.

aPDT—Antimicrobial Photodynamic Therapy; AV—Aloe Vera; B_2—Vitamin B_2 (Riboflavin); CFU—Colony-Forming Unit(s); CHX—Chlorhexidine; FMN—Flavin Mononucleotide; H_2O_2—Hydrogen Peroxide; J—Joule; LED—Light-Emitting Diode; MD—Mechanical Debridement; MBL—Marginal Bone Level; PD—Probing Depth; PGA—Poly-L-Glycolic Acid; PI—Plaque Index; PDT—Photodynamic Therapy; P−L−—No Photosensitizer and No Light; P+L−—Photosensitizer Only; P−L+—Light Only; P+L+—Photoactivated Disinfection; PS—Photosensitizer; RF—Riboflavin; TBO—Toluidine Blue O; Tf—*Tannerella forsythia*; BoP—Bleeding on Probing; PGA/RF/AV—Riboflavin-Loaded Poly-L-Glycolic Acid Nanoparticles in Aloe Vera Gel; PI—Plaque Index; MBL—Marginal Bone Level.

Table 5. Summary of light source parameters from each study.

Light Source	Author/Year	Operating Mode	Wavelength (nm)	Energy Density (Fluence) (J/cm^2)	Power Output (mW)	Irradiation Time (s)
Blue diode laser (Pioon, China)	Afrasiabi et al., 2023 [25]	Continuous	445 nm	12, 18, 24, and 30	-	30 s
FotoSan460; CMS Dental ApS, Copenhagen, Denmark	Bärenfaller et al., 2016 [26]	Continuous	460 ± 10	120	1	30, 60

Table 5. *Cont.*

Light Source	Author/Year	Operating Mode	Wavelength (nm)	Energy Density (Fluence) (J/cm^2)	Power Output (mW)	Irradiation Time (s)
BioLight (Department of Physics and Astronomy at the University of British Columbia, Vancouver, BC, Canada)	Comeau et al., 2022 [27]	Continuous	440–460	1.3	830	60
LED (DY400-4, Denjoy, China)	Etemadi et al., 2023 [28]	Continuous	390–480	300–420	1000 ± 100	-
QLF-D (s digital, Inspektor Research Systems, Amsterdam, The Netherlands)	Kang et al., 2019 [29]	Continuous	405	25.3	84.5	-
FotoSan460; CMS Dental ApS, Copenhagen, Denmark).	Kunz et al., 2019 [30]	Continuous	460 ± 10	-	1	30, 60
FotoSan® BLUE LAD; (CMS Dental, Denmark)	Leelanarathiwata et al., 2020 [31]	Continuous	450–470	37–40	29.1−31.4	10
Diode laser (SiroLaser Blue, Dentsply Sirona, Bensheim, Germany)	Morelato et al., 2022 [32]	Pulsed mode (100 Hz)	445	1.24	100	60
FotoSan 630 LAD pen FlashMax P3 460 (CMS Dental, Denmark)	Nielsen et al., 2015 [33]	Continuous	630 460	37.7	0.4	60
Diode laser system (Periowave™ Vancouver, BC, Canada)	Qamar et al., 2023 [24]	Continuous	670	-	280	60

LED—Light-Emitting Diode; QLF-D—Quantitative Light-Induced Fluorescence Device.

Table 6. Summary of photosynthesizer concentrations and incubation times.

Author and Year	Concentration/s of Riboflavin Used
Afrasiabi et al., 2023 [25]	100 µM
Bärenfaller et al., 2016 [26]	0.1%
Comeau et al., 2022 [27]	0.1–1.5%
Etemadi et al., 2023 [28]	0.5%
Kang et al., 2019 [29]	10 µg/mL
Kunz et al., 2019 [30]	0.1%
Leelanarathiwata et al., 2020 [31]	0.18 FMN
Morelato et al., 2022 [32]	0.1%
Nielsen et al., 2015 [33]	133 µmol/L inplanktonic microbial suspension
Qamar et al., 2023 [24]	0.1%

FMN-riboflavin-5′-phosphate.

3.3. General Characteristics of the Included Studies

The general characteristics of the 10 included studies are shown in Tables 3–6.

3.4. Main Study Outcomes

The reviewed studies underscore the significant potential of riboflavin-mediated PDT for managing microbial biofilms and infections in various periodontal and dental applications. Riboflavin, a biocompatible photosensitizer, generates ROS such as singlet oxygen and hydrogen peroxide when activated by UV or blue light, effectively disrupting microbial cells and biofilms [25,26]. In orthodontic treatments, riboflavin-mediated PDT notably reduced microbial populations around brackets, thereby addressing challenges posed by conventional biofilm management strategies [25]. On implant surfaces, riboflavin-mediated PDT significantly decreased *Aggregatibacter actinomycetemcomitans* biofilms, though its efficacy was slightly lower than chlorhexidine or curcumin-mediated PDT [28,29]. In addition, studies have demonstrated its dose-dependent ability to reduce *Enterococcus faecalis* biofilm formation, with higher riboflavin concentrations and optimized laser parameters improving disinfection outcomes [25]. While results suggest that riboflavin-mediated PDT may be less potent than sodium hypochlorite in some cases, it has the advantage of causing minimal discolouration, indicating its potential as a safer alternative for root canal disinfection [25]. Furthermore, riboflavin-loaded dental resins exhibit enhanced mechanical stability and antimicrobial properties, offering avenues for further optimization [27]. Similar findings on titanium implants indicate that riboflavin-mediated PDT, activated with a 445 nm diode laser, achieves comparable biofilm reductions to methylene blue–based PDT and chlorhexidine, with the added benefit of minimal staining—an important consideration for aesthetic zones [32]. Overall, these results support riboflavin-PDT as a promising adjunctive therapy in periodontology, providing safety, biocompatibility, and material preservation. However, additional research is required to refine its antimicrobial efficacy and determine its value as a standalone clinical treatment.

4. Discussion

4.1. Results in the Context of Other Evidence

Riboflavin-mediated PDT, activated by blue diode lasers or LEDs, has shown significant antimicrobial effects, particularly at higher light power densities [25]. Although it effectively reduces single-species bacterial counts, its efficacy decreases in complex multi-species biofilms—especially when serum is present—underscoring the importance of adjunctive mechanical biofilm removal [26]. In comparison to the gold standard treatment for periodontitis, which typically involves systemic and local antibiotic administration alongside root planing, riboflavin-mediated PDT offers a targeted antimicrobial strategy that is minimally invasive and may reduce the risk of antibiotic resistance [26–28]. Riboflavin-loaded resin systems may facilitate integration into restorative dentistry by providing both antimicrobial activity and mechanical stability [27]. However, their limited penetration into deeper biofilms suggests that additional strategies are required to enhance treatment efficacy in more complex microbial environments. They offer limited penetration into deeper biofilms, which could indicate a need for a photosensitizer that can be excited at a longer wavelength [28]. Riboflavin-mediated PDT also exhibits selective antimicrobial action, effectively reducing certain pathogens such as *Veillonella parvula* but not others, including *Lactobacillus gasseri* [29]. Pre-treatment with hydrogen peroxide significantly boosts its effectiveness, particularly when coupled with mechanical debridement [30]. This combination was particularly effective in reducing complex multi-species biofilms, which are typically more resistant to single-agent treatments. In peri-implantitis, riboflavin-based PDT achieves bacterial reductions comparable to methylene blue–based PDT with red lasers, thus offering a promising option in aesthetically sensitive areas [31,32]. Nonetheless, alternative photosensitizers like toluidine blue O (TBO) under red light may provide more comprehensive microbial eradication in certain clinical scenarios [33]. More recent strategies, such as combining riboflavin-loaded nanoparticles in aloe vera gel with mechanical debridement, further improve clinical outcomes by reducing probing depth and microbial load more effectively than PDT alone [24]. These combinatory approaches highlight the potential for enhanced therapeutic protocols that integrate riboflavin-mediated PDT with other adjunctive treatments to overcome existing limitations. While riboflavin-mediated PDT presents a non-invasive alternative with a lower risk of antibiotic resistance, additional research is necessary to refine treatment protocols, enhance effectiveness in complex biofilms, and assess long-term clinical applications [24–34].

Several recent studies underscore the broad potential of riboflavin-mediated PDT across various dental and medical applications. Łopaciński et al. [14] demonstrated its effectiveness against oral candidiasis, whereas Etemadi et al. [35] found that riboflavin, when photoactivated by blue light, could substantially reduce periodontitis-related bacteria. Notably, Etemadi et al. also reported that blue light alone produced significant bacterial reductions in some cases, highlighting the need for further investigations to delineate riboflavin's specific contribution as a photosensitizer. In the orthodontic context, Alqerban et al. [36] reported that applying 0.1% riboflavin in PDT effectively bonded orthodontic brackets and conferred considerable antibacterial benefits. Increasing the riboflavin concentration to 0.5% enhanced antimicrobial efficacy yet compromised bonding strength, indicating a trade-off. Kamran et al. [37] similarly confirmed that riboflavin-mediated PDT markedly reduced *Streptococcus mutans* and *Streptococcus sanguinis* levels around orthodontic brackets, underscoring its promise for improving antimicrobial control in orthodontic treatments. Moradi et al. [38] showed that antimicrobial PDT using curcumin or riboflavin significantly reduced *Enterococcus faecalis* biofilms in root canals, achieving comparable results to 5.25% NaOCl. While NaOCl produced the highest bacterial reduction, these findings support PDT as a viable adjunct for root canal disinfection. Beyond oral applications, Najari et al. [39] suggested that riboflavin-mediated PDT, when combined with antibiotics such as colistin, could be valuable for difficult-to-treat *Pseudomonas aeruginosa* infections. Additionally, Alshehri et al. [40] showed that riboflavin-mediated PDT offered the highest antifungal efficacy against *Candida albicans* on acrylic denture surfaces without damaging the denture material. Arboleda et al. [41], however, found that rose bengal–mediated PDT, rather than riboflavin-mediated PDT, effectively inhibited the growth of three fungal species in a corneal infection model. Finally, Kashiwabuchi et al. emphasized that continued refinement in riboflavin preparation and light delivery could further enhance the therapeutic outcomes of riboflavin-mediated PDT, reinforcing the need for additional in vitro and clinical trial [42]. While in situ gels like Atridox provide sustained doxycycline release without the need for additional equipment, riboflavin-mediated PDT requires photoactivation but offers selective antimicrobial action and potential integration into restorative dental materials, and further research is needed to fully evaluate and optimize both approaches for managing complex periodontal infections [43–47]. The integration of riboflavin-mediated PDT into various clinical practices demonstrates significant potential, yet highlights the necessity for ongoing optimization and validation through further research [23–44].

4.2. Limitations of the Evidence

Despite the promising outcomes reported, several limitations in the current body of evidence constrain a definitive assessment of riboflavin-mediated PDT in periodontology. First, the marked heterogeneity in study protocols, ranging from the type and intensity of light sources to the concentration of riboflavin and the duration of exposure, makes direct comparisons challenging and precludes the establishment of standardized guidelines [21,24–33]. Additionally, most of the included studies were in vitro, limiting the generalizability of their findings to clinical practice [24–33]. Even among the few in vivo or clinical trials, sample sizes were frequently small and follow-up times relatively short, raising questions about long-term efficacy and safety [24–33]. Moreover, outcome measures often relied on colony-forming units or visually assessed biofilm reduction without consistent use of advanced or standardized diagnostic tools [24–33]. Two major issues are the scattering of short-wavelength light, which limits efficacy, and the possibility that photokilling a portion of the cell population could lead to the development of an unresponsive group of cells, which were not addressed by the studies analysed [29,33]. Finally, potential biases, such as the lack of blinding and reliance on subjective endpoints, further highlight the need for more robust, controlled clinical trials with uniform protocols, larger cohorts, and longer observation periods [21–23].

4.3. Limitations of the Review Process

A key limitation of the review process relates to the marked heterogeneity of study designs, intervention protocols, and outcome measures, which necessitated a largely narrative synthesis rather than a quantitative meta-analysis. While PRISMA guidelines were followed to enhance transparency, the exclusion of non-English studies and grey literature potentially narrowed the scope, increasing the risk of missing relevant data. Furthermore, although study selection and data extraction were conducted in duplicate, the reliance on authors' subjective judgments may introduce inadvertent bias. Finally, the decision not to apply the GRADE framework, due to substantial variability in parameters and methodologies, limits the ability to draw definitive conclusions about the overall certainty of the evidence. These factors highlight the need for more uniform protocols and comprehensive strategies in future systematic reviews of riboflavin-mediated photodynamic therapy in periodontology.

4.4. Implications for Practice, Policy, and Future Research

Riboflavin-mediated PDT shows considerable promise as an adjunctive or alternative strategy in periodontal care, especially for managing biofilm-related infections and potentially reducing reliance on conventional antimicrobials. Clinically, practitioners could integrate riboflavin-mediated PDT into existing protocols for periodontal debridement or implant maintenance, leveraging its generally low toxicity and minimal staining profile compared to other photosensitizers. From a policy perspective, regulatory bodies and professional organizations should consider supporting standardized protocols and guidelines to facilitate consistent implementation across different clinical settings. This includes establishing optimal light parameters, riboflavin concentrations, and treatment durations to maximize therapeutic efficacy. In parallel, future research must focus on high-quality randomized controlled trials with robust sample sizes and longer follow-up to validate riboflavin-mediated PDT's effectiveness in vivo. Investigations into combination therapies, such as pairing PDT with other antimicrobial or anti-inflammatory agents and innovations in photosensitizer delivery methods (e.g., nanoparticles or bioactive materials) may further enhance treatment outcomes. Through these combined efforts, riboflavin-mediated PDT stands to gain broader acceptance and become an integral component of evidence-based periodontal care.

5. Conclusions

The findings of this systematic review suggest that riboflavin-mediated PDT holds considerable promise for enhancing antimicrobial efficacy and clinical outcomes in periodontology. Although the heterogeneity in study designs and outcome measures precludes a definitive consensus, the cumulative evidence indicates that riboflavin-mediated PDT often compares favourably, or at least equivalently, to conventional interventions such as mechanical debridement. Consequently, while the results do not uniformly or unequivocally refute the null hypothesis, which posits no significant difference in effectiveness between riboflavin-mediated PDT and established non-surgical therapies, they do increasingly challenge it. Notably, riboflavin-mediated PDT demonstrated advantages in reducing biofilm mass, minimizing staining, and potentially lowering the risk of antibiotic resistance.

To provide more conclusive guidance for clinical practice, future well-designed randomized controlled trials with standardized protocols, larger cohorts, and extended follow-up periods are needed to fully determine whether riboflavin-mediated PDT indeed offers a superior or distinct therapeutic benefit in periodontal care.

Author Contributions: Conceptualization, M.Ł. and R.W.; methodology, J.F-R. and R.W.; software, M.Ł. and J.F.-R.; formal analysis, J.F.-R., A.L. and M.Ł.; investigation, J.F.-R. and M.Ł.; writing—original draft preparation, J.F-R., A.L., R.W. and M.Ł.; writing—review and editing, A.L., J.F.-R., M.Ł., R.W. and D.S.; supervision, R.W. and D.S.; funding acquisition, R.W. and D.S. All authors have read and agreed to the published version of the manuscript.

Funding: This research received no external funding.

Conflicts of Interest: The authors declare no conflicts of interest.

References

1. Peechakara, B.V.; Sina, R.E.; Gupta, M. Vitamin B2 (Riboflavin) [Updated 1 February 2024]. In *StatPearls [Internet]*; StatPearls Publishing: Treasure Island, FL, USA, 2025. Available online: https://ncbi.nlm.nih.gov/books/NBK525977/ (accessed on 4 February 2025).
2. Averianova, L.A.; Balabanova, L.A.; Son, O.M.; Podvolotskaya, A.B.; Tekutyeva, L.A. Production of Vitamin B2 (Riboflavin) by Microorganisms: An Overview. *Front. Bioeng. Biotechnol.* **2020**, *8*, 570828. [CrossRef]
3. Powers, H.J. Riboflavin (vitamin B2) health. *Am. J. Clin. Nutr.* **2003**, *77*, 1352–1360. [CrossRef]
4. Insińska-Rak, M.; Sikorski, M.; Wolnicka-Glubisz, A. Riboflavin and Its Derivates as Potential Photosensitizers in the Photodynamic Treatment of Skin Cancers. *Cells* **2023**, *12*, 2304. [CrossRef] [PubMed] [PubMed Central]
5. Niculescu, A.G.; Grumezescu, A.M. Photodynamic Therapy—An Up-to-Date Review. *Appl. Sci.* **2021**, *11*, 3626. [CrossRef]
6. Correia, J.H.; Rodrigues, J.A.; Pimenta, S.; Dong, T.; Yang, Z. Photodynamic Therapy Review: Principles, Photosensitizers, Applications, and Future Directions. *Pharmaceutics* **2021**, *13*, 1332. [CrossRef] [PubMed] [PubMed Central]
7. Alfei, S.; Schito, G.C.; Schito, A.M.; Zuccari, G. Reactive Oxygen Species (ROS)-Mediated Antibacterial Oxidative Therapies: Available Methods to Generate ROS and a Novel Option Proposal. *Int. J. Mol. Sci.* **2024**, *25*, 7182. [CrossRef] [PubMed] [PubMed Central]
8. Azizi, A.; Shohrati, P.; Goudarzi, M.; Lawaf, S.; Rahimi, A. Comparison of the effect of photodynamic therapy with curcumin and methylene Blue on streptococcus mutans bacterial colonies. *Photodiagnosis Photodyn. Ther.* **2019**, *27*, 203–209. [CrossRef] [PubMed]
9. Pordel, E.; Ghasemi, T.; Afrasiabi, S.; Benedicenti, S.; Signore, A.; Chiniforush, N. The Effect of Different Output Powers of Blue Diode Laser along with Curcumin and Riboflavin against *Streptococcus mutans* around Orthodontic Brackets: An In Vitro Study. *Biomedicines* **2023**, *11*, 2248. [CrossRef] [PubMed] [PubMed Central]
10. Schlafer, S.; Vaeth, M.; Hørsted-Bindslev, P.; Frandsen, E.V. Endodontic photoactivated disinfection using a conventional light source: An in vitro and ex vivo study. *Oral Surg. Oral Med. Oral Pathol. Oral Radiol. Endodontology* **2010**, *109*, 634–641. [CrossRef] [PubMed]
11. Abrahamse, H.; Hamblin, M.R. New photosensitizers for photodynamic therapy. *Biochem. J.* **2016**, *473*, 347–364. [CrossRef] [PubMed] [PubMed Central]
12. Kashef, N.; Hamblin, M.R. Can microbial cells develop resistance to oxidative stress in antimicrobial photodynamic inactivation? *Drug Resist. Updat.* **2017**, *31*, 31–42. [CrossRef] [PubMed] [PubMed Central]
13. Chen, H.; Sun, G.; Wang, H.; Yu, S.; Tian, Z.; Zhu, S. Effect of collagen cross-linkers on dentin bond strength: A systematic review and network meta-analysis. *Front. Bioeng. Biotechnol.* **2023**, *10*, 1100894. [CrossRef] [PubMed] [PubMed Central]
14. Łopaciński, M.; Fiegler-Rudol, J.; Niemczyk, W.; Skaba, D.; Wiench, R. Riboflavin- and Hypericin-Mediated Antimicrobial Photodynamic Therapy as Alternative Treatments for Oral Candidiasis: A Systematic Review. *Pharmaceutics* **2025**, *17*, 33. [CrossRef]
15. Khoury, R.D.; de Carvalho, L.S.; do Nascimento, M.F.R.; Alhussain, F.; Abu Hasna, A. Endodontic irrigants from a comprehensive perspective. *World J. Clin. Cases* **2024**, *12*, 4460–4468. [CrossRef] [PubMed] [PubMed Central]
16. Pashley, D.H.; Tay, F.R.; Breschi, L.; Tjäderhane, L.; Carvalho, R.M.; Carrilho, M.; Tezvergil-Mutluay, A. State of the art etch-and-rinse adhesives. *Dent. Mater.* **2011**, *27*, 1–16. [CrossRef] [PubMed] [PubMed Central]
17. De Silva, P.; Saad, M.A.; Thomsen, H.C.; Bano, S.; Ashraf, S.; Hasan, T. Photodynamic therapy, priming and optical imaging: Potential co-conspirators in treatment design and optimization—A Thomas Dougherty Award for Excellence in PDT paper. *J. Porphyr. Phthalocyanines* **2020**, *24*, 1320–1360. [CrossRef] [PubMed] [PubMed Central]
18. de Moraes, I.Q.S.; do Nascimento, T.G.; da Silva, A.T.; de Lira, L.M.S.S.; Parolia, A.; Porto, I.C.C.M. Inhibition of matrix metalloproteinases: A troubleshooting for dentin adhesion. *Restor. Dent. Endod.* **2020**, *45*, e31. [CrossRef] [PubMed] [PubMed Central]

19. Alrefeai, M.; Aljamhan, A.; Al Habdan, A.H.; Alzehiri, M.; Naseem, M.; Alkhudhairy, F. Influence of methylene blue, riboflavin and indocyanine green on the bond strength of caries-affected dentin when bonded to resin-modified glass ionomer cement. *Photodiagnosis Photodyn. Ther.* **2022**, *38*, 102792. [CrossRef]
20. Schardt, C.; Adams, M.B.; Owens, T.; Keitz, S.; Fontelo, P. Utilization of the PICO Framework to Improve Searching PubMed for Clinical Questions. *BMC Med. Inform. Decis. Mak.* **2007**, *7*, 16. [CrossRef] [PubMed]
21. Page, M.J.; McKenzie, J.E.; Bossuyt, P.M.; Boutron, I.; Hoffmann, T.C.; Mulrow, C.D.; Shamseer, L.; Tetzlaff, J.M.; Akl, E.A.; Brennan, S.E.; et al. The PRISMA 2020 statement: An updated guideline for reporting systematic reviews. *BMJ* **2021**, *372*, n71. [CrossRef] [PubMed]
22. Watson, P.F.; Petrie, A. Method Agreement Analysis: A Review of Correct Methodology. *Theriogenology* **2010**, *73*, 1167–1179. [CrossRef]
23. Higgins, J.P.T.; Thomas, J.; Chandler, J.; Cumpston, M.; Li, T.; Page, M.J.; Welch, V.A. (Eds.) *Cochrane Handbook for Systematic Reviews of Interventions*, 2nd ed.; Wiley-Blackwell: Chichester, UK, 2019. [CrossRef]
24. Qamar, Z.; Sayed Abdul, N.; Soman, C.; Shenoy, M.; Bamousa, B.; Rabea, S.; Albahkaly, H.S. Clinical and radiographic peri-implant outcomes with riboflavin-loaded Poly-L-glycolic acid nanoparticles incorporated in aloe-vera gel treating peri-implantitis in chronic hyperglycemic patients. *Photodiagnosis Photodyn. Ther.* **2023**, *44*, 103752. [CrossRef]
25. Afrasiabi, S.; Entezari, S.; Etemadi, A.; Chiniforush, N. The influence of different modes of power density during antimicrobial photodynamic therapy for photokilling of *Streptococcus mutans*. *Photodiagnosis Photodyn. Ther.* **2023**, *44*, 103770. [CrossRef] [PubMed]
26. Bärenfaller, V.; Clausen, C.; Sculean, A.; Eick, S. Effect of photoactivated disinfection using light in the blue spectrum. *J. Photochem. Photobiol. B* **2016**, *158*, 252–257. [CrossRef]
27. Comeau, P.; Burgess, J.; Rezqi Qomi, N.; Lee, A.; Manso, A. The antimicrobial, physical, and chemical properties of a riboflavin-loaded dental resin intended for antimicrobial photodynamic therapy. *Photodiagnosis Photodyn. Ther.* **2022**, *40*, 103124. [CrossRef]
28. Etemadi, A.; Hashemi, S.S.; Chiniforush, N. Evaluation of the effect of photodynamic therapy with curcumin and riboflavin on implant surface contaminated with *Aggregatibacter actinomycetemcomitans*. *Photodiagnosis Photodyn. Ther.* **2023**, *44*, 103833. [CrossRef]
29. Kang, S.M.; Jung, H.I.; Kim, B.I. Susceptibility of oral bacteria to antibacterial photodynamic therapy. *J. Oral Microbiol.* **2019**, *11*, 1644111. [CrossRef]
30. Kunz, D.; Wirth, J.; Sculean, A.; Eick, S. In-vitro activity of additive application of hydrogen peroxide in antimicrobial photodynamic therapy using LED in the blue spectrum against bacteria and biofilm associated with periodontal disease. *Photodiagnosis Photodyn. Ther.* **2019**, *26*, 306–312. [CrossRef]
31. Leelanarathiwata, K.; Katsuta, Y.; Katsuragi, H.; Watanabe, F. Antibacterial activity of blue high-power light-emitting diode-activated flavin mononucleotide against *Staphylococcus aureus* biofilm on a sandblasted and etched surface. *Photodiagnosis Photodyn. Ther.* **2020**, *31*, 101855. [CrossRef] [PubMed]
32. Morelato, L.; Budimir, A.; Smojver, I.; Katalinić, I.; Vuletić, M.; Ajanović, M.; Gabrić, D. A novel technique for disinfection treatment of contaminated dental implant surface using 0.1% riboflavin and 445 nm diode laser—An in vitro study. *Bioengineering* **2022**, *9*, 308. [CrossRef] [PubMed]
33. Nielsen, H.K.; Garcia, J.; Væth, M.; Schlafer, S. Comparison of riboflavin and toluidine blue O as photosensitizers for photoactivated disinfection on endodontic and periodontal pathogens in vitro. *PLoS ONE* **2015**, *10*, e0140720. [CrossRef]
34. Fiegler-Rudol, J.; Zięba, N.; Turski, R.; Misiołek, M.; Wiench, R. Hypericin-Mediated Photodynamic Therapy for Head and Neck Cancers: A Systematic Review. *Biomedicines* **2025**, *13*, 181. [CrossRef] [PubMed]
35. Etemadi, H.; Parker, S.; Chiniforush, N. Blue light photodynamic therapy with curcumin and riboflavin in the management of periodontitis: A systematic review. *J. Lasers Med. Sci.* **2021**, *12*, e15. [CrossRef] [PubMed]
36. Alqerban, A. Effectiveness of Riboflavin and Rose Bengal Photosensitizer Modified Adhesive Resin for Orthodontic Bonding. *Pharmaceuticals* **2021**, *14*, 48. [CrossRef] [PubMed] [PubMed Central]
37. Kamran, M.A.; Qasim, M.; Udeabor, S.E.; Hameed, M.S.; Mannakandath, M.L.; Alshahrani, I. Impact of riboflavin mediated photodynamic disinfection around fixed orthodontic system infected with oral bacteria. *Photodiagnosis Photodyn. Ther.* **2021**, *34*, 102232. [CrossRef] [PubMed]
38. Moradi, M.; Fazlyab, M.; Pourhajibagher, M.; Chiniforush, N. Antimicrobial action of photodynamic therapy on Enterococcus faecalis biofilm using curing light, curcumin and riboflavin. *Aust. Endod. J.* **2022**, *48*, 274–282. [CrossRef] [PubMed]
39. Najari, E.; Zamani, S.; Arabi, M.S.; Ardebili, A. Antimicrobial photodynamic effect of the photosensitizer riboflavin, alone and in combination with colistin, against pandrug-resistant *Pseudomonas aeruginosa* clinical isolates. *J. Infect. Chemother.* **2024**, *30*, 892–898. [CrossRef]
40. Alshehri, A.H. Mechanical and antimicrobial effects of riboflavin-mediated photosensitization of in vitro Candida albicans formed on polymethyl methacrylate resin. *Photodiagnosis Photodyn. Ther.* **2021**, *36*, 102488. [CrossRef]

41. Arboleda, A.; Miller, D.; Cabot, F.; Taneja, M.; Aguilar, M.C.; Alawa, K.; Amescua, G.; Yoo, S.H.; Parel, J.-M. Assessment of rose bengal versus riboflavin photodynamic therapy for inhibition of fungal keratitis isolates. *Am. J. Ophthalmol.* **2014**, *158*, 64–70.e2. [CrossRef]
42. Kashiwabuchi, R.T.; Carvalho, F.R.; Khan, Y.A.; Hirai, F.; Campos, M.S.; McDonnell, P.J. Assessment of fungal viability after long-wave ultraviolet light irradiation combined with riboflavin administration. *Graefes Arch. Clin. Exp. Ophthalmol.* **2013**, *251*, 521–527. [CrossRef]
43. Sholapurkar, A.; Sharma, D.; Glass, B.; Miller, C.; Nimmo, A.; Jennings, E. Professionally Delivered Local Antimicrobials in the Treatment of Patients with Periodontitis—A Narrative Review. *Dent. J.* **2020**, *9*, 2. [CrossRef] [PubMed] [PubMed Central]
44. Büchtner, A.; Meyer, U.; Kruse-Lösler, B.; Joos, U.; Kleinheinz, J. Sustained release of doxycycline for the treatment of peri-implantitis: Randomised controlled trial. *Br. J. Oral Maxillofac. Surg.* **2004**, *42*, 439–444. [CrossRef]
45. Micu, I.C.; Muntean, A.; Roman, A.; Stratul, Ș.I.; Pall, E.; Ciurea, A.; Soancă, A.; Negucioiu, M.; Barbu Tudoran, L.; Delean, A.G. A Local Desiccant Antimicrobial Agent as an Alternative to Adjunctive Antibiotics in the Treatment of Periodontitis: A Narrative Review. *Antibiotics* **2023**, *12*, 456. [CrossRef] [PubMed] [PubMed Central]
46. Tomasi, C.; Koutouzis, T.; Wennström, J. Locally Delivered Doxycycline as an Adjunct to Mechanical Debridement at Retreatment of Periodontal Pockets. *J. Periodontol.* **2008**, *79*, 431–439. [CrossRef]
47. Toledano, M.; Osorio, M.T.; Vallecillo-Rivas, M.; Toledano-Osorio, M.; Rodríguez-Archilla, A.; Toledano, R.; Osorio, R. Efficacy of local antibiotic therapy in the treatment of peri-implantitis: A systematic review and meta-analysis. *J. Dent.* **2021**, *113*, 103790. [CrossRef]

pharmaceutics

MDPI

Article

Enhanced Nanogel Formulation Combining the Natural Photosensitizer Curcumin and *Pectis brevipedunculata* (Asteraceae) Essential Oil for Synergistic Daylight Photodynamic Therapy in Leishmaniasis Treatment

Lara Maria Oliveira Campos [1], Estela Mesquita Marques [1], Daniele Stéfanie Sara Lopes Lera-Nonose [2], Maria Julia Schiavon Gonçalves [2], Maria Valdrinez Campana Lonardoni [2], Glécilla Colombelli de Souza Nunes [3], Gustavo Braga [4] and Renato Sonchini Gonçalves [1,*]

1 Laboratory of Chemistry of Natural Products, Department of Chemistry, Federal University of Maranhão (UFMA), São Luís 65080-805, Brazil; lara.moc@discente.ufma.br (L.M.O.C.); estela.marques@discente.ufma.br (E.M.M.)
2 Department of Clinical Analysis and Biomedicine, State University of Maringá (UEM), Maringá 87020-900, Brazil; dsslInonose2@uem.br (D.S.S.L.L.-N.); pg405366@uem.br (M.J.S.G.); mvclonrdoni@uem.br (M.V.C.L.)
3 Research Nucleus in Pharmaceutical Sciences Program, State University of Maringá (UEM), Maringá 87020-900, Brazil; gcsnunes2@uem.br
4 University College (COLUN), Federal University of Maranhão (UFMA), São Luís 65080-805, Brazil; gustavo.braga@ufma.br
* Correspondence: renato.sg@ufma.br; Tel.: +55-98-9851-49235

Abstract: Background/Objectives: Neglected tropical diseases (NTDs), such as leishmaniasis, remain a global health challenge due to limited therapeutic options and rising drug resistance. In this study, we developed an advanced nanogel formulation incorporating curcumin (CUR) and *Pectis brevipedunculata* essential oil (EO*Pb*) within an F127/Carbopol 974P matrix to enhance bioavailability and therapeutic efficacy against *Leishmania (Leishmania) amazonensis* (*LLa*) promastigotes. **Methods**: The chemical profile of EO*Pb* was determined through GC-MS and NMR analyses, confirming the presence of key bioactive monoterpenes such as neral, geranial, α-pinene, and limonene. The nanogel formulation (nG*PC*) was optimized to ensure thermosensitivity, and stability, exhibiting a sol–gel transition at physiological temperatures. Rheological analysis revealed that nG*PC* exhibited Newtonian behavior at 5 °C, transitioning to shear-thinning and thixotropic characteristics at 25 and 32 °C, respectively. This behavior facilitates its application and controlled drug release, making it ideal for topical formulations. Dynamic light scattering (DLS) analysis demonstrated that nG*PC* maintained a stable nanoscale structure with hydrodynamic radius below 300 nm, while Fourier-transform infrared spectroscopy (FTIR) confirmed strong molecular interactions between EO*Pb*, CUR, and the polymer matrix. Biological assays demonstrated that nG*PC* significantly enhanced anti-promastigote activity compared to free CUR and OE*Pb*. **Results**: At the highest tested concentration (50 μg/mL EO*Pb* and 17.5 μg/mL CUR) nG*PC* induced over 88% mortality in *LLa* promastigotes across 24, 48, and 72 h, indicating sustained efficacy. Even at lower concentrations, nG*PC* retained dose-dependent activity, suggesting a synergistic effect between CUR and EO*Pb*. These findings highlight the potential of nG*PC* as an innovative nanocarrier for daylight photodynamic therapy (dPDT) in the treatment of leishmaniasis. Future studies will investigate the underlying mechanisms of this synergism and explore the potential application of photodynamic therapy (PDT) to further enhance therapeutic outcomes.

Keywords: leishmaniasis; *Pectis brevipedunculata* essential oil; curcumin

https://doi.org/10.3390/pharmaceutics17030286

1. Introduction

Neglected tropical diseases (NTDs) represent a critical global health challenge, disproportionately affecting populations in tropical and subtropical regions, often living under conditions of extreme poverty [1]. Over one billion individuals are estimated to be impacted by NTDs, including conditions such as leishmaniasis, Chagas disease, and lymphatic filariasis [2]. These diseases are associated with significant morbidity, prolonged disability, and substantial economic costs. Despite their widespread prevalence and the immense burden they impose, NTDs remain largely neglected in the global health agenda, facing barriers such as limited funding, insufficient drug development, the rise in drug resistance, and challenges in vector control [3–5]. These complexities underscore the urgent need for novel therapeutic strategies to address conventional treatments' limitations, particularly through innovative delivery systems that provide targeted, accessible, and effective solutions [6,7].

Leishmania (Leishmania) amazonensis (*LLa*) is one of the most prevalent protozoan parasites responsible for cutaneous leishmaniasis in the Americas, including Brazil, Peru, and other Latin American countries [8,9]. Transmitted by the bite of infected Lutzomyia, *LLa* primarily affects the skin, causing the formation of painful lesions or ulcers. If left untreated, these lesions can progress into chronic wounds, leading to irreversible scarring and, in some cases, mucocutaneous leishmaniasis [10]. The parasite's ability to invade and replicate within macrophages, which are essential for immune defense, complicates the host's immune response, allowing the infection to persist. While conventional therapies like pentavalent antimonials and miltefosine are available, their effectiveness is often limited by increasing drug resistance, side effects, and the need for prolonged treatment [10]. As a result, there is a pressing demand for alternative therapeutic strategies, particularly those leveraging advanced drug delivery systems such as nanogels, which can enhance drug efficacy and target the parasite more specifically [11–13].

Natural products, particularly essential oils (EOs) from plants native to the Amazon rainforest, have gained significant attention as promising therapeutic agents for NTDs. These oils, rich in bioactive molecules such as terpenoids and phenolic compounds, exhibit potent antimicrobial, antiparasitic, and anti-inflammatory properties, making them ideal candidates for addressing diseases like leishmaniasis [14,15]. The combination of EOs from different plant species or the incorporation of plant extracts into EO formulations has been shown to create synergistic or complementary effects, amplifying their therapeutic potential while minimizing the adverse side effects associated with conventional drugs. By utilizing the complex array of bioactive compounds in these natural products, researchers can develop more robust, effective, and targeted treatments for NTDs [16–21].

Accordingly, we hypothesize that a nanogel formulation based on the F127 copolymer and carbopol 974P, loaded with low concentrations of EO of *Pectis brevipedunculata* (EO*Pb*) and curcumin (CUR), will exhibit synergistic effects in vitro against *LLa* promastigote cells. *Pb* (Asteraceae), a plant native to the tropical and subtropical regions of the Americas, is known for its anti-inflammatory, antimicrobial, and antiparasitic properties [13,22]. The EO, characterized by a high content of monoterpenes like neral, geranial, α-pinene, and limonene, demonstrates significant antimicrobial properties, underscoring its potential as a natural resource for developing treatments against parasitic infections [23,24]. Previous studies from our group have demonstrated that EO*Pb*-loaded nanogels possess effective larvicidal, leishmanicidal, and anti-inflammatory activities, without cytotoxic effects [12,13]. In parallel, CUR, derived from *Curcuma longa*, is a well-established compound with proven leishmanicidal effects and has been extensively studied for its ability to inhibit parasite growth, modulate immune responses, and reduce inflammation. CUR's low toxicity and antioxidant properties further enhance its potential as a therapeutic agent [25–27].

In this study, we designed a semi-solid nanoplatform following Green Chemistry (GC) principles, employing FDA-approved excipients while minimizing energy consumption [12,13]. A thermosensitive nanogel based on F127/974P was selected for EO*Pb*/CUR delivery due to its rapid sol–gel transition, stability, and suitability for topical applications. Unlike liposomes, micelles, or nanoemulsions, this system was developed through a low-energy, eco-friendly approach without the use of organic solvents. Its semi-solid nature enhances spreadability, bioadhesion, and skin permeation, making it an effective platform for cutaneous disease treatment [28]. To investigate its therapeutic potential, EO*Pb*/CUR was incorporated into the nanogel matrix at low concentrations and assessed for its efficacy against *LLa* promastigotes. The cytotoxicity of these compounds was specifically assessed at concentrations below 50 μg/mL of EO*Pb* and 20 μg/mL of CUR, both as isolated bioactive compounds and in combination within the nanogel. These concentrations were selected based on their biological activity against *LLa*, as reported in the literature on EO*Pb* and CUR [26,27,29]. Notably, while nanogels containing individual compounds (EO*Pb*- and CUR-loaded nanogels) exhibited limited activity, the combined formulation (EO*Pb*/CUR-loaded nanogel) demonstrated significant anti-promastigote effects, inducing dose-dependent mortality in *LLa* promastigotes. This study not only introduces a sustainable alternative for leishmanicidal therapies but also establishes nanogels as efficient carriers for dPDT without the need for high-energy light sources. The dPDT approach thus emerges as an environmentally friendly, cost-effective, and operationally viable strategy, paving the way for more efficient and sustainable therapeutic systems.

2. Materials and Methods

2.1. Materials

Carbopol 974P NF polymer was supplied by IMCD114 Brasil (São Paulo, SP, Brazil). Ultrapure water, sodium chloride, anhydrous sodium sulfate (≥99%), curcumin (≥99%), XTT (2,3-bis(2-methoxy-4-nitro-5-sulfophenyl)-5-[(phenylamino)carbonyl]-2H-tetrazolium hydroxide), PMS (N-methyl dibenzopyrazine methyl sulfate), penicillin, streptomycin, fetal bovine serum, and amphotericin B (AmB) were procured from Merck (Rahway, NJ, USA). Pluronic F127, a triblock copolymer of poly(ethylene oxide)-poly(propylene oxide)-poly(ethylene oxide) (MW = 12,600 g/mol; $EO_{99}PO_{67}EO_{99}$), was also acquired from Merck.

2.2. Plant Material

The herbaceous species *Pb* was obtained from the Universidade Federal do Maranhão (UFMA) campus in São Luís, Maranhão, Brazil, at coordinates 2°33′20.5″ S and 44°18′32.7″ W. Following collection, a voucher specimen (No. 5287) was cataloged and preserved in the Rosa Mochel Herbarium (SLUI) at the Universidade Estadual do Maranhão (UEMA) in São Luís, MA, Brazil. The sampling adhered to Brazilian regulations for biodiversity protection and was officially recorded under SisGen code AAFB38B.

2.3. Extraction Procedure

The (EO*Pb*) was extracted through hydrodistillation using a Clevenger-type apparatus [12]. For this process, 300 g of air-dried plant material was finely cut with pruning shears to optimize extraction. The prepared material was then immersed in 500 mL of distilled water within a flask, and hydrodistillation was carried out for 2.5 h after reflux initiation. Following extraction, the obtained oil/water (O/W) mixture was centrifuged at 3500 rpm for 10 min at 25 °C. To remove any remaining moisture, the oil phase was dried over anhydrous sodium sulfate. The extraction yield of EO*Pb*, calculated relative to the dry weight of the plant material, was determined to be 0.81%.

2.4. CG-MS Analyses of EOPb

The chemical characterization of EO*Pb* was conducted using GC-MS and NMR techniques, following standardized methodologies [12]. For gas chromatography and mass spectrometry analyses, a Shimadzu system equipped with an RXi-1MS fused capillary column was employed, using helium as the carrier gas. The temperature gradient was carefully adjusted, and sample solutions (10 mg/mL in CH_2Cl_2) were injected with a 1:50 split ratio. Retention indices were established through a homologous series of n-alkanes, while peak areas and retention times were recorded to determine the relative composition of the constituents. GC-MS analyses were performed using a Shimadzu QP2010 SE system with an AOC-20i auto-injector under the same conditions applied in GC. Component identification was based on retention times, retention indices, and mass spectral comparison against reference libraries (ADAMS and FFNSC) and literature data.

For NMR spectroscopy, ^{1}H, ^{13}C, and DEPT-^{13}C spectra were recorded using a BRUKER Avance III HD spectrometer (11.75 Tesla), operating at 500.13 MHz for ^{1}H and 125.76 MHz for ^{13}C. The samples were dissolved in deuterated chloroform ($CDCl_3$), and chemical shifts were reported in ppm, with tetramethylsilane (TMS) as the internal reference.

2.5. Preparation of Nanogels

The nanostructured formulations were prepared according to the methodology described by Schmolka, using a cold procedure [12,13]. A portion of the F127 copolymer was slowly incorporated into distilled water and kept in an ice bath at 5–10 °C. The solution was maintained under slow stirring to ensure the hydration of the F127 polymer chains. Subsequently, the 974P polymer was added in small portions until complete solubility was achieved, leading to the formation of the nanogel. Following this, the EO*Pb* was added, and the system was stirred for 30 min. To finalize the organization of the polymer chains, the final solution was refrigerated (5 °C) overnight, resulting in the nanogel containing EO*Pb*. The preparation of the nanogel containing CUR followed the same methodology, except for the process of incorporating CUR molecules into the F127 copolymeric micelles, where a direct addition process was employed. In this case, a small amount of F127 was placed in a round-bottom flask containing distilled water at a temperature of 40 °C with constant stirring. After solubilizing the F127, a quantity of CUR was added to the system and stirred at 40 °C for 30 min. After cooling the system, the preparation process described for the nanogel containing EO*Pb* was followed to obtain the final material containing both EO*Pb* and CUR (nGPC) as shown in Figure 1A. The empty nanogel (nG) was prepared using the same steps, except the addition of EO*Pb* and/or CUR.

2.6. Stability Assay of Nanogels

To evaluate the influence of temperature on the physical and chemical stability of the nanogel formulations, accelerated stability studies were performed following ANVISA guidelines for cosmetics and the US Pharmacopeia [30]. Each formulation (1 mL) was subjected to centrifugation at 3000 rpm for 30 min at 25 ± 1 °C. The samples were then stored under two distinct conditions—ambient temperature (25 ± 3 °C) and refrigerated storage (5 ± 3 °C)—with continuous temperature monitoring throughout the experiment. Additionally, the formulations underwent a thermal stress test involving seven alternating cycles of 24 h at 5 °C followed by 24 h at 25 °C. Physical stability was assessed based on homogeneity, phase separation, and organoleptic properties, including visual appearance, color, and odor.

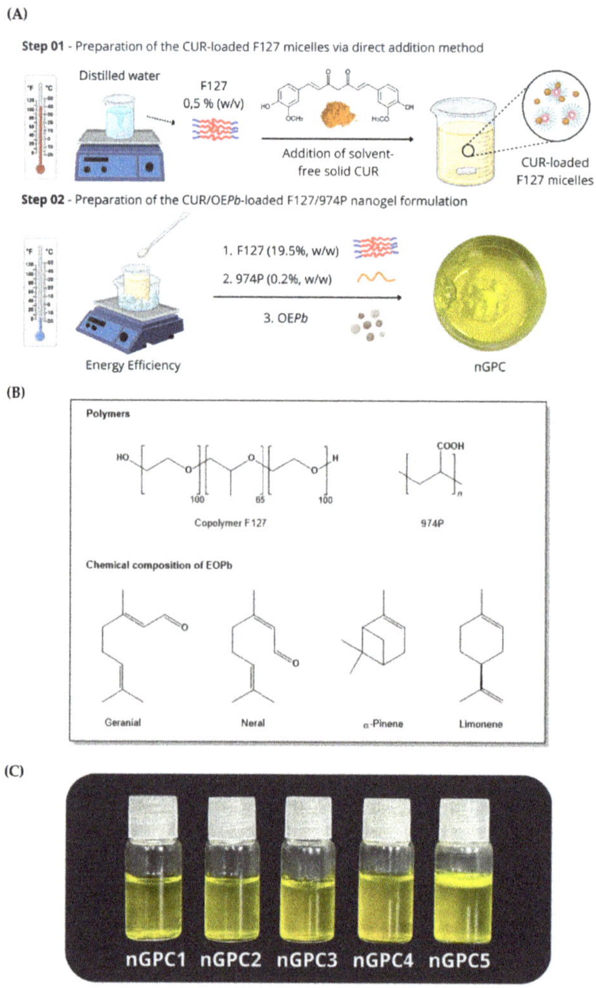

Figure 1. (**A**) Stages of preparation of nG*P*C (nanogel loaded with EO*Pb* and CUR), involving the addition of curcumin (CUR) to the solution under controlled temperature conditions to ensure its uniform dispersion within the polymeric matrix, followed by the incorporation of *Pectis brevipedunculata* essential oil (EO*Pb*). (**B**) Molecular structure of the polymers utilized in nanogel formulation and primary chemical constituents composing EO*Pb*. (**C**) Photographs of the nG*P*C1–nG*P*C5 formulations following the accelerated stability test, where the nG*P*C5 nanogel exhibits a reaming effect.

2.7. FTIR Analysis

FTIR analysis was carried out in reflectance mode using a Shimadzu FTIR Tracer-100 spectrophotometer (Kyoto, Japan). Lyophilized samples of nG, nG*P*, and nG*P*C were prepared as KBr pellets, whereas pure EO*Pb* was examined in Attenuated Total Reflectance (ATR) mode. ATR-FTIR measurements utilized a ZnSe crystal window (PIKE Technologies, Madison, WI, USA). Spectral data were recorded within the 400–4000 cm^{-1} range, maintaining a resolution of 8 cm^{-1} and averaging 50 scans per sample. To optimize spectral accuracy, samples were evenly spread on the ATR crystal surface, and the crystal window was meticulously cleaned with hexane and acetone before each measurement.

2.8. Scanning Electron Microscope (SEM)

The morphological characterization of nanogels nG and nGPC was conducted via SEM. The samples were initially flash-frozen in liquid nitrogen at −196 °C and subsequently lyophilized for 24 h using a Thermo Micro Modulyo freeze dryer (Thermo Electron Corporation, Pittsburgh, PA, USA). To improve imaging contrast, a fine metallic coating was deposited using a BAL-TEC SCD 050 Sputter Coater (Balzers, Liechtenstein). The morphology of the lyophilized samples was then examined at 100× and 50× magnifications using a FEI Quanta 250 microscope (Thermo Fisher Scientific, Karlsruhe, Germany).

2.9. DLS Analysis

The assessment of particle size, polydispersity index (PDI), and diffusional thermodynamic activation parameters was carried out through DLS using a Litesizer™ 500 analyzer (Anton Paar GmbH, Graz, Austria) equipped with a BM 10 module. The mean hydrodynamic radius (R_h) of nanogels nG and nGPC were measured in ultrapure water at four different temperatures: 25, 32, 37, and 45 °C. A 40 mW semiconductor laser operating at a 658 nm wavelength was employed for analysis. R_h values were recorded using a 3.0 mL quartz cuvette. Each measurement was performed in triplicate, and results were expressed as mean ± standard deviation (SD). The diffusion coefficients (D_{if}) were calculated from the R_h values using the Stokes–Einstein equation, assuming the formation of non-interacting spherical particles (Equation (1)) [31].

$$D_{i_f} = \frac{k_B T}{6\pi\eta R_h} \tag{1}$$

where k_B is the Boltzmann constant ($1.3806503 \times 10^{-23}$ J K^{-1}), T is the absolute temperature (K), and η is the viscosity of the medium (Pa s^{-1}). To obtain the values of the diffusional activation energy (E_{ad}), as well as the diffusional entropy ($\Delta S_d^\ddagger$) and enthalpy ($\Delta H_d^\ddagger$), the Arrhenius and Eyring models, adapted for the diffusion process, were employed. The E_{ad} was determined using the following Arrhenius equation (Equation (2)) [32,33]:

$$D_{i_f} = Ae^{-\frac{E_{ad}}{RT}} \tag{2}$$

where D_{if} is the diffusion coefficient, A is the pre-exponential Arrhenius factor, R is the gas constant (8.314 J K^{-1} mol^{-1}), and T is the absolute temperature in K. The plot of $\ln D_{i_f} = \ln A - \frac{E_{ad}}{RT}$ gives E_{ad} by means of the slope. The calculations of $\Delta S_d^\ddagger$ and $\Delta H_d^\ddagger$ are obtained by the adapted Eyring model for diffusion (Equation (3)):

$$D_{i_f} = \frac{RT}{Nh} e^{\frac{\Delta S_d^\ddagger}{R}} e^{-\frac{\Delta H_d^\ddagger}{RT}} \tag{3}$$

where $N = 6.02 \times 10^{23}$ mol^{-1}, and $h = 6.626 \times 10^{-34}$ J s. The plot of $\ln D_{i_f} = \ln\left(\frac{RT}{Nh} e^{\frac{\Delta S_d^\ddagger}{R}} - \frac{\Delta H_d^\ddagger}{RT}\right)$ gives the $\Delta H_d^\ddagger$ using the angular coefficient, and the linear coefficient gives the $\Delta S_d^\ddagger$. The enthalpy of activation ($\Delta H_d^\ddagger$) is obtained from the slope of the plot of $\ln D_{i_f} T$, while the entropy of activation ($\Delta S_d^\ddagger$) is obtained from the linear coefficient. Finally, the variation in the diffusive Gibbs free energy ($\Delta G_d^\ddagger$) is calculated using Equation (4) [34,35]:

$$\Delta G_d^\ddagger = \Delta H_d^\ddagger - T\Delta S_d^\ddagger \tag{4}$$

2.10. Rheological Analysis

The rheological behavior of nG*P*C was analyzed using a Thermo Scientific HAAKE MARS II controlled-stress rheometer (Waltham, MA, EUA). The instrument was configured with a parallel plate system, incorporating a titanium-coated steel cone (C35/2° Ti) with a diameter of 35 mm and a fixed gap of 0.105 mm to ensure precise measurements. All measurements were conducted at a controlled temperature of 5, 25, and 32 °C. Before analysis, the samples were equilibrated for 1 min to ensure thermal and structural stabilization. Flow curves were obtained by applying shear rates in two phases: an upward ramp from 0 to 500 s^{-1} and a downward ramp from 500 to 0 s^{-1}. Each phase lasted 150 s, ensuring steady-state conditions were reached before transitioning between ramps. This protocol allowed the assessment of the shear-thinning behavior and any potential hysteresis effects in the nG*P*C.

2.11. In Vitro Assay Against LLa Promastigote Cells

LLa strain PH8 promastigotes were maintained in 199 culture medium supplemented with 10% heat-inactivated fetal bovine serum and antibiotics (100 UI/mL penicillin and 0.1 mg/mL streptomycin). Cultures were incubated at 27 °C and routinely subcultured to ensure parasite viability. For experimental assays, *LLa* promastigotes were seeded in 96-well plates containing RPMI 1640 medium, reaching a final concentration of 2×10^7 parasites/mL after compound addition. The nG*P*C nanogel was prepared by incorporating 2 mg of EO*Pb* and 0.7 mg of CUR, subsequently diluted in RPMI 1640 medium. The final tested concentrations ranged from 50 to 6.25 μg/mL for EO*Pb* and from 17.5 to 2.19 μg/mL for CUR. For evaluating the nanogel containing the EO*Pb*/CUR combination, the same concentration range and dilution scheme were applied. The nG, nG*P*, and nGC were evaluated to assess the toxicity of the bioactive compounds in their non-combined forms, using the same concentration ranges.

An untreated *LLa* control was included to assess parasite viability, while AmB at 1.95 μg/mL served as a positive control. The plates were incubated at 27 °C for 24, 48, and 72 h to evaluate *LLa* promastigote viability. The colorimetric XTT assay (2,3-bis(2-methoxy-4-nitro-5-sulfophenyl)-5-[(phenylamino)carbonyl]-2H-tetrazolium hydroxide) was employed for this purpose. A reaction mixture containing 20% XTT, PMS (N-methyl dibenzopyrazine methyl sulfate), and 60% saline solution (0.9%) was added to each well. Following a 4 h incubation at 37 °C with 5% CO_2, absorbance was measured at 450/620 nm using a spectrophotometer. The percentage of inhibition was calculated by comparing treated samples to untreated controls, with AmB as the reference drug.

All experiments were conducted in triplicate under conditions appropriate for dPDT, ensuring controlled light exposure parameters during the assay. Mortality rates were determined using logarithmic regression, based on a control curve generated from serial dilutions of Leishmania in culture medium, starting at 2×10^7 parasites/mL and being progressively diluted by a factor of two until reaching 6.25×10^5 parasites/mL.

2.12. Statistical Analysis

For the in vitro experiments, the half-maximal inhibitory concentration (IC_{50}) of the tested compounds was calculated using logistic regression analysis based on the mean mortality at each tested concentration, employing Microsoft Excel (Microsoft Corporation, Redmond, WA, USA). All graphical representations were performed using Prism 9 (GraphPad, San Diego, CA, USA) and Origin Pro (version 8.5).

3. Results and Discussion

3.1. Development of Nanogels

Prior to the nanogel formulation, the chemical profile of EO*Pb* was characterized through GC-MS analysis, revealing a total of nineteen components, which account for 92.66% of the oil's composition. Of these, 64.58% are oxygenated monoterpenes, represented by the isomers geranial (36.06%) and neral (28.52%), while the remaining compounds include α-pinene (15.72%) and limonene (8.28%). The chemical structures of the major compounds were confirmed through ^{1}H and ^{13}C NMR [13] and are represented in Figure 1B. According to previous studies, various combinations of F127 and 974P percentages were tested to find the optimal formulation that would allow the thermoresponsive behavior of the nanogel, particularly a rapid sol–gel transition [12,13].

Formulations with concentrations of 5–10/0.1–0.3% remained in a liquid state at both 5 and 30 °C, indicating an absence of thermoresponsive behavior. Conversely, those containing 20/0.1–0.3% remained liquid at 5 °C but exhibited a sol–gel transition at 30 °C within approximately 10 min. The 20/0.1 formulation displayed low viscosity, whereas 20/0.3 resulted in a highly viscous system. The optimal composition, determined as 20/0.2, was selected as the basis for incorporating EO*Pb* into the nG system due to its rapid sol–gel transition properties.

Furthermore, stability tests showed that adding up to 1% EO*Pb* resulted in stable and transparent formulations, with no phase separation observed after the accelerated stability tests. However, concentrations above this threshold led to formulations with low stability, exhibiting creaminess and phase separation [12]. For this study, the F127/974P/EO*Pb* ratio was fixed at 20/0.2/1% (*w*/*w*) and CUR was added at concentrations ranging from 0.01 to 0.05% (*w*/*w*), resulting in the formulations outlined in Table 1. This was accomplished by testing the maximum amount of CUR that could be incorporated into the gel matrix containing 1% (*w*/*w*) EO*Pb*, followed by an evaluation of the system's accelerated stability. Formulations containing up to 0.03% CUR (nG*P*C1-nG*P*C4) remained stable even after being subjected to accelerated stability testing (seven cycles) and shelf-life testing over 180 days. However, when the CUR content exceeded 0.04%, creaming effect was observed in nanogel nG*P*C5 within 48 h of preparation (Figure 1C). Therefore, the nG*P*C4 formulation, which exhibited the highest percentage of the bioactive EO*Pb*/CUR compounds, was selected for further characterization and referred to throughout the study as nG*P*C.

Table 1. Optimized nanogel formulations (nG*P*C1–nG*P*C5) with varying CUR and water (% *w*/*w*) concentrations, combined with a fixed composition of F127, 974P, and EO*Pb*.

			Component % (*w*/*w*)			
Code	**Water**	**F127**	**974P**	**EO*Pb***	**CUR**	**Stability** [a]
nG*P*C 1	78.99	20	0.2	1	0.01	S
nG*P*C 2	78.78	20	0.2	1	0.02	S
nG*P*C 3	78.47	20	0.2	1	0.03	S
nG*P*C 4	78.36	20	0.2	1	0.04	S
nG*P*C 5	78.25	20	0.2	1	0.05	C

[a] S: Stable; C: Creaming.

3.2. Characterization of Nanogels

3.2.1. FTIR

Figure 2 displays the FTIR spectra of the nanogels nG, nGP, and nG*P*C. The analysis of the nG spectrum (Figure 2A) reveals a broad and intense absorption band at 3384 cm^{-1}, overlapping with the band at 3564 cm^{-1}. Due to the miscibility of 0.2% 974P in 20% (*w*/*w*) F127, part of the 974P-974P and F127-F127 intermolecular interactions is replaced by the formation of F127-974P crosslinked hydrogen bonds. The band observed at 3384 cm^{-1} in the nG spectrum is related to a higher-energy O–H stretch, with a blue shift ($\Delta\nu = 180\ cm^{-1}$). However, a relatively large proportion of F127-F127 hydrogen bonds remain present, as indicated by the strong and broad absorption band at 3564 cm^{-1}, which justifies the coexistence of micellar structures of F127 in the nanogel composition. Figure 2B shows the FTIR spectrum of the nG*P* nanogel.

The incorporation of 1% EO*Pb* into the nG matrix induces notable changes in the absorption bands characteristic of the F127/974P system. A prominent and sharp band at 3676 cm^{-1} emerges due to a significant red shift ($\Delta\nu = 112\ cm^{-1}$) from the original 3564 cm^{-1} band observed in the nG spectrum. This shift suggests a reduction in the energy required for O–H stretching, likely attributed to EO*Pb* molecules disrupting some F127-974P interactions to occupy the pores of the nG*P* matrix. Additionally, the band at 3384 cm^{-1} in nG undergoes a blue shift to 3340 cm^{-1} ($\Delta\nu = 44\ cm^{-1}$), possibly indicating the formation of new hydrogen bonds between F127/974P and the geranial and neral isomers. However, it is likely that most EO*Pb* molecules preferentially associate with the hydrophobic PPO chains of F127. This hypothesis is reinforced by the higher energy demand for asymmetric C–H stretching, evidenced by the observed blue shift ($\Delta\nu = 19$ cm^{-1}) from 2904 cm^{-1} (nG) to 2885 cm^{-1} in the nG*P* spectrum (Figure 2B), suggesting a significant increase in hydrophobic interactions within the system.

Figure 2C,D show the spectra of the nG*P*C material. The intense band related to O–H stretching is split into three signals. The signals at 3550 and 3475 cm^{-1} are attributed to free O–H stretches of CUR molecules and intermolecular hydrogen bonds between F127/974P and CUR molecules, respectively. The signal at 3414 cm^{-1} is attributed to F127/974P intermolecular hydrogen bonds. The presence of the band at 2885 cm^{-1}, assigned to C–H stretching, suggests that the highly hydrophobic CUR molecules preferentially associate with the PPO chains of F127.

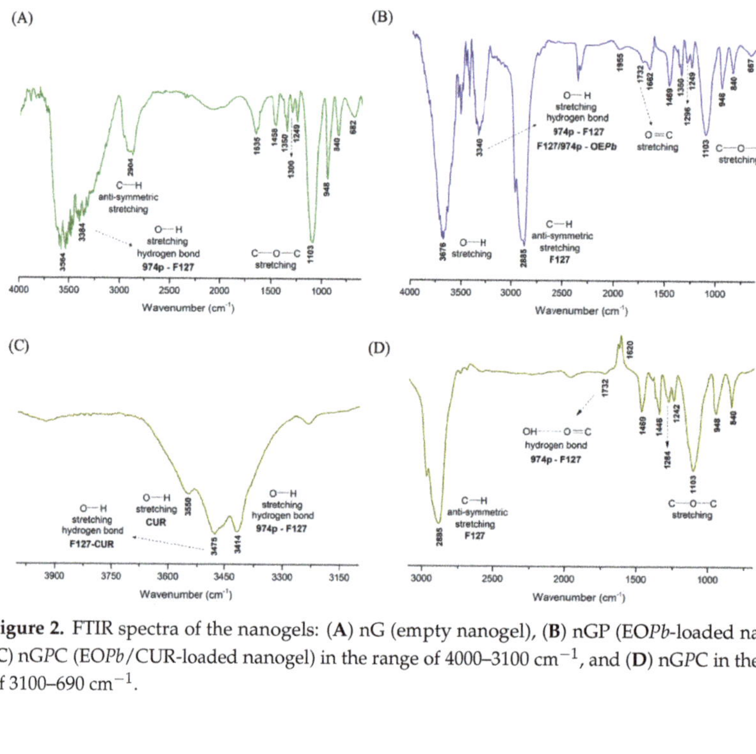

Figure 2. FTIR spectra of the nanogels: (**A**) nG (empty nanogel), (**B**) nG*P* (EO*Pb*-loaded nanogel) (**C**) nG*P*C (EO*Pb*/CUR-loaded nanogel) in the range of 4000–3100 cm^{-1}, and (**D**) nG*P*C in the range of 3100–690 cm^{-1}.

3.2.2. SEM

SEM is widely recognized as a crucial technique for examining the intricate architectures of nano- and microstructured formulations. Its superior high-resolution imaging capability makes it indispensable for characterizing materials at scales essential to pharmaceutical applications, providing valuable insights into their structural attributes and functional potential. In this study, SEM was utilized to assess both the surface and internal morphology of the lyophilized nG nanogel.

nG micrographs (Figure 3A,B) reveal that the nG nanogel matrix exhibits a porous architecture, featuring interconnected channel-like structures characteristic of crosslinked F127/974P polymer chains due to intermolecular hydrogen bonding. These morphological characteristics offer valuable insight into the properties of nG, suggesting that its porous network effectively retains the liquid phase containing EO*Pb*/CUR molecules, thereby increasing viscosity through strong hydrogen-bonding interactions with water. In fact, the incorporation of EO*Pb*/CUR into nG induces notable morphological modifications in the nanoformulation. SEM micrographs of nGPC reveal a rougher surface texture, suggesting that the pores have been filled, as evidenced by their less defined appearance (Figure 3C–F). In agreement with the FTIR findings, the robust intermolecular interactions between EO*Pb*/CUR and the PEO polymer chains restrict the development of pores throughout the lyophilization process.

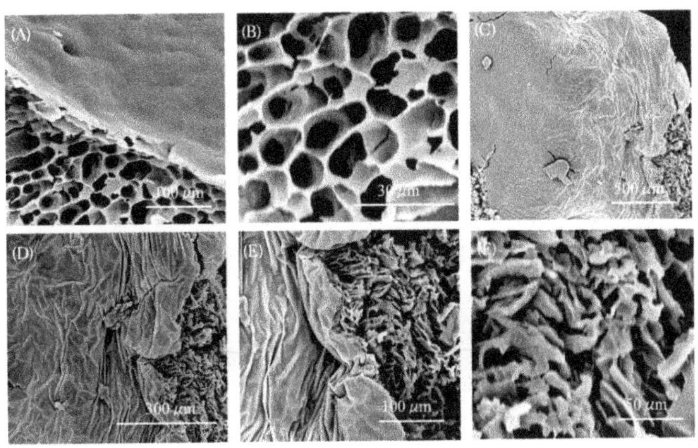

Figure 3. SEM micrographs of nanogels after the freeze-drying process: (**A**) and (**B**) nG (empty nanogel) at magnifications of 1000× and 5000×, respectively; (**C**), (**D**), (**E**), and (**F**) nGPC (EO*Pb*-loaded nanogel) at magnifications of 200×, 500×, 1000×, and 2000×, respectively.

3.2.3. DLS

The DLS technique is widely used in nanogel characterization due to its ability to accurately measure particle sizes in suspension at the nanoscale [36]. In addition to evaluating the particle size distribution and providing valuable insights into the colloidal stability and intrinsic properties of nanogels, DLS was also fundamental in determining the diffusional thermodynamic parameters of activation. This highlights the crucial role of DLS not only in assessing nanogel stability but also in obtaining key activation parameters that govern their diffusion behavior. This technique is particularly effective in monitoring changes in hydrodynamic radius (R_h) in response to variations in temperature, pH, and other environmental factors, providing crucial data for developing nanomaterials designed for pharmaceutical and medicinal applications. Analysis of the R_h values for nG reveals a marked reduction in particle size with increasing temperature (Table 2).

DLS measurements were performed on solutions diluted to below 1% (m/v). At concentrations lower than the critical micelle concentration (CMC) of F127, the demicellization process is promoted, resulting in a decreased population of smaller particles. This phenomenon arises due to the system's overall entropy, which drives the aggregation of smaller particles into more polydisperse structures (R_h = 661 nm ± 6 and PDI = 0.34). However, since the micellization process of triblock copolymers is highly temperature-dependent, as the temperature of the nG system is increased from 25 to 32 °C, the critical micelle temperature (TMC) compensates for the CMC [37–40]. This results in the formation of smaller particles with reduced polydispersity (R_h = 124 nm ± 5 and PDI = 0.24), indicating an increase in the system's total entropy and promoting enhanced particle diffusion, as shown in the analysis of the Diffusivity (D_{if}) as a function of temperature in Figure 4A. This behavior highlights the thermoresponsive nature of the nanogel. At higher temperatures of 32 and 37 °C, the diffusion processes of nG become even more pronounced, leading to a substantial reduction in nanoparticle sizes (R_h = 17 nm ± 3 and PDI = 0.25).

Table 2. DLS measurements as a function of temperature for the nG (empty nanogel) and nG*PC* (EO*Pb*/CUR-loaded nanogel). Measurements were conducted in quintuplicate, and results are expressed as mean ± SD.

Temperature (°C)	nG	nG*PC*
	R_h (nm)/PDI	
25	661.00 ± 6.00/0.34	288.00 ± 74.00/0.29
32	124.00 ± 5.00/0.24	296.00 ± 24.00/0.44
37	17.00 ± 3.00/0.25	237.00 ± 17.00/0.42
45	16.93 ± 3.00/0.26	333.50 ± 22.00/0.45

The decrease in R_h with increasing temperature may be attributed to the dehydration of the PEO groups in the hydrophilic corona and the PPO core at higher temperatures, which leads to a reduction in R_h [40,41]. This process occurs because the rise in thermal energy induces gradual dehydration in non-ionic surfactants, increasing the tendency for separation between the pseudo-phases in the aqueous environment due to shifts in the dynamic equilibrium of micellization. As the temperature increases, the dehydration of both the core and the PEO groups intensifies, causing structural changes in the copolymer. In addition to dehydration, the higher temperature promotes a more efficient entanglement between the PEO and PPO groups, leading to a notable decrease in the size of the diffusing species within the medium [40,42]. Furthermore, the reduction in R_h could be related to the fact that copolymers with lower molar mass remain as unimers at elevated temperatures. Triblock architecture copolymers, such as F127, exhibit a dynamic equilibrium between unimers and micelles through an insertion–expulsion mechanism, and between micelles of various geometries and sizes via fusion–fragmentation processes [43].

These characteristics, along with the temperature increase, lead to greater friction between the terminal groups due to water molecule extrusion, ultimately promoting an equilibrium shift toward smaller micelles. As the temperature rises, the F127 copolymer undergoes structural reorganization driven by dehydration and heightened friction between the copolymer's terminal groups, favoring fragmentation processes and altering the micellization equilibrium [40]. This phenomenon is mainly driven by the copolymer's structural arrangement in solution, where the hydrophilic PEO segments extend beyond the micelle core, contributing to increased fluidity compared to copolymers with a higher hydrophobic content. Additionally, F127 exhibits anomalies related to macromolecular relaxations, primarily due to the conformational changes of the methyl groups in the PPO blocks. These changes are induced by the extrusion of water molecules from the PPO segments as temperature increases. These unique properties of F127 are responsible for its self-diffusion behavior and characteristic micellization equilibria when compared to more hydrophobic copolymers.

The assessment of R_h values for the nGPC material demonstrates a distinct behavior when compared to the nG formulation. Unlike nG, the increase in temperature does not significantly reduce the particle size of the nGPC material. The observed particle sizes for nGPC, ranging from 237 ± 17 nm to 333 ± 22 nm, are consistent with the stability studies. However, the self-organization dynamics of these materials diverge from those of nG, with the inclusion of EOPb/CUR leading to a reduction in diffusion coefficients (D_{if}) within the system (Figure 4B). The observed decrease in the D_{if} values for nGPC can be attributed to the impact of the EOPb/CUR on the self-organization behavior of the nanogel system. The reduction in the diffusion coefficients reflects shifts in the dynamic micellization equilibria, which are influenced by the multicomponent nature of the system. Additionally, copolymers with concentrations $\leq$0.05 g/mL exhibit different aggregation equilibria compared to those at concentrations near or above 0.1 g/mL. These changes in aggregation behavior and thermodynamic properties under varying temperature conditions explain the observed variations in the material's behavior in solution [44].

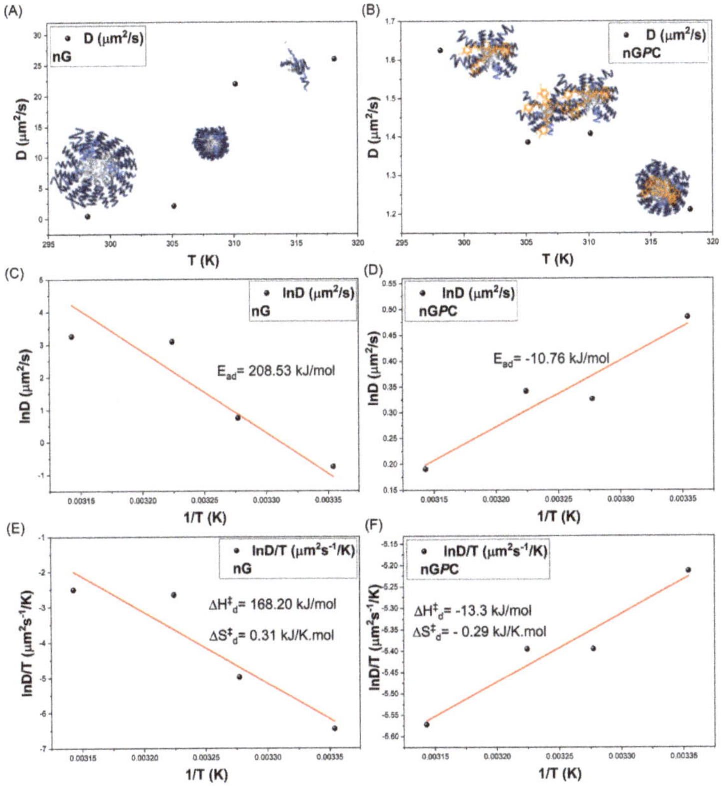

Figure 4. Comparative analysis of the diffusion coefficient D_{if} as a function of temperature (K): (**A**,**C**,**E**) nG (empty nanogel) and (**B**,**D**,**F**) nGPC (EOPb/CUR-loaded nanogel).

To gain deeper insights into the effects of temperature, the diffusional activation energy (E_{ad}) and the thermodynamic parameters of diffusion ($\Delta H_d^{\ddagger}$ and $\Delta S_d^{\ddagger}$) were calculated using the Arrhenius law (Equation (2)) (Figure 4C,D) and Eyring's theory (Equation (3)) (Figure 4E,F), both adapted for diffusion processes [33,44,45]. Activation parameters play a critical role in elucidating the mechanisms underlying diffusion, as they provide insights into the energy required for these processes to occur. For the nG system, the calculated value E_{ad} (greater than zero, as shown in Table 3 confirms the temperature dependence of the diffusion process. Specifically, an E_{ad} of 208.53 kJ/mol indicates that the system utilizes thermal energy to facilitate the diffusion of species in solution. This is accompanied by an enthalpy change ($\Delta H_d^{\ddagger}$) of 168.20 kJ/mol, signifying energy absorption, and an entropy change ($\Delta S_d^{\ddagger}$) of 0.31 kJ/K·mol, reflecting an increase in system disorder.

The temperature rise enhances the hydrophobicity of the copolymer and increases system entropy, leading to the formation of micelles and copolymeric pre-aggregates with smaller hydrodynamic radius (R_h). This, in turn, increases the excluded volume of the copolymer in solution, which refers to the geometric space occupied by the macromolecular segments. As thermal energy is absorbed, the number of possible configurations available to the system expands, allowing for a broader distribution of species within the nG system and promoting diffusion in the medium. This thermodynamic behavior highlights the adaptability of the system to temperature variations and its potential for temperature-sensitive applications.

The nG*PC* system exhibited a reversal in thermal behavior, with an E_{ad} value of −10.76 kJ/mol, contrasting sharply with the nG system. This shift highlights the impact of incorporating EO*Pb*/CUR, which significantly disrupt the micellization equilibria of the material. At this stage, the thermal energy provided to the system is predominantly utilized in alternative processes, such as structural reorganization, rather than in mass transport via diffusion. This is evident from the exothermic nature of the process, reflected by a $\Delta H_d^{\ddagger}$ value of −13.30 kJ/mol. The exothermic nature of the diffusion process reveals two key points. First, incorporating EO*Pb*/CUR introduces strong intermolecular interactions between components, resulting in energy release as the system reorganizes itself. This finding was further supported by FTIR analysis, which revealed that the more hydrophobic EO*Pb* molecules predominantly associate with the PPO segments of F127. This interpretation is reinforced by the observed increase in energy required for the anti-symmetric C–H stretching, as evidenced by the enhanced intensity and blue shift ($\Delta\nu = 19$ cm^{-1}) of the absorption band, shifting from 2904 cm^{-1} (nG) to 2885 cm^{-1} in the nG*PC* spectrum (Figure 2). This shift suggests a notable enhancement in the system's hydrophobic interactions, consistent with the enthalpic interaction processes identified.

Second, the decrease in diffusional entropy ($\Delta S_d^{\ddagger} = -0.29$ kJ/K·mol) indicates a reduction in the configurational possibilities of the system. As energy is released, the system becomes more ordered, restricting the range of diffusional configurations.

The synergistic effect of these changes is further validated by in vitro applications in cutaneous leishmaniasis. The nG*PC* system demonstrated superior efficacy compared to the control material, underscoring the role of EO*Pb*/CUR in altering the dynamic organization of the nanogel. These incorporations were pivotal in inducing shifts in activation patterns, resulting in an inversion of the diffusional mechanistic behavior. The influence of temperature on the nG and nG*PC* systems is further emphasized by the values of the diffusional Gibbs free energy function ($\Delta G_d^{\ddagger}$) as a function of temperature, presented in Table 3, illustrating the thermodynamic distinctions between the two systems.

The increase in temperature for the nG system leads to a progressive decrease in $\Delta G_d^{\ddagger}$ values, as shown in Figure 5A. This trend indicates that higher temperatures promote diffusion processes, as less energy is required for the micellar systems to diffuse within the solution. This observation aligns with reductions in R_h, $\Delta H_d^{\ddagger}$, and $\Delta S_d^{\ddagger}$, reflecting enhanced micellar dynamics and greater diffusional efficiency at elevated temperatures. In contrast, the nG*PC* system exhibits a thermodynamic inversion with increasing temperature, as previously discussed. This is characterized by negative E_{ad} values and a monotonically increasing trend in $\Delta G_d^{\ddagger}$ (Figure 5B). The system also shows a decrease in $\Delta S_d^{\ddagger}$, indicating molecular reorganization and an increased ordering of water molecules to solvate monomeric micelles, micellar pre-aggregates, micelles, and EO*Pb*/CUR as temperature rises. The exothermic $\Delta H_d^{\ddagger}$ values observed with increasing temperature suggest that the transfer of unimers, micellar pre-aggregates, and EO*Pb* from the solution into the micelle formation is a thermodynamically favorable process. The hydrophobic PPO segments of the copolymer predominantly drive this phenomenon. This complex thermodynamic mechanism explains the monotonically increasing $\Delta H_d^{\ddagger}$ values: as the system undergoes self-association and structural reorganization, greater energy is required for these processes to progress.

The diffusion mass transfer profiles of both the nG and nG*PC* systems reveal complex behaviors. The intrinsic properties of F127, combined with the incorporation of EO*Pb*/CUR, amplify the hydrophobic driving forces within the system. These interactions are responsible for the observed structural changes and thermodynamic inversions, further highlighting the intricate relationship between molecular architecture, temperature, and diffusion dynamics.

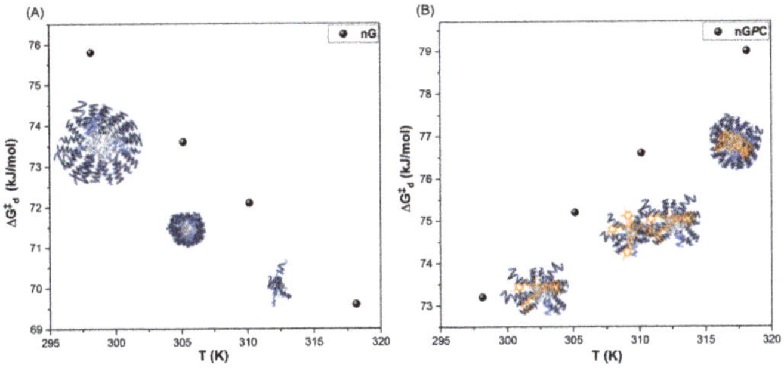

Figure 5. Plot of $\Delta G_d^{\ddagger}$ as a function of temperature for the (**A**) nG (empty nanogel) and (**B**) nG*PC* (EO*Pb*/CUR-loaded nanogel).

Table 3. Thermodynamic parameters of diffusional process for nG and nG*PC*.

nG		nGPC	
Parameter	**Value**	**Parameter**	**Value**
E_{ad} (kJ mol^{-1})	208.53	E_{ad} (kJ mol^{-1})	−10.76
$\Delta S_d^{\ddagger}$ (kJ K^{-1} mol^{-1})	0.31	$\Delta G_d^{\ddagger}$ (kJ K^{-1} mol^{-1})	−0.29
$\Delta H_d^{\ddagger}$ (kJ mol^{-1})	168.20	$\Delta H_d^{\ddagger}$ (kJ mol^{-1})	−13.30
$\Delta G_d^{\ddagger}$ (kJ mol^{-1}) at different temperatures			
Temperature (K)	nG	Temperature (K)	nG*PC*
298.15	75.80	298.15	73.20
303.15	73.60	303.15	75.20
305.15	72.10	305.15	76.60
310.15	69.60	310.15	79.00

3.3. *Rheological Analysis*

The flow curve analysis of the nG*PC* sample, evaluated up to a shear rate of 1500 s^{-1} at 5 °C, revealed characteristic Newtonian fluid behavior (Figure 6A). The shear stress versus shear rate curve was linear, starting at the origin, and reaching 250 Pa at 1500 s^{-1}. Notably, the forward and backward curves overlapped completely, indicating the absence of hysteresis. This reinforces the rheological stability of the material and rules out thixotropic or rheopectic effects. The constant viscosity, calculated at 0.167 Pa·s, suggests that nG*PC* maintains uniform rheological properties even at low temperatures such as 5 °C. At 25 °C, the rheological analysis of the nG*P*C sample demonstrated non-Newtonian behavior, contrasting with the Newtonian characteristics observed at 5 °C (Figure 6B). The shear stress versus shear rate curve exhibited shear-thinning behavior, where viscosity decreased with increasing shear rate. This indicates an internal fluid structure that reorganizes under high shear forces, a common characteristic of suspensions or nanogels. The forward curve showed a decrease in shear stress from 200 s^{-1} to 1500 s^{-1}, suggesting viscoelastic or thixotropic responses, while the backward curve was nearly linear, indicating incomplete structural recovery of the fluid.

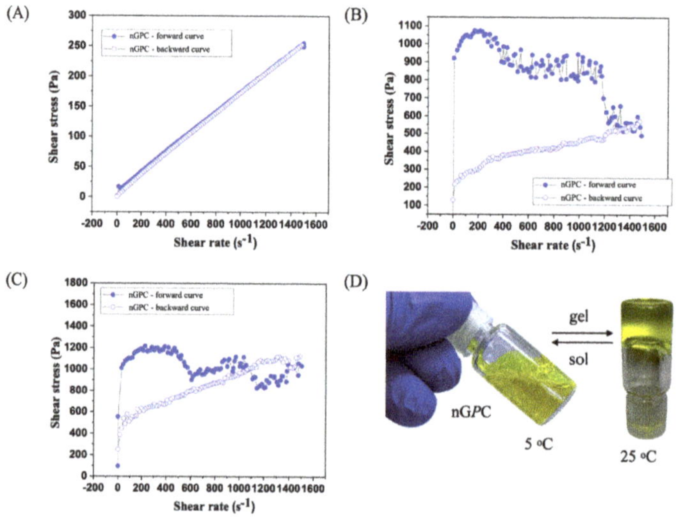

Figure 6. Rheological behavior of the nG*P*C (EO*Pb*/CUR-loaded nanogel) sample at varying temperatures: (**A**) Newtonian fluid behavior at 5 °C with a linear shear stress versus shear rate curve; (**B**) shear-thinning behavior at 25 °C, demonstrating viscosity decrease with increasing shear rate; (**C**) pronounced thixotropic pattern at 32 °C, with viscosity reduction and incomplete structural recovery after shear. The curves demonstrate the nanogel's dynamic response to shear forces, highlighting its suitability for topical applications; (**D**) real image of the nG*P*C nanogel during the sol–gel transition, showing sol at 5 °C and gel at 25 °C. The curves demonstrate the nanogel's dynamic response to shear forces, highlighting its suitability for topical applications.

At 32 °C, the nG*P*C sample displayed rheological behavior characteristic of non-Newtonian systems, with a pronounced thixotropic pattern (Figure 6C). During the test, the nanogel's viscosity decreased as the shear rate increased, but it did not fully recover after the removal of shear forces. This suggests that the internal structure of the nanogel reorganizes and becomes more fluid under high-shear conditions. Such behavior is typical of materials where viscosity depends on shear history, as observed in many viscoelastic or thixotropic systems. The forward curve exhibited three peaks followed by drops in viscosity, indicating continuous structural changes within the nanogel as the shear rate increased. However, the structure did not fully restore itself after each peak. This highlights the nanogel's dynamic response to shear, making it easier to apply at high shear rates but with viscosity not returning to its initial state. On the other hand, the backward curve was almost linear but showed a steeper slope than experiments conducted at 25 °C. This indicates that after shear, the sample remained more fluid, with a partially reorganized structure that did not entirely return to its previous condition.

This rheological behavior has significant implications for the topical applications of nG*P*C, particularly at temperatures ranging from 25 to 32 °C, which correspond to typical human skin temperatures. The reduction in viscosity with increasing shear rate facilitates the application of the nanogel, enhancing its spreadability over the skin. The thixotropic behavior, characterized by variations in shear stress, is advantageous for the controlled release of bioactive compounds, enabling a more effective and gradual therapeutic delivery. This profile is especially desirable in topical treatments, as it ensures prolonged and targeted action. Furthermore, the observed rheological stability suggests that the nanogel nG*P*C (Figure 6D) maintains its efficacy under physiological conditions, underscoring its strong potential for dermatological applications where stable and controlled performance is critical under varying skin temperatures.

3.4. In Vitro Assay Against LLa Promastigotes

Leishmaniasis remains a major global health challenge, particularly in tropical and subtropical regions where access to effective treatments is limited. Conventional therapies, such as pentavalent antimonials, AmB, and miltefosine, suffer from significant drawbacks, including high toxicity, elevated costs, prolonged treatment duration, and emerging drug resistance. These limitations highlight the urgent need for novel therapeutic approaches that offer improved efficacy, safety, and accessibility. In this context, the nG*P*C represents a significant advancement by leveraging the synergistic effects of EO*Pb*/CUR within a thermosensitive system. The use of FDA-approved excipients and GC principles enhances its economic viability and sustainability, reducing production costs and improving accessibility. Notably, the nG*P*C is compatible with dPDT, eliminating the need for high-energy artificial light sources and expanding its clinical potential.

To evaluate its therapeutic potential, in vitro assays were conducted to assess its antileishmanial activity against *LLa* promastigotes. The primary objective of this study was to evaluate the therapeutic potential of EO*Pb*/CUR when incorporated into an F127/974P nanogel matrix at low concentrations [26,27,29]. Specifically, the study aimed to determine whether these concentrations would maintain their biological efficacy upon encapsulation, considering that the nanogel matrix could modulate the therapeutic performance of the EO*Pb*/CUR compounds. It is crucial to acknowledge that the excipients used in nanogel preparation may influence the cytotoxic profile of the bioactives. This aspect becomes particularly relevant when analyzing the concentration range of EO*Pb*/CUR within nanogel formulations, as elevated concentrations could enhance cytotoxicity, potentially compromising the safety and therapeutic index of the final formulation.

To test this hypothesis, the efficacy of nanogel formulations, including empty nanogels, those containing CUR, those containing EO*Pb*, and the combination of both compounds, was evaluated. This experimental design allowed for a comprehensive comparison of the effects of each formulation, both in isolation and in combination, thereby providing critical insights into the potential synergistic or additive effects of the EO*Pb*/CUR combination. Furthermore, this setup allowed for the assessment of the influence of the nanogel matrix itself on the bioactivity of the encapsulated compounds. While the encapsulation within the nanogel was hypothesized to reduce the immediate bioavailability of OE*Pb*/CUR due to its controlled release mechanism, it was also expected that the sustained-release properties of the nanogel could provide significant therapeutic advantages. By prolonging the release of active compounds over time, the nanogel system has the potential to enhance overall therapeutic efficacy, particularly for the treatment of chronic or relapsing diseases such as leishmaniasis. This balance between a possible initial reduction in potency and a prolonged therapeutic effect forms the foundation for investigating the effectiveness of these nanogel-based delivery systems.

The effect of the nanogel formulations on *LLa* promastigote cell viability was evaluated at three different time points: 24, 48, and 72 h. Interestingly, the nanogels nG, nGC, and nG*P* showed no anti-promastigote activity at any concentration or time point tested. In contrast, the nanogel n*GPC* demonstrated significant activity, as shown in Figure 7. At the highest concentration tested (17.5 µg/mL of EO*Pb* and 50 µg/mL of CUR), the combination formulation induced over 88% mortality of the promastigotes across all time points (24, 48, and 72 h). This strong effect was observed consistently at each time interval, suggesting a robust and sustained action of the combined compounds. At the lowest concentration tested (2.19 µg/mL of EO*Pb* and 6.25 µg/mL of CUR), the combination formulation still exhibited notable activity, with mortality rates of 24.15%, 21.35%, and 10.40% at 24, 48, and 72 h, respectively. The data also indicate a potential synergistic or additive effect between the two compounds, as the combined formulation exhibited greater efficacy than the individual compounds.

For comparison, AmB (1.95 µg/mL), a standard treatment for leishmaniasis, exhibited mortality rates of 97.67, 96.33, and 96.67% at 24, 48, and 72 h, respectively, indicating sustained high efficacy with minimal variation across time. While the highest concentration of n*GPC* did not reach the mortality levels observed with AmB, it still demonstrated significant activity, particularly considering its advantages in formulation stability, targeted delivery, and reduced toxicity. Furthermore, the progressive decline in mortality rates at the lowest concentration of n*GPC* suggests that sustained drug release or enhanced bioavailability strategies could further optimize its efficacy. Moreover, despite AmB's well-established effectiveness, its clinical use is limited by high toxicity, particularly nephrotoxicity, necessitating careful monitoring and hospitalization. Additionally, prolonged treatment durations contribute to patient non-compliance and increase the risk of relapse, reinforcing the need for alternative therapies with improved safety and therapeutic profiles [46].

This synergistic effect can be attributed to the complementary properties of the bioactives. EO*Pb*, derived from a scarcely studied species, presents a promising therapeutic approach, while CUR, known for its broad phototherapeutic spectrum, remains underexplored as a leishmanicidal agent in the absence of UV–visible light ($\lambda_{max} \approx$ 420–430 nm). The dPDT strategy adopted here harnesses the cytotoxic effects of both compounds while eliminating the need for high-energy light sources, thus aligning with GC and sustainability principles [25]. Building upon our previous research, we observed a remarkable improvement in efficacy with the combined formulation. Whereas the EO*Pb*-loaded nanogel previously required 280 µg/mL to achieve ≈ 80% mortality of *LLa* [13], the n*GPC* attained the same effect with just 25/8.75 µg/mL of EO*Pb*/CUR.

Interestingly, the reduction in cell mortality at 72 h in the C3 treatment was also observed with C4, both representing the lowest tested concentrations of the combined compounds. In contrast, the highest concentrations (C1 and C2) exhibited a more pronounced cellular effect, independent of time. This suggests that the potential synergistic effect is primarily concentration-dependent rather than time-dependent, indicating that the drug's efficacy does not progressively increase over time. This phenomenon may be attributed to a reduction in the availability of compounds due to cellular uptake, highlighting the need for an optimal minimal effective dose. According to Kuti (2016), antimicrobial activity depends on concentration, minimal effective concentration, and exposure time [47]. When the concentration effect is more significant than the time effect, the drug is classified as concentration-dependent, with efficacy determined by the ratio of maximum free drug concentration to the minimal effective concentration. Conversely, when time predominates, efficacy depends on how long the drug concentration remains above the minimal effective dose. Given that n*GPC* demonstrated sustained activity over time at its highest concentration but a progressive reduction at lower concentrations, its efficacy likely follows a concentration-dependent profile. This underscores the importance of optimizing drug delivery to maintain effective concentrations for prolonged periods. Further studies on the mechanism of action are necessary to better elucidate this phenomenon.

Since the experimental conditions of this study included the application of dPDT, the findings strongly support its role in enhancing the therapeutic efficacy of the nGPC system. The use of dPDT probably increased the observed leishmanicidal effects, reinforcing the importance of photodynamic activation in this therapeutic strategy. Given that CUR is a potent photosensitizer, its incorporation into the nanogel system alongside EOPb under dPDT conditions may provide a synergistic effect, enhancing the leishmanicidal potential of nGPC. These results underscore the relevance of dPDT as an integral component of this approach, suggesting that future optimizations should continue to explore its role in maximizing the therapeutic potential of nanogel-based treatments for leishmaniasis.

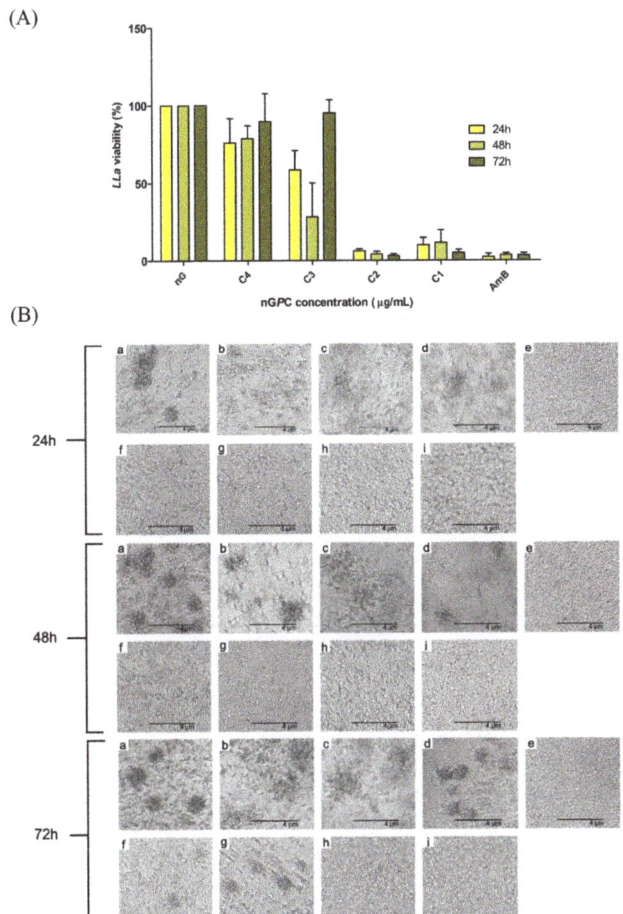

Figure 7. (**A**) in vitro viability (%) of *LLa* promastigote cells in response to different concentrations of nG*P*C (EO*Pb*/CUR-loaded nanogel). The concentrations C4–C1 represent the combination of EO*Pb*/CUR as follows: C4 = 6.65/2.19, C3 = 12.5/4.38, C2 = 25/8.75 and C1 = 50/17.5 (µg/mL). The nG (empty nanogel) and AmB (amphotericin B) were used as negative and positive controls, respectively. nG*P* (EO*Pb*-loaded nanogel) and nGC (CUR-loaded nanogel) did not exhibit cytotoxicity against *LLa* at any of the tested concentrations; therefore, their results were not included in the graph. (**B**) Representative images of *LLa* cultures treated with nanogel formulations at different time points: (a) untreated; (b) nG; (c) nGC (50 µg/mL); (d) nG*P* (17.5 µg/mL); (e) AmB (1.95 µg/mL); (f–i) nG*P*C (C4–C1).

4. Conclusions

This study demonstrates the potential of the nanogel formulation nG*P*C incorporating EO*Pb*/CUR as a promising therapeutic strategy against *LLa* promastigotes under dPDT conditions. The physicochemical characterization confirmed the stability and thermosensitivity of nG*P*C, ensuring its suitability for topical application. Rheological analysis revealed a transition from Newtonian to shear-thinning and thixotropic behavior, facilitating its application in topical treatment. Spectroscopic analyses confirmed molecular interactions that facilitated improved diffusional properties. Furthermore, DLS measurements revealed that EO*Pb*/CUR incorporation influenced R_h and thermodynamic parameters, indicating strong intermolecular interactions. The negative diffusional activation energy and entropy suggested enhanced system stability and structural reorganization rather than mere diffusion, reinforcing the efficacy of the formulation. These findings underscore the importance of DLS as a powerful tool for evaluating the synergistic behavior of EO*Pb*/CUR in nanogels. Biological evaluations demonstrated that nG*P*C significantly enhanced anti-promastigote activity compared to free EO*Pb* or CUR, with over 88% mortality at the highest tested concentration and a dose-dependent response at lower concentrations. These findings suggest a synergistic interaction between EO*Pb* and CUR, likely mediated by the nanogel matrix, which improves bioavailability and therapeutic efficacy. Furthermore, the experimental conditions confirmed the relevance of dPDT in enhancing the leishmanicidal effects of nG*P*C, reinforcing its potential as a light-activated therapeutic approach.

The results underscore the potential of nG*P*C in overcoming the limitations of conventional leishmaniasis treatments, particularly by enhancing drug stability, reducing toxicity, and enabling controlled release. Future studies should focus on elucidating the molecular mechanisms underlying the observed synergism, as well as evaluating the impact of dPDT to further enhance therapeutic outcomes. Overall, nG*P*C represents an innovative and effective platform for delivering bioactive compounds against*LLa* promastigotes, reinforcing the relevance of nanotechnology and natural product-based therapies in addressing neglected tropical diseases.

Author Contributions: Conceptualization, data curation, methodology, investigation, writing—original draft, and writing—review and editing, L.M.O.C., E.M.M., D.S.S.L.L.-N., M.J.S.G., M.V.C.L. and G.B.; conceptualization, data curation, methodology, and formal analysis, G.C.d.S.N.; conceptualization, data curation, methodology, investigation, writing—original draft, writing—review and editing, visualization, supervision, and project administration, R.S.G. All authors have read and agreed to the published version of the manuscript.

Funding: This research was funded by the Postgraduate Program in Chemistry (PPGQuim), Federal University of Maranhão (UFMA), São Luís, MA, Brazil. The authors thank the Coordination for the Improvement of Higher Education Personnel (CAPES) and the National Council for Scientific and Technological Development (CNPq) for their financial support through the Master's scholarships provided to the students of the PPGQuim (grant: PVCET3179-2022). They also thank the Foundation for the Support of Research and Scientific and Technological Development of Maranhão (FAPEMA) for funding the research initiation grant for the Institutional Scientific Initiation Scholarship Program (PIBIC/AGEUFMA Grant: PVCET3179-2022).

Institutional Review Board Statement: Not applicable.

Informed Consent Statement: Not applicable.

Data Availability Statement: The original contributions presented in this study are included in the article. Further inquiries can be directed to the corresponding author.

Acknowledgments: The authors would like to extend their special thanks to IMCD Brazil (São Paulo, SP, Brazil) for kindly providing the 974P NF polymer used in this study, and the Federal University of Technology–Paraná (UTFPR) and the Multi-User Research Support Laboratory at the Apucarana Campus (Lamap) for the DLS analyses.

Conflicts of Interest: The authors declare no conflicts of interest.

References

1. World Health Organization (WHO). *Neglected Tropical Diseases*. World Health Organization: Geneva, Switzerland, 2025. Available online: https://www.who.int/news-room/fact-sheets/detail/neglected-tropical-diseases (accessed on 2 February 2025).
2. Hotez, P.J.; Kamath, A. Neglected tropical diseases in sub-Saharan Africa: Review of their prevalence, distribution, and disease burden. *PLoS Negl. Trop. Dis.* **2009**, *3*, e412. [CrossRef]
3. Molyneux, D.H.; Savioli, L.; Engels, D. Neglected tropical diseases: Progress towards addressing the chronic pandemic. *Lancet* **2017**, *389*, 312–325. [CrossRef] [PubMed]
4. Fitzpatrick, C.; Nwankwo, U.; Lenk, E.; de Vlas, S.J.; Bundy, D.A.P. An Investment Case for Ending Neglected Tropical Diseases. In *Major Infectious Diseases*, 3rd ed.; Holmes, K.K., Bertozzi, S., Bloom, B.R., Jha, P., Eds.; The International Bank for Reconstruction and Development/The World Bank: Washington, DC, USA, 2017; Chapter 17.
5. Hotez, P.; Aksoy, S. PLOS Neglected Tropical Diseases: Ten years of progress in neglected tropical disease control and elimination ... More or less. *PLoS Negl. Trop. Dis.* **2017**, *11*, e0005355. [CrossRef] [PubMed]
6. Ezike, T.C.; Okpala, U.S.; Onoja, U.L.; Nwike, C.P.; Ezeako, E.C.; Okpara, O.J.; Okoroafor, C.C.; Eze, S.C.; Kalu, O.L.; Odoh, E.C.; et al. Advances in drug delivery systems, challenges and future directions. *Heliyon* **2023**, *9*, e17488. [CrossRef] [PubMed]
7. Zhang, Y.; Chan, H.F.; Leong, K.W. Advanced materials and processing for drug delivery: The past and the future. *Adv. Drug Deliv. Rev.* **2013**, *65*, 104–120. [CrossRef]
8. Cupolillo, E.; Grimaldi, G., Jr.; Momen, H. A general classification of New World Leishmania using numerical zymotaxonomy. *Am. J. Trop. Med. Hyg.* **1994**, *50*, 296–311. [CrossRef]
9. Kato, H.; Uezato, H.; Gomez, E.A.; Terayama, Y.; Calvopiña, M.; Iwata, H.; Hashiguchi, Y. Establishment of a mass screening method of sand fly vectors for Leishmania infection by molecular biological methods. *Am. J. Trop. Med. Hyg.* **2007**, *77*, 324–329. [CrossRef]
10. Mann, S.; Frasca, K.; Scherrer, S.; Henao-Martínez, A.F.; Newman, S.; Ramanan, P.; Suarez, J.A. A Review of Leishmaniasis: Current Knowledge and Future Directions. *Curr. Trop. Med. Rep.* **2021**, *8*, 121–132. [CrossRef]
11. da Costa, C.S.; Marques, E.M.; do Nascimento, J.R.; Lima, V.A.S.; Santos-Oliveira, R.; Figueredo, A.S.; de Jesus, C.M.; de Souza Nunes, G.C.; Brandão, C.M.; de Jesus, E.T.; et al. Design of Liquid Formulation Based on F127-Loaded Natural Dimeric Flavonoids as a New Perspective Treatment for Leishmaniasis. *Pharmaceutics* **2024**, *16*, 252. [CrossRef]
12. Marques, E.M.; Rocha, R.L.; Brandão, C.M.; Xavier, J.K.A.M.; Camara, M.B.P.; Mendonça, C.J.S.; de Lima, R.B.; Souza, M.P.; Costa, E.V.; Gonçalves, R.S. Development of an Eco-Friendly Nanogel Incorporating Pectis brevipedunculata Essential Oil as a Larvicidal Agent Against *Aedes aegypti*. *Pharmaceutics* **2024**, *16*, 1337. [CrossRef]
13. Marques, E.M.; Santos Andrade, L.G.; Rebelo Alencar, L.M.; Dias Rates, E.R.; Ribeiro, R.M.; Carvalho, R.C.; de Souza Nunes, G.C.; Sara Lopes Lera-Nonose, D.S.; Gonçalves, M.J.S.; Lonardoni, M.V.C.; et al. Nanotechnological formulation incorporating Pectis brevipedunculata (Asteraceae) essential oil: An ecofriendly approach for leishmanicidal and anti-inflammatory therapy. *Polymers* **2025**, *17*, 379. [CrossRef] [PubMed]
14. Carvalho, C.E.; Sobrinho-Junior, E.P.; Brito, L.M.; Nicolau, L.A.; Carvalho, T.P.; Moura, A.K.; Rodrigues, K.A.; Carneiro, S.M.; Arcanjo, D.D.; Citó, A.M.; et al. Anti-Leishmania activity of essential oil of Myracrodruon urundeuva (Engl.) Fr. All.: Composition, cytotoxicity and possible mechanisms of action. *Exp. Parasitol.* **2017**, *175*, 59–67. [CrossRef] [PubMed]
15. Ferreira, O.O.; Cruz, J.N.; de Moraes, Â.A.B.; de Jesus Pereira Franco, C.; Lima, R.R.; Anjos, T.O.D.; Siqueira, G.M.; Nascimento, L.D.D.; Cascaes, M.M.; de Oliveira, M.S.; et al. Essential oil of the plants growing in the Brazilian Amazon: Chemical composition, antioxidants, and biological applications. *Molecules* **2022**, *27*, 4373. [CrossRef] [PubMed]
16. de Lara da Silva, C.E.; Oyama, J.; Ferreira, F.B.P.; de Paula Lalucci-Silva, M.P.; Lordani, T.V.A.; de Lara da Silva, R.C.; de Souza Terron Monich, M.; Teixeira, J.J.V.; Lonardoni, M.V.C. Effect of essential oils on *Leishmania amazonensis*: A systematic review. *Parasitology* **2020**, *147*, 1392–1407. [CrossRef]
17. Alves, A.B.; da Silva Bortoleti, B.T.; Tomiotto-Pellissier, F.; Ganaza, A.F.M.; Gonçalves, M.D.; Carloto, A.C.M.; Rodrigues, A.C.J.; Silva, T.F.; Nakazato, G.; Kobayashi, R.K.T.; et al. Synergistic Antileishmanial Effect of Oregano Essential Oil and Silver Nanoparticles: Mechanisms of Action on *Leishmania amazonensis*. *Pathogens* **2023**, *12*, 660. [CrossRef]
18. Alanazi, A.D.; Alghabban, A.J. Antileishmanial and synergic effects of *Rhanterium epapposum* essential oil and its main compounds alone and combined with glucantime against *Leishmania major* infection. *Int. J. Parasitol. Drugs Drug Resist.* **2024**, *26*, 100571. [CrossRef]

19. Monzote, L.; Geroldinger, G.; Tonner, M.; Scull, R.; De Sarkar, S.; Bergmann, S.; Bacher, M.; Staniek, K.; Chatterjee, M.; Rosenau, T.; et al. Interaction of ascaridole, carvacrol, and caryophyllene oxide from essential oil of *Chenopodium ambrosioides* L. with mitochondria in *Leishmania* and other eukaryotes. *Phytother. Res.* **2018**, *32*, 1729–1740. [CrossRef]
20. Essid, R.; Damergi, B.; Fares, N.; Jallouli, S.; Limam, F.; Tabbene, O. Synergistic combination of *Cinnamomum verum* and *Syzygium aromaticum* treatment for cutaneous leishmaniasis and investigation of their molecular mechanism of action. *Int. J. Environ. Health Res.* **2024**, *34*, 2687–2701. [CrossRef]
21. Santana, R.C.; Rosa, A.D.S.; Mateus, M.H.D.S.; Soares, D.C.; Atella, G.; Guimarães, A.C.; Siani, A.C.; Ramos, M.F.S.; Saraiva, E.M.; Pinto-da-Silva, L.H. In vitro leishmanicidal activity of monoterpenes present in two species of *Protium* (Burseraceae) on *Leishmania amazonensis*. *J. Ethnopharmacol.* **2020**, *259*, 112981. [CrossRef]
22. Pereira, S.L.; Marques, A.M.; Sudo, R.T.; Kaplan, M.A.; Zapata-Sudo, G. Vasodilator Activity of the Essential Oil from Aerial Parts of *Pectis brevipedunculata* and Its Main Constituent Citral in Rat Aorta. *Molecules* **2013**, *18*, 3072–3085. [CrossRef]
23. Santos, S.R.; Melo, M.A.; Cardoso, A.V.; Santos, R.L.; de Sousa, D.P.; Cavalcanti, S.C. Structure-Activity Relationships of Larvicidal Monoterpenes and Derivatives against *Aedes aegypti* Linn. *Chemosphere* **2011**, *84*, 150–153. . [CrossRef] [PubMed]
24. Limane, B.B.; Ezzine, O.; Dhahri, S.; Ben Jamaa, M.L. Essential Oils from Two Eucalyptus from Tunisia and Their Insecticidal Action on *Orgyia trigotephras* (Lepidoptera, Lymantriidae). *Biol. Res.* **2014**, *47*, 29. [CrossRef]
25. Varzandeh, M.; Mohammadinejad, R.; Esmaeilzadeh-Salestani, K.; Dehshahri, A.; Zarrabi, A.; Aghaei-Afshar, A. Photodynamic therapy for leishmaniasis: Recent advances and future trends. *Photodiagn. Photodyn. Ther.* **2021**, *36*, 102609. [CrossRef] [PubMed]
26. Dourado, D.; Silva Medeiros, T.; do Nascimento Alencar, É.; Matos Sales, E.; Formiga, F.R. Curcumin-loaded nanostructured systems for treatment of leishmaniasis: A review. *Beilstein J. Nanotechnol.* **2024**, *15*, 37–50. [CrossRef] [PubMed]
27. Khan, M.; Nadhman, A.; Sehgal, S.A.; Siraj, S.; Yasinzai, M.M. Formulation and Characterization of a Self-Emulsifying Drug Delivery System (SEDDS) of Curcumin for the Topical Application in Cutaneous and Mucocutaneous Leishmaniasis. *Curr. Top. Med. Chem.* **2018**, *18*, 1603–1609. [CrossRef]
28. Suhail, M.; Rosenholm, J.M.; Minhas, M.U.; Badshah, S.F.; Naeem, A.; Khan, K.U.; Fahad, M. Nanogels as drug-delivery systems: A comprehensive overview. *Ther. Deliv.* **2019**, *10*, 697–717. [CrossRef]
29. Camara, M.B.P.; Lima, A.S.; Jumbo, L.O.V.; Tavares, C.P.; Mendonça, C.J.S.; Monteiro, O.S.; Araújo, S.H.C.; Oliveira, E.E.; Lima Neto, J.S.; Maia, J.G.S.; et al. Seasonal and Circadian Evaluation of the Essential Oil from *Pectis brevipedunculata* and Its Acaricidal Activity against *Rhipicephalus microplus* (Acari: Ixodidae). *J. Braz. Chem. Soc.* **2023**, *34*, 1020–1029.
30. *United States Pharmacopeia and National Formulary (USP 41-NF 36)*; United States Pharmacopeial Convention: Rockville, MD, USA, 2016.
31. Alexander, S.; Cosgrove, T.; Prescott, S.W.; Castle, T.C. Flurbiprofen Encapsulation Using Pluronic Triblock Copolymers. *Langmuir* **2011**, *27*, 8054–8060. [CrossRef]
32. Haillant, O.; Dumbleton, D.; Zielnik, A. An Arrhenius Approach to Estimating Organic Photovoltaic Module Weathering Acceleration Factors. *Sol. Energy Mater. Sol. Cells* **2011**, *95*, 1889–1895. [CrossRef]
33. Griffiths, P.C.; Stilbs, P.; Yu, G.E.; Booth, C. Role of Molecular Architecture in Polymer Diffusion: A PGSE-NMR Study of Linear and Cyclic Poly(ethylene Oxide). *J. Phys. Chem.* **1995**, *99*, 16752–16756. [CrossRef]
34. De, M.; Bhattacharya, S.C.; Moulik, S.P.; Panda, A.K. Interfacial Composition, Structural and Thermodynamic Parameters of Water/(Surfactant+n-Butanol)/n-Heptane Water-in-Oil Microemulsion Formation in Relation to the Surfactant Chain Length. *J. Surfactants Deterg.* **2010**, *13*, 475–484. [CrossRef]
35. Hwang, D.; Ramsey, J.D.; Kabanov, A.V. Polymeric micelles for the delivery of poorly soluble drugs: From nanoformulation to clinical approval. *Adv. Drug Deliv. Rev.* **2020**, *156*, 80–118. [CrossRef] [PubMed]
36. Chakraborty, M.; Panda, A.K. Spectral Behaviour of Eosin Y in Different Solvents and Aqueous Surfactant Media. *Spectrochim. Acta Part Mol. Biomol. Spectrosc.* **2011**, *81*, 458–465. [CrossRef] [PubMed]
37. Alexandridis, P.; Hatton, T.A. Poly(ethylene Oxide)-poly(propylene Oxide)-poly(ethylene Oxide) Block Copolymer Surfactants in Aqueous Solutions and at Interfaces: Thermodynamics, Structure, Dynamics, and Modeling. *Colloids Surfaces Physicochem. Eng. Asp.* **1995**, *96*, 1–46. [CrossRef]
38. Wanka, G.; Hoffmann, H.; Ulbricht, W. Phase Diagrams and Aggregation Behavior of Poly(oxyethylene)-Poly(oxypropylene)-Poly(oxyethylene) Triblock Copolymers in Aqueous Solutions. *Macromolecules* **1994**, *27*, 4145–4159. [CrossRef]
39. Alexander, S.; Cosgrove, T.; Castle, T.C.; Grillo, I.; Prescott, S.W. Effect of Temperature, Cosolvent, and Added Drug on Pluronic–Flurbiprofen Micellization. *J. Phys. Chem. B* **2012**, *116*, 11545–11551. [CrossRef]
40. Brown, W.; Schillin, K. Triblock Copolymers in Aqueous Solution Studied by Static and Dynamic Light Scattering and Oscillatory Shear Measurements: Influence of Relative Block Sizes. *Am. Chem. Soc.* **1992**, *6044*, 6038–6044. [CrossRef]
41. Sharma, P.K.; Bhatia, S.R. Effect of Anti-Inflammatories on Pluronic® F127: Micellar Assembly, Gelation and Partitioning. *Int. J. Pharm.* **2004**, *278*, 361–377. [CrossRef]
42. Nilsson, M.; Håkansson, B.; Söderman, O.; Topgaard, D. Influence of Polydispersity on the Micellization of Triblock Copolymers Investigated by Pulsed Field Gradient Nuclear Magnetic Resonance. *Macromolecules* **2007**, *40*, 8250–8258. [CrossRef]

43. Landazuri, G.; Fernandez, V.V.A.; Soltero, J.F.A.; Rharbi, Y. Kinetics of the Sphere-to-Rod like Micelle Transition in a Pluronic Triblock Copolymer. *J. Phys. Chem. B* **2012**, *116*, 11720–11727. [CrossRef]
44. Brown, W.; Stilbs, P. On the Solution Conformation of Poly(ethylene Oxide): An FT-Pulsed Field Gradient NMR Self-Diffusion Study. *Polymer* **1982**, *23*, 1780–1784. . [CrossRef]
45. Espenson, J.H. *Chemical Kinetics and Reaction Mechanisms*, 2nd ed.; McGraw-Hill Series in Advanced Chemistry; McGraw-Hill: New York, NY, USA, 1995.
46. Dash, S.K.; Benival, D.; Jindal, A.B. Formulation strategies to overcome amphotericin B-induced toxicity. *Mol. Pharm.* **2024**, *21*, 5392–5412. [CrossRef] [PubMed]
47. Kuti, J.L. Optimizing Antimicrobial Pharmacodynamics: A Guide for Your Stewardship Program. *Rev. Med. Clin. Condes* **2016**, *27*, 615–624. [CrossRef]

pharmaceutics

MDPI

Systematic Review

The Role of Photodynamic Therapy Mediated by Natural Photosensitisers in the Management of Peri-Implantitis: A Systematic Review

Aleksandra Warakomska [1], Jakub Fiegler-Rudol [1,*], Magdalena Kubizna [2], Dariusz Skaba [1] and Rafał Wiench [1,*]

[1] Department of Periodontal Diseases and Oral Mucosa Diseases, Faculty of Medical Sciences in Zabrze, Medical University of Silesia, 40-055 Katowice, Poland; awarakomska@sum.edu.pl (A.W.); dskaba@sum.edu.pl (D.S.)

[2] Department of Oral Surgery, Faculty of Medical Sciences in Zabrze, Medical University of Silesia, 40-055 Katowice, Poland; mkubizna@acstom.bytom.pl

* Correspondence: jakub.fiegler@gmail.com (J.F.-R.); rwiench@sum.edu.pl (R.W.)

Abstract: Background: Peri-implantitis, an inflammatory condition leading to progressive bone loss around dental implants, represents a significant challenge in modern implant dentistry. Conventional mechanical debridement and adjunctive antibiotics or antiseptics often fail to fully eradicate complex biofilms and may promote antibiotic resistance. Photodynamic therapy (PDT) mediated by natural photosensitizers (e.g., curcumin, riboflavin, and 5-aminolevulinic acid) has emerged as a potential adjunctive strategy for peri-implantitis management due to its targeted antimicrobial and anti-inflammatory effects. **Objectives**: This systematic review aimed to evaluate the antimicrobial efficacy, clinical outcomes, and safety of PDT mediated by natural photosensitizers in the treatment of peri-implantitis and to identify optimal protocols regarding photosensitizer concentrations, light source parameters, and application techniques. Methods: Following PRISMA 2020 guidelines, databases (PubMed/Medline, Embase, Scopus, and Cochrane Library) were searched from 1 January 2015 to 3 January 2025 for English-language publications. Studies assessing naturally based PDT interventions for peri-implantitis or in vitro biofilms from diseased implant surfaces were included. Quality assessment used the Revised Cochrane Risk of Bias tool (RoB 2) for randomized controlled trials and a tailored nine-item framework for in vitro studies. Eleven studies met the inclusion criteria. **Results**: Despite heterogeneity in methodologies, especially regarding light wavelengths, energy densities, and photosensitizer formulations, most studies reported notable reductions in bacterial viability, biofilm mass, and clinical indices (probing depth and bleeding on probing). Curcumin and riboflavin frequently demonstrated comparable antimicrobial efficacy to standard disinfectants, while 5-aminolevulinic acid (5-ALA)-based PDT also showed promising clinical and microbiological improvements. However, complete biofilm eradication was rarely achieved. **Conclusions**: Natural-photosensitizer-based PDT appears to be a valuable adjunct to mechanical debridement for peri-implantitis, enhancing microbial control and clinical outcomes. Standardization of PDT protocols and further well-designed clinical trials with extended follow-up periods are warranted to confirm long-term efficacy and inform evidence-based guidelines.

Keywords: peri-implantitis; photodynamic therapy; curcumin; riboflavin; 5-ALA; antimicrobial therapy; dental implants; biofilm

1. Introduction

1.1. Rationale

Peri-implant diseases are inflammatory conditions around dental implants, such as peri-implant mucositis and peri-implantitis [1]. They involve inflammation that may lead to supporting bone loss [2] and are a growing concern in implant dentistry [1,2]. Peri-implant mucositis is a reversible condition marked by redness, swelling, and bleeding on probing without further bone loss [3], whereas peri-implantitis is irreversible, showing similar inflammatory signs with progressive bone loss and increased probing depths [2,4–9]. This progression parallels the transition from gingivitis to periodontitis in natural teeth, highlighting the need for early intervention [2–9]. The primary etiological factor is the oral biofilm [10]; however, systemic and local factors, including diabetes mellitus, tobacco use, genetic predisposition, insufficient keratinized gingiva, poor oral hygiene, and prosthetic design flaws, also play a role [11,12]. Furthermore, metallosis from titanium particles and ions released due to tribocorrosion and fretting can elicit an inflammatory response that exacerbates bone loss [13–17]. Management typically relies on mechanical debridement to disrupt biofilms [18–20], but this method often fails to eradicate biofilm from the implant's surface. Adjunctive antiseptics and antibiotics have been used to improve outcomes; however, they are associated with antibiotic resistance, adverse side effects, and limited long-term efficacy [19–21]. Consequently, alternative strategies are being explored, such as photodynamic therapy (PDT), which uses light, a photosensitizer, and oxygen to generate reactive oxygen species that destroy microbial cells [22,23]. PDT's distinct mechanism reduces resistance risk and allows for targeted microbial killing [24]. Recent attention has focused on natural photosensitizers like curcumin and riboflavin for antimicrobial photodynamic therapy (aPDT) [25,26]. These agents are biocompatible, exhibit broad-spectrum antimicrobial activity and possess anti-inflammatory and antioxidant properties, making them suitable for managing peri-implant diseases [22–26]. Curcumin, a polyphenol, disrupts biofilm integrity and has potent antimicrobial effects [26,27], while riboflavin, upon light activation, produces singlet oxygen and other reactive oxygen species that target bacterial membranes and DNA [25,28,29]. Both also promote wound healing and reduce inflammation, aiding in the management of peri-implant tissue damage [28,29].

1.2. Objectives

The primary objective of this systematic review is to evaluate the clinical efficacy, antimicrobial potential, and safety of aPDT mediated by natural photosensitisers in the management of peri-implantitis. Additionally, it seeks to identify optimal treatment protocols, including light source parameters, photosensitizer concentrations, and application techniques, to provide evidence-based recommendations for clinical use. By addressing these aspects, this review intends to bridge the gap between experimental findings and practical applications, offering insights into the potential of these natural photosensitizers as adjunctive therapies in peri-implantitis management.

2. Materials and Methods

2.1. Focused Question

A systematic review was conducted following the PICO framework [30], structured as follows: in patients with clinically diagnosed peri-implantitis or ex vivo specimens (biofilms) derived from the diseased implant surfaces—reflecting the true polymicrobial biofilm complexity observed in peri-implantitis (population), does treatment with antimicrobial photodynamic therapy mediated by natural photosensitisers (intervention), compared to traditional mechanical debridement, the use of natural photosensitisers alone, or other non-surgical therapies (comparison), result in more effective management or reduction of peri-implantitis symptoms (outcome)?

2.2. Search Strategy

This systematic review was registered with PROSPERO under the registration number CRD42025635967. The review process was aligned with the PRISMA 2020 (Preferred Reporting Items for Systematic Reviews and Meta-Analyses) guidelines to ensure comprehensive and transparent reporting [31]. An extensive literature search was executed across several databases, including PubMed/Medline, Embase, Scopus, and the Cochrane Library, using the specific search terms detailed in Table 1. Three researchers independently conducted the database searches employing identical search strategies to maintain consistency. To refine the search results, inclusion criteria were set to encompass studies published from 1 January 2015 to 3 January 2025 and limited to articles published in English. Following the initial retrieval, studies were screened based on their titles and abstracts to ascertain their relevance and adherence to the inclusion criteria outlined in Section 2.3. Subsequently, two authors performed a comprehensive full-text assessment of the shortlisted articles to extract pertinent data systematically. In addition to the primary search, a snowballing technique was employed by reviewing the reference lists of eligible studies to identify any further relevant research that might have been missed initially. This review proposes that photodynamic therapy utilizing natural photosensitizers may offer a superior or supplementary approach to the management of peri-implantitis, potentially enhancing treatment outcomes compared to traditional non-surgical interventions. Studies incorporated into this analysis were meticulously selected based on defined inclusion and exclusion criteria to ensure the relevance and quality of the evidence gathered. Figure 1 shows the selection process.

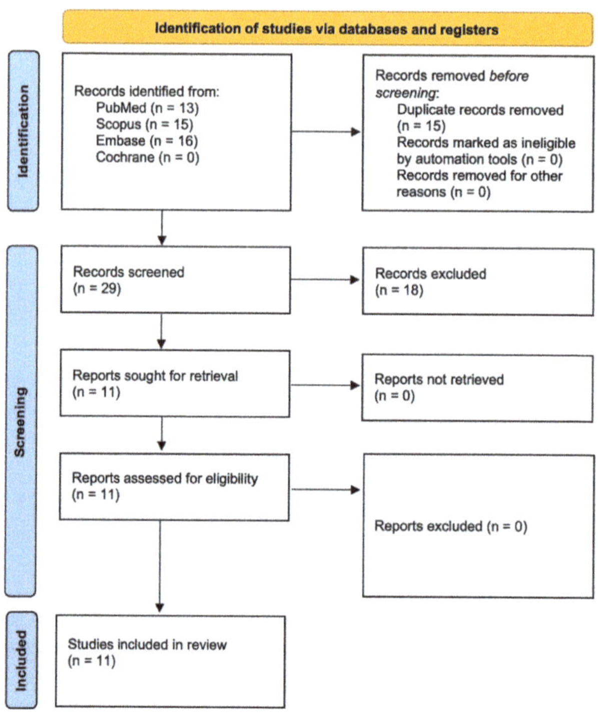

Figure 1. Prisma 2020 flow diagram.

Table 1. Search syntax used in the study.

Source	Search Term	Number of Results
Medline via PubMed	(("Curcumin"[MeSH] OR "Curcumin") OR ("Riboflavin"[MeSH] OR "Riboflavin" OR "Vitamin B2") OR ("Hypericin"[MeSH] OR "Hypericin") OR ("Chlorophyll"[MeSH] OR "Chlorophyll" OR "Chlorophyllin") OR ("Carotenoids"[MeSH] OR "Carotenoids" OR "Lycopene") OR ("Hematoporphyrins"[MeSH] OR "Hematoporphyrin Derivatives") OR ("5-Aminolevulinic Acid"[MeSH] OR "5-ALA" OR "Aminolevulinic Acid") OR ("Phthalocyanines"[MeSH] OR "Phthalocyanines" OR "ZnPc" OR "AlPc" OR "AlClPc") OR ("Protoporphyrins"[MeSH] OR "Protoporphyrin IX" OR "Natural porphyrins")) AND (("Photodynamic Therapy"[MeSH] OR "Photodynamic Therapy" OR "PDT")) AND (("Peri-implantitis"[MeSH] OR "Peri-implantitis"))	13
Scopus	(TITLE-ABS-KEY("Curcumin") OR TITLE-ABS-KEY("Riboflavin") OR TITLE-ABS-KEY("Vitamin B2") OR TITLE-ABS-KEY("Hypericin") OR TITLE-ABS-KEY("Chlorophyll") OR TITLE-ABS-KEY("Chlorophyllin") OR TITLE-ABS-KEY("Carotenoids") OR TITLE-ABS-KEY("Lycopene") OR TITLE-ABS-KEY("Hematoporphyrin Derivatives") OR TITLE-ABS-KEY("5-Aminolevulinic Acid") OR TITLE-ABS-KEY("5-ALA") OR TITLE-ABS-KEY("Aminolevulinic Acid") OR TITLE-ABS-KEY("Phthalocyanines") OR TITLE-ABS-KEY("ZnPc") OR TITLE-ABS-KEY("AlPc") OR TITLE-ABS-KEY("AlClPc") OR TITLE-ABS-KEY("Protoporphyrin IX") OR TITLE-ABS-KEY("Natural porphyrins")) AND (TITLE-ABS-KEY("Photodynamic Therapy") OR TITLE-ABS-KEY("PDT")) AND (TITLE-ABS-KEY("Peri-implantitis"))	15
Embase	(("curcumin"/exp OR "curcumin") OR ("riboflavin"/exp OR "riboflavin" OR "vitamin B2") OR ("hypericin"/exp OR "hypericin") OR ("chlorophyll"/exp OR "chlorophyllin" OR "chlorophyll") OR ("carotenoid"/exp OR "carotenoids" OR "lycopene") OR ("hematoporphyrin derivative"/exp OR "hematoporphyrin derivatives") OR ("5-aminolevulinic acid"/exp OR "5-ALA" OR "aminolevulinic acid") OR ("phthalocyanine"/exp OR "phthalocyanines" OR "ZnPc" OR "AlPc" OR "AlClPc") OR ("protoporphyrin"/exp OR "protoporphyrin IX" OR "natural porphyrins")) AND ("photodynamic therapy"/exp OR "photodynamic therapy" OR "PDT") AND ("periimplantitis"/exp OR "peri-implantitis" OR "periimplantitis")	16
Cochrane data base	((MH "Curcumin" OR "Curcumin") OR (MH "Riboflavin" OR "Riboflavin" OR "Vitamin B2") OR (MH "Hypericin" OR "Hypericin") OR (MH "Chlorophyll" OR "Chlorophyllin" OR "Chlorophyll") OR (MH "Carotenoids" OR "Carotenoids" OR "Lycopene") OR (MH "Hematoporphyrins" OR "Hematoporphyrin Derivatives") OR (MH "5-Aminolevulinic Acid" OR "5-ALA" OR "Aminolevulinic Acid") OR (MH "Phthalocyanines" OR "Phthalocyanines" OR "ZnPc" OR "AlPc" OR "AlClPc") OR (MH "Protoporphyrins" OR "Protoporphyrin IX" OR "Natural porphyrins")) AND (MH "Photodynamic Therapy" OR "Photodynamic Therapy" OR "PDT") AND (MH "Peri-implantitis" OR "Peri-implantitis")	0

2.3. Selection of Studies

In the selection phase of this systematic review, each reviewer individually assessed the titles and abstracts of the retrieved articles to ensure impartiality. When disagreements arose concerning a study's eligibility, the reviewers engaged in collective discussions until they reached unanimous consensus. This meticulous approach, in line with PRISMA guidelines, guaranteed that only the most relevant and high-quality studies were incorporated into the analysis, thereby enhancing the review's reliability and reproducibility [31]. The following inclusion and exclusion were used to decide which studies to include.

Inclusion criteria are shown as follows:

- Investigations utilizing natural photosensitizers in photodynamic therapy for the treatment of peri-implantitis, encompassing both in vitro and animal studies.
- Randomized controlled trials where natural photosensitizers serve as the primary photosensitizer in PDT for managing peri-implantitis.
- Research evaluating the combined effects of natural photosensitizers in PDT with other antimicrobial or anti-inflammatory treatments.
- Studies incorporating control groups that compare aPDT mediated by natural photosensitisers against standard mechanical debridement, alternative non-surgical therapies, or no treatment.
- Studies directly comparing the effectiveness of aPDT mediated by natural photosensitisers with other non-surgical treatment modalities for peri-implantitis.
- Research featuring extended follow-up periods to assess the sustained impact of naturally mediated aPDT on peri-implantitis management.
- Articles that meet predefined quality standards and specifically address the reduction or management of peri-implantitis symptoms using naturally mediated aPDT.

Exclusion criteria are shown as follows:

- Unpublished theses, conference abstracts, dissertations, and other non-peer-reviewed materials.
- Articles published in languages other than English.
- No full text available.
- Multiple reports of the same study or those sharing identical ethical approval numbers.
- Research focused on dental or medical issues unrelated to peri-implantitis.
- Studies utilizing synthetic photosensitizing agents.
- Laboratory studies that do not replicate oral conditions pertinent to peri-implantitis or fail to address relevant microbial strains.
- Case reports, case series, narrative reviews, systematic reviews, editorials, books, and other formats that do not provide original research data.
- Studies that do not include a control or comparison group.
- Applications of PDT not intended as a therapeutic method for peri-implantitis.

Limiting the review to English-language publications and excluding the grey literature was a deliberate choice to ensure methodological rigor and manage resource constraints, as English-language studies typically represent the bulk of high-quality, peer-reviewed research and the grey literature often lacks a comprehensive peer review needed for reliable data extraction. This approach enhances the consistency, reproducibility, and overall reliability of the review, though it may introduce language and publication biases by potentially overlooking relevant studies published in other languages or in non-peer-reviewed formats.

2.4. Data Extraction

At the beginning of the study selection, each reviewer separately evaluated the titles and abstracts of the retrieved articles to reduce the risk of bias. The agreement between reviewers was quantified using Cohen's kappa statistic to ensure consistent decision-making [32]. In cases where reviewers disagreed on the eligibility of a study, thorough discussions were conducted among the authors until a unanimous consensus was reached. After finalizing the selection of relevant studies, the three reviewers systematically extracted comprehensive data from each included article. The data encompassed bibliographic information such as the first author and publication year, study design, specific peri-implantitis cases addressed, and the types of test and control groups used. Additionally, they recorded the duration of follow-up periods and measured outcomes related to peri-implantitis management. They detailed the specifications of the light sources employed, including type, wavelength, and power parameters. Information on the concentrations of photosensitizers, the incorporation of nanocarriers or other adjunctive substances, as well as the incubation and irradiation times during photodynamic therapy, was also meticulously documented. This thorough data extraction process ensured that all relevant variables were captured, enabling a robust and comprehensive analysis of the efficacy and parameters of naturally mediated photodynamic therapy in the treatment of peri-implantitis. Our systematic review identified significant clinical heterogeneity among studies evaluating naturally mediated photodynamic therapy for peri-implantitis. Variability in photosensitizer concentrations, light source parameters, incubation times, and study designs complicates direct comparisons and efficacy interpretation. Standardized protocols and further high-quality trials are needed to optimize aPDT for clinical use. Outcome measurements in this systematic review primarily include microbial load reduction (colony-forming units per milliliter, CFU/mL), biofilm mass reduction (crystal violet assay, scanning electron microscopy), changes in microbial viability and metabolic activity, reactive oxygen species (ROS) generation, downregulation of biofilm-related genes, and clinical improvements such as bleeding on probing (BoP), probing depth (PD), plaque index (PI), and marginal bone level (MBL), providing a comprehensive evaluation of the efficacy of naturally mediated photodynamic therapy in managing peri-implantitis.

3. Results

3.1. Study Selection

Figure 1 presents the comprehensive research process aligned with the PRISMA guidelines [31]. The initial literature search identified 44 articles, which were subsequently reduced to 29 after removing duplicates. Upon reviewing the titles and abstracts, 11 studies were selected for full-text assessment. 2 Studies were excluded, as they were reviews [33,34]. Ultimately, 11 studies were included in the final analysis.

3.2. Quality Assessment Presentation and Risk of Bias in Individual Studies

For clinical studies, the quality assessment was conducted using the Revised Cochrane Risk of Bias Tool (RoB 2) for randomized controlled trials (RCTs) [35,36]. We applied the RoB2 by evaluating key domains—randomization, deviations from intended interventions, missing outcome data, outcome measurement, and selective reporting—assigning ratings of low risk, some concerns, or high risk to inform our overall assessment. For the in vitro studies, we developed a tailored framework based on nine essential criteria: clear specification of photosensitizer concentration and origin, defined incubation period, detailed light source parameters (wavelength, power, fluence, and power density), use of a calibrated power meter, inclusion of a negative control group, presentation of statistical analyses, completeness of outcome data, and independence from funding sources. These criteria were chosen to ensure methodological consistency, reproducibility, and reliability of findings, thereby strengthening the rigor of our review. The results of this test is shown in Table 2.

Table 2. Results of the RoB2 test for RCTs.

Study	Study Type	Randomization Process	Deviations from Intended Interventions	Missing Outcome Data	Measurement of Outcomes	Selective Reporting	Overall RoB 2 Rating
Qamar et al., 2023 [37]	RCT	Low risk	Some concerns	Low risk	Low risk	Low risk	Some concerns

The methodological quality of the other study types was independently evaluated by three reviewers, focusing on key aspects of PDT protocols, including study design, implementation, and data analysis, to ensure objectivity and result reliability. Potential biases were identified by assigning a score of 1 for each affirmative ("yes") response and 0 for each negative ("no") response based on predefined evaluation criteria: (1) specification of photosensitizer concentration, (2) disclosure of the photosensitizer's origin or source, (3) clear definition of the incubation period, (4) provision of detailed light source specifications (type, wavelength, output power, fluence, and power density), (5) use of a power meter to measure light parameters, (6) inclusion of a negative control group in the experimental design, (7) presentation of numerical results with relevant statistical analyses, (8) absence of missing data regarding study outcomes, and (9) independence of the study from its funding sources. Extracted data were systematically analyzed and categorized based on the total number of affirmative responses, with the risk of bias classified as high (0–3 points), moderate (4–6 points), or low (7–9 points). Each study's total score determined its corresponding bias risk level according to the guidelines in *The Cochrane Handbook for Systematic Reviews of Interventions* [38]. This rigorous quality assessment ensured that only studies with robust and reliable methodologies were included in the systematic review, thereby enhancing the overall validity and credibility of the findings. The results of this quality assessment are presented in Table 3.

Table 3. The results of the quality assessment for the in vitro studies.

Author and Year	1	2	3	4	5	6	7	8	9	Total Score	Risk
Etemadi et al., 2023 [39]	1	1	1	1	0	1	1	1	0	7	Low
Leelanarathiwatat et al., 2020 [40]	1	0	1	1	0	1	1	1	1	7	Low
Mahdizade-Ari et al., 2019 [41]	1	0	1	1	1	1	1	1	1	8	Low
Morelato et al., 2022 [42]	1	1	1	1	0	1	1	1	1	8	Low
Pourhajibagher et al., 2019 [43]	1	1	1	1	1	1	1	1	1	9	Low
Tonon et al., 2022 [44]	1	0	0	1	0	1	1	1	0	5	Moderate
Wenzler et al., 2024 [45]	1	0	1	1	0	1	1	1	1	7	Low
Rossi et al., 2022 [46]	1	1	1	1	0	1	1	1	0	7	Low
Petrini et al., 2022 [47]	1	1	1	1	0	1	1	1	0	7	Low
Radunović et al., 2020 [48]	1	1	1	1	0	1	1	1	0	7	Low

3.3. Data Presentation

Tables 4–11 present a comprehensive summary of the data extracted from the eight studies that satisfied the inclusion criteria and were incorporated into the review. The tables detail the general characteristics of the studies, the properties of the light sources utilized, and the specific features of employed photosensitizers in aPDT protocols.

Table 4. A general overview of the studies.

Author and Year	Country	Study Design
Qamar et al., 2023 [37]	Saudi Arabia	Clinical study
Etemadi et al., 2023 [39]	Iran and Italy	In vitro
Leelanarathiwatat et al., 2020 [40]	Thailand and Japan	In vitro
Mahdizade-Ari et al., 2019 [41]	Iran	In vitro
Morelato et al., 2022 [42]	Croatia, Bosnia, and Herzegovina	In vitro
Pourhajibagher et al., 2019 [43]	Iran and Italy	In vitro
Tonon et al., 2022 [44]	Brazil and USA	In vitro
Wenzler et al., 2024 [45]	Germany	In vitro
Rossi et al., 2022 [46]	Italy	Retrospective Analysis
Petrini et al., 2022 [47]	Italy	In vitro
Radunović et al., 2020 [48]	Serbia and Italy	In vitro

Table 5. Main details from RCTs.

Author and Year	Species	Photosensitizer Concentration	Outcome Measures
Qamar et al., 2023 [37]	*Porphyromonas gingivalis* and *Tannerella forsythia*	Riboflavin loaded on poly-L-glycolic acid nanoparticles incorporated in aloe vera gel (PGA/RF/AV) 0.1% riboflavin concentration in the PGA/RF/AV gel	Significant reduction in microbial counts of *P. gingivalis* and *T. forsythia* Improvement in clinical parameters: BoP, PD, PI, and MBL; Enhanced treatment outcomes compared to PDT alone.

Table 6. Main details from each in vitro study.

Author and Year	Species	Photosensitizer Concentration	Outcome Measures
Etemadi et al., 2023 [39]	*A. actinomycetemcomitans*	Curcumin (5 mg/mL); Riboflavin (0.5%)	CFU/mL: quantitative measure of bacterial reduction. Groups were analyzed to determine the efficacy of treatments in reducing A.a biofilm.
Leelanarathiwatat et al., 2020 [40]	*Staphylococcus aureus*	MB: 10 mg/mL FMN: 0.18 mg/mL	Log reduction in CFU/mL (colony-forming units); Biofilm mass reduction measured by crystal violet assay; Direct observation using SEM and fluorescent stereomicroscopy.
Mahdizade-Ari et al., 2019 [41]	*A. actinomycetemcomitans*	Curcumin: 80 µg/mL	Reduction in microbial cell survival; Decrease in metabolic activity; Reduction in quorum sensing; No significant change in efflux capacity.
Morelato et al., 2022 [42]	*Staphylococcus aureus* and *Candida albicans*	Riboflavin (0.1%) MB (0.1%)	Reduction in CFU of *Staphylococcus aureus* and *Candida albicans*. Antimicrobial effect was comparable between 445 nm riboflavin and 660 nm methylene blue photodynamic therapy protocols. SEM analysis showed reduced biofilm, but some microorganisms remained visible.
Pourhajibagher et al., 2019 [43]	*Aggregatibacter actinomycetemcomitans*, *Porphyromonas gingivalis*, and *Prevotella intermedia*	GQD-Cur: 100 µg/mL	Reduction in microbial cell viability; Reduction in biofilm biomass; Significant ROS generation in a dose-dependent manner; Downregulation of biofilm-related genes: rcpA (8.1-fold), fimA (9.6-fold), and inpA (11.8-fold).
Tonon et al., 2022 [44]	*Porphyromonas gingivalis*, *Fusobacterium nucleatum*, and *Streptococcus oralis*	Curcumin-loaded polymeric nanoparticles (Curcumin-NP) Concentration: 500 µg/mL	Reduction in bacterial viability in planktonic cultures (log reduction values); Limited antibiofilm activity on multispecies biofilms; Significant antimicrobial effects when photoactivated with blue light (420 nm); Non-cytotoxic to human periodontal ligament fibroblast cells.

Table 6. *Cont.*

Author and Year	Species	Photosensitizer Concentration	Outcome Measures
Wenzler et al., 2024 [45]	*Aggregatibacter actinomycetemcomitans*, *Campylobacter rectus*, *Eikenella corrodens*, *Fusobacterium nucleatum*, *Porphyromonas gingivalis*, *Prevotella intermedia*, *Parvimonas micra*, *Treponema denticola*, and *Tannerella forsythia*	PDT: HELBO® Blue Photosensitizer; PTT: EmunDo® dye; Curcumin/DMSO solution: curcumin: 100 mg/L with 0.5% DMSO.	PDT: bacterial reduction; PTT: bacterial reduction; Curcumin/DMSO + laser: bacterial reduction.
Petrini et al., 2022 [47]	*Streptococcus oralis*	ALAD 5%	Reduction in bacterial biofilm on infected titanium surfaces
Radunović et al., 2020 [48]	*Enterococcus faecalis*, *Escherichia coli*, *Staphylococcus aureus*, *Veillonella parvula*, and *Porphyromonas gingivalis*	ALAD 10%, 25%, and 50%	Reductions in CFU

CFU—colony-forming units; MB—methylene blue; FMN—flavin mononucleotide; GQD-Cur—curcumin doped with graphene quantum dots; ROS—reactive oxygen species; BoP—bleeding on probing; PD—probing depth; PI—plaque index; MBL—marginal bone level; PDT—photodynamic therapy; PTT—photothermal therapy; SEM—scanning electron microscopy; DMSO—dimethyl sulfoxide; NP—nanoparticles; ALAD—5-aminolevulinic acid.

Table 7. Main details from the retrospective study.

Author and Year	Species	Photosensitizer Concentration	Outcome Measures
Rossi et al., 2022 [46]	*Porphyromonas gingivalis*, *Prevotella intermedia*, *Aggregatibacter actinomycetemcomitans*, *Fusobacterium nucleatum*, *Tannerella forsythia*, *Streptococcus* spp., *Staphylococcus* spp., and *Enterococcus faecalis*	ALAD 5%	PPD, BOP, MOB, REC, and VAS

PPD—probing pocket depth; BOP—bleeding on probing; MOB—mobility; VAS—visual analogue scale; REC—recession.

Table 8. Main outcomes and study groups from the RCT.

Author/Year	Study Groups	Main Results
Qamar et al., 2023 [37]	Riboflavin-loaded nanoparticles in aloe vera gel (PGA/RF/AV) + MD. Treated with riboflavin-mediated PDT combined with MD. Treated with MD alone.	Riboflavin-loaded nanoparticles incorporated into aloe vera gel (PGA/RF/AV) both showed effectiveness in treating peri-implantitis in diabetic patients, with the PGA/RF/AV complex achieving superior clinical and microbiological outcomes. While both treatment approaches significantly reduced microbial counts of *Porphyromonas gingivalis* and *Tannerella forsythia* and improved parameters like probing depth, plaque index, and marginal bone levels, the PGA/RF/AV complex was particularly effective in reducing bleeding on probing and minimizing microbial loads over six months. This highlights the potential of combining riboflavin with aloe vera for enhanced antimicrobial and anti-inflammatory effects.

PGA—poly(γ-glutamic acid); RF—riboflavin; AV—aloe vera; MD—mechanical debridement; PDT—photodynamic therapy; PD—probing depth; PI—plaque index; BOP—bleeding on probing.

Table 9. Main outcomes and study groups for non-RCT studies.

Reference	Author/Year	Study Groups	Main Results
[39]	Etemadi et al., 2023	Negative control: sterile PBS wash only. Positive Control: 0.12% chlorhexidine. Curcumin alone: moderate antibacterial effect, comparable to PDT with curcumin. Riboflavin alone: lesser antibacterial effect than curcumin. LED alone: minimal effect on CFU/mL reduction. PDT with curcumin + LED: highly effective, second only to chlorhexidine. PDT with riboflavin + LED: moderately effective but less than curcumin-based PDT.	PDT with curcumin + LED was significantly more effective than PDT with riboflavin + LED, showing greater reductions in bacterial colonies (CFU/mL) compared to riboflavin-based PDT, LED alone, and the negative control. Curcumin-based PDT exhibited antimicrobial properties comparable to CHX, the gold standard, highlighting its potential as a non-invasive disinfection method. In contrast, PDT with riboflavin + LED achieved moderate reductions in CFU/mL, though it was less effective than curcumin-based PDT. These results suggest that curcumin is a more promising photosensitizer for PDT due to its superior bactericidal activity and potential as a safe alternative for implant surface decontamination.
[40]	Leelanarathiwatat et al., 2020	Control group Light groups: biofilm exposed to light sources only. Red diode laser: applied for 60 s. Blue LED: applied for 10 s. Photosensitizer groups: biofilm treated with photosensitizers only. Methylene blue: no light activation. FMN: no light activation. Photoactivated PS groups (aPDT): MB with a red diode laser (MB*R): activated for 60 s. FMN with blue LED (FMN*B): activated for 10 s.	Riboflavin-mediated photodynamic therapy using FMN activated by blue LED light demonstrated significant antibacterial effects against Staphylococcus aureus biofilms, achieving a log reduction of 1.23 (approximately 93% reduction in viable bacteria) and a 52–62% decrease in biofilm mass. The blue LED alone showed no antibacterial activity, confirming the essential role of FMN activation. FMN-mediated PDT was as effective as MB-mediated PDT activated by a red diode laser but required only 10 s of irradiation compared to 60 s for MB, offering a faster and more practical treatment option. Additionally, FMN's light yellow color was noted for cosmetic ease of removal. However, while effective, FMN-PDT did not completely eradicate bacteria, particularly in deeper biofilm layers, suggesting it is best used in combination with other therapies. These findings highlight FMN-PDT as a promising and efficient method for biofilm reduction with potential clinical advantages.
[41]	Mahdizade-Ari et al., 2019	Whole bacterial cell suspension from *A. actinomycetemcomitans* treated with Cur-aPDT. Whole bacterial cell suspension from untreated *A. actinomycetemcomitans*. Cell-free supernatant fluid from *A. actinomycetemcomitans* treated with Cur-aPDT. Cell-free supernatant fluid from untreated *A. actinomycetemcomitans*. Bacterial cell pellet from *A. actinomycetemcomitans* treated with Cur-aPDT. Bacterial cell pellet from untreated *A. actinomycetemcomitans*.	Cur-aPDT significantly reduces microbial cell survival, metabolic activity, and QS abilities in *Aggregatibacter actinomycetemcomitans*, with bystander effects playing a critical role. The therapy decreased cell survival by up to 82.7%, metabolic activity by 42.6%, and QS mediator production by 83.2%, particularly when using treated whole bacterial cell suspensions and cell-free supernatant fluids. These effects suggest that Cur-aPDT generates metabolites with antimicrobial properties that influence neighboring untreated cells, thereby enhancing the overall efficacy of the treatment. However, the therapy showed no significant impact on bacterial efflux pump activity. These findings indicate that the combined direct and bystander effects of Cur-aPDT could make it a potent adjunct therapy for managing localized infections such as periodontitis and peri-implantitis.

Table 9. *Cont.*

Reference	Author/Year	Study Groups	Main Results
[42]	Morelato et al., 2022	Negative control: no surface treatment was applied to the implants. Positive control: surface treatment with 0.2% CHX using a sterile cotton pellet for 60 s. Photodynamic therapy group 1: treatment using a 660 nm diode laser (red light) with 0.1% methylene blue as the photosensitizer. Photodynamic therapy group 2: Treatment using a 445 nm diode laser (blue light) with 0.1% riboflavin as the photosensitizer.	Riboflavin-mediated photodynamic therapy using a 445 nm diode laser for disinfecting contaminated dental implant surface was evaluated against a conventional PDT protocol involving methylene blue with a 660 nm laser and CHX treatment. Results revealed that both PDT approaches significantly reduced Staphylococcus aureus and Candida albicans biofilms, showing comparable efficacy to CHX. The riboflavin-445 nm combination offered aesthetic advantages over methylene blue, as it did not cause discoloration. However, no approach achieved complete microbial eradication, highlighting PDT as a complementary method to mechanical cleaning for peri-implantitis treatment. This study suggests the potential of riboflavin-based PDT as a safe, effective adjunctive therapy, particularly suitable for the aesthetic zone. Further in vivo studies are needed to validate these findings.
[43]	Pourhajibagher et al., 2019	Biofilms treated with GQD. Biofilms treated with curcumin. Biofilms treated with GQD-Cur. Biofilms exposed to blue LED. Biofilms treated with GQD and exposed to blue LED. Biofilms treated with curcumin and exposed to blue LED. Biofilms treated with GQD-Cur and exposed to blue LED. Control: untreated biofilms.	Cur-aPDT using GQD-Cur effectively suppresses perio-pathogens in both planktonic and biofilm forms. GQD-Cur composites were successfully synthesized and characterized using various techniques, confirming their structural and chemical properties, with minimal cytotoxicity to human gingival fibroblasts. Under blue LED irradiation, photoexcited GQD-Cur significantly reduced bacterial viability (93%) and biofilm formation capacity (76%), showing superior antimicrobial effects compared to other treatment groups. The treatment also induced a concentration-dependent increase in ROS production and markedly downregulated key biofilm-related gene expressions, including rcpA, fimA, and inpA, by 8.1-, 9.6-, and 11.8-fold, respectively. These findings highlight GQD-Cur as a promising, non-cytotoxic, nanoscale platform for enhanced antimicrobial photodynamic therapy in periodontitis management.
[44]	Tonon et al., 2022	Curcumin (free): with light activation (L+); without light activation (L−). Curcumin-loaded nanoparticles (Curcumin-NP): with light activation (L+); without light activation (L−). Controls: positive control: 0.12% CHX; negative control: ultrapure water (L−). Nanoparticles without curcumin (NP L+ and L−). 10% DMSO.	Curcumin-NP were successfully synthesized, showing stability, homogeneity, a size of 189 nm, and a 67.5% encapsulation efficiency. Curcumin-NP demonstrated enhanced antimicrobial effects when activated by blue light, particularly against planktonic cultures of *Porphyromonas gingivalis*, *Fusobacterium nucleatum*, and *Streptococcus oralis* but showed limited efficacy against mature multispecies biofilms on titanium surfaces. Blue-light activation improved the photodynamic effects, with curcumin-NP exhibiting higher activity against Gram-negative bacteria like *P. gingivalis* and *F. nucleatum* compared to Gram-positive *S. oralis*. Importantly, the curcumin-NP and free curcumin were non-cytotoxic to human periodontal ligament fibroblast cells. These findings suggest that while curcumin-NP shows promise in antimicrobial PDT, further improvements in biofilm penetration and activity are needed to optimize its therapeutic potential.

Table 9. *Cont.*

Reference	Author/Year	Study Groups	Main Results
[45]	Wenzler et al., 2024	PDT: HELBO® Blue Photosensitizer + laser application. PDT dye: HELBO® Blue. Photosensitizer without laser application. Curcumin/DMSO + laser. Curcumin/DMSO only. DMSO: DMSO solution only, without laser application. PTT: EmunDo® dye + 810 nm laser irradiation. PTT Dye: EmunDo® dye without laser application. Control: untreated group.	Cur-aPDT using 445 nm laser irradiation did not show significant antibacterial improvement compared to curcumin/DMSO without laser activation, suggesting the antibacterial effect was primarily due to the solvent DMSO. DMSO alone demonstrated significant bacterial reduction, highlighting its inherent antimicrobial properties, though its efficacy was slightly reduced when combined with curcumin, possibly due to dilution effects. Compared to conventional PDT or PTT, curcumin-based PDT with 445 nm laser irradiation was less effective, potentially due to suboptimal absorption at this wavelength, indicating a need for further optimization of laser parameters, solvents, and curcumin concentrations.
[46]	Rossi et al., 2022	Periodontitis group (n = 10) and peri-implantitis group (n = 10)	PDT using 5-ALA demonstrated significant clinical benefits in the treatment of periodontitis and peri-implantitis. A retrospective analysis of 20 patients revealed that adjunctive PDT with 5% 5-ALA gel significantly reduced probing PPD and BOP at 3 and 6 months post-treatment. In periodontal sites, PPD showed a significant reduction ($p < 0.001$), while BOP also decreased significantly ($p = 0.001$). Similarly, in peri-implantitis cases, PPD reduction was statistically significant ($p < 0.001$), though other improvements, such as decreased BOP and slight increases in exposed implant threads, were noted without reaching statistical significance. Patients reported no pain and perceived sustained benefits. These findings support 5-ALA PDT as a promising adjunct to non-surgical therapy for managing periodontal and peri-implant infections
[47]	Petrini et al., 2022	MACHINED (control group), MACHINED + ALAD (experimental group), and DAE (control group)	PDT using 5-ALA demonstrated significant antibacterial and antibiofilm activity against *Streptococcus oralis* biofilm on titanium implant surfaces. The study showed that applying a 5% 5-ALA gel followed by red LED light irradiation (630 nm) significantly reduced bacterial CFUs and biofilm biomass on both machined and DAE titanium surfaces. CFU counts decreased by 89% on machined surfaces and 77% on DAE surfaces compared to unexposed controls ($p < 0.050$). Live/dead staining confirmed 100% bacterial cell death in PDT-treated samples, and SEM revealed a significant reduction in biofilm accumulation. These findings support 5-ALA-mediated PDT as an effective strategy for implant decontamination and peri-implant disease management.

Table 9. *Cont.*

Reference	Author/Year	Study Groups	Main Results
[48]	Radunović et al., 2020	*Enterococcus faecalis* (1-h incubation with 10% and 50% ALAD); *Enterococcus faecalis* (25 min incubation with 10%, 25%, and 50% ALAD); *Escherichia coli* (25 min incubation with 10%, 25%, and 50% ALAD); *Staphylococcus aureus* (25 min incubation with 10%, 25%, and 50% ALAD); *Veillonella parvula* (25 min incubation with 10%, 25%, and 50% ALAD); *Porphyromonas gingivalis* (25 min incubation with 10%, 25%, and 50% ALAD).	PDT using ALAD gel and red LED irradiation demonstrated a significant antibacterial effect across all tested bacterial species. Enterococcus faecalis showed total inactivation with 50% ALAD + 7 min LED, while lower ALAD concentrations (25%) combined with 5 min LED were effective in reducing CFUs. Escherichia coli and *Porphyromonas gingivalis* required 50% ALAD for significant reduction, with LED irradiation enhancing bacterial eradication at lower concentrations. Staphylococcus aureus and *Veillonella parvula* exhibited intrinsic sensitivity to ALAD alone, but LED irradiation amplified the bactericidal effect. Overall, 25 min of 50% ALAD incubation followed by 5 min LED irradiation was the most effective protocol, achieving substantial bacterial reduction, with implications for treating oral infections and antibiotic-resistant bacteria.

PBS—phosphate-buffered saline; CFU/mL—colony-forming units per milliliter; PDT—photodynamic therapy; LED—light-emitting diode; PS—photosensitizer; MB—methylene blue; FMN—flavin mononucleotide); aPDT—antimicrobial photodynamic therapy; WBCST—whole bacterial cell suspension treated; WBCSU—whole bacterial cell suspension untreated; CFSFT—cell-free supernatant fluid treated; CFSFU—cell-free supernatant fluid untreated; BCPT—bacterial cell pellet treated; BCPU—bacterial cell pellet untreated; QS—quorum sensing; CHX—chlorhexidine; GQD—graphene quantum dots; GQD-Cur—graphene quantum dots with curcumin; ROS—reactive oxygen species; PGA/RF/AV—poly(glycolic acid)/riboflavin/aloe vera; MD—mechanical debridement; NP—nanoparticles; DMSO—dimethyl sulfoxide; HELBO®—a specific brand of Blue Photosensitizer for PDT; PTT—photothermal therapy; Curcumin-NP—curcumin-loaded polymeric nanoparticles; Cur-aPDT—curcumin-mediated antimicrobial photodynamic therapy; DAE—double-acid-etched; ALAD—5-aminolevulinic acid.

Table 10. Light sources physical parameters of the RCT that fulfilled the eligibility criteria.

Author/Year	Light Source	Operating Mode	Wavelength (nm)	Energy Density (J/cm^2)	Power Output (mW)	Powermeter Used	Energy Output (J)	Irradiation Time (s)	Power Density (mW/cm^2)
Qamar et al., 2023 [37]	Diode laser (670 nm)	Continuous wave	670	1.1	280	Not specified	Not specified	60	1100

Table 11. Light sources physical parameters of studies that fulfilled the eligibility criteria.

Author/Year	Light Source	Operating Mode	Wavelength (nm)	Energy Density (J/cm^2)	Power Output (mW)	Powermeter Used	Energy Output (J)	Irradiation Time (s)	Power Density (mW/cm^2)
Etemadi et al., 2023 [39]	LED (DY400-4, Denjoy, China)	Continuous wave	390–480	300–420	1000 ± 100	LaserPoint s.r.l, Milano, Italy		300	
Leelanarathiwatat et al., 2020 [40]	Blue LED and red diode laser	Pulsed wave	450–470, 670	37–40, 4.24	291–314 12	Not specified	29.1–31.4 0.2	10 60	3700–4000 75
Mahdizade-Ari et al., 2019 [41]	Blue LED	Continuous wave	435 ± 20	300–420	Not specified	Not specified		300	1000–1400
Morelato et al., 2022 [42]	Diode laser	660 nm laser: Continuous-wave mode 445 nm laser: Pulsed mode (100 Hz)	445 660	1.24 1240	100	Not specified	1.24	60	124.34
Pourhajibagher et al., 2019 [43]	Blue LED	Continuous wave	60–420	Not specified	1000–1400	LaserPoint s.r.l, Milan	Not specified	60	1000–1400

Table 11. *Cont.*

Author/Year	Light Source	Operating Mode	Wavelength (nm)	Energy Density (J/cm²)	Power Output (mW)	Powermeter Used	Energy Output (J)	Irradiation Time (s)	Power Density (mW/cm²)
Tonon et al., 2022 [44]	Blue Light	Fixed output power	420	72	-	Not specified	Not specified	720	95.5
Wenzler et al., 2024 [45]	HELBO® TheraLite laser SIROLaserBlue FOX Q810plus laser	Continuous wave	660 445 810	Not specified	100 600 200	Not specified	Not specified	10 (per point × 6)	70.74 373.02 565.90
Petrini et al., 2022 [47]	AlGaAs power LED device (TL-01)	Not specified	630 ± 10	100	380	Not specified	Not specified	420	380
Radunović et al., 2020 [48]	AlGaAs power LED (TL-01)	Continuous	630 ± 10	23	Not specified	Not specified	Not specified	Not specified	380

LED—light-emitting diode.

3.4. General Characteristics of the Included Studies

Table 4 outlines the general characteristics of the eight studies included in the analysis.

3.5. Characteristics of Light Sources Used in aPDT

Table 6 provides details on the physical parameters of the light sources utilized in the studies meeting the inclusion criteria.

The significant heterogeneity in photodynamic therapy protocols—including variations in light wavelength, energy density, photosensitizer concentration, and incubation time—poses a challenge in drawing definitive conclusions from the aggregated data. To address this, we meticulously extracted and tabulated key methodological parameters from each study, enabling us to identify both commonalities and critical differences. We then employed a narrative synthesis. Additionally, rigorous quality assessments allowed us to weight findings from studies with more standardized protocols more heavily. Ultimately, while our findings support the potential of naturally mediated aPDT as promising adjunctive treatments for peri-implantitis, the observed variability underscores the need for standardized protocols and further research to ensure more precise, comparable, and clinically translatable results.

4. Discussion

4.1. Results in the Context of Other Evidence

The systematic review highlights the promising potential of naturally mediated aPDT in managing peri-implantitis, offering significant antimicrobial efficacy and clinical benefits [38–47]. Curcumin-mediated aPDT, activated by LED light, demonstrated comparable antimicrobial properties to chlorhexidine, the gold standard for implant decontamination [38]. Riboflavin-aPDT, activated by blue LED, effectively reduced Staphylococcus aureus biofilms with aesthetic advantages due to its light-yellow colour [39]. Cur-aPDT also showed significant impacts on quorum sensing and bystander effects, enhancing its overall efficacy against *Aggregatibacter actinomycetemcomitans* [40]. Riboflavin-based PDT with a 445 nm laser reduced biofilm on titanium surfaces, proving particularly suitable for aesthetic zones [41]. Graphene quantum dots combined with curcumin enhanced ROS production and antimicrobial activity [42]. Riboflavin-loaded nanoparticles in aloe vera gel significantly improved clinical parameters in peri-implantitis treatment, particularly in diabetic patients [43]. Curcumin-loaded nanoparticles showed high efficacy against planktonic bacteria but limited effects on biofilms [44]. However, curcumin/DMSO-based aPDT revealed limited antibacterial effects when combined with a 445 nm laser, emphasizing the need for optimized protocols [45]. Additionally, three studies evaluating 5-ALA-mediated photodynamic therapy (5-ALA PDT) have underscored its potential in peri-implantitis management [46–48]. Rossi et al. reported that applying a 5% 5-ALA gel significantly reduced probing pocket depth and bleeding on probing at 3 and 6 months post-treatment, showing promise as an adjunctive therapy [46]. Petrini et al. demonstrated that 5-ALA-based PDT effectively curtailed *Streptococcus oralis* biofilm formation on titanium surfaces [47]. Similarly, Radunović et al. found that 5-ALA gel, particularly at higher concentrations, exerted a strong bactericidal effect against multiple bacterial strains relevant to peri-implantitis [48]. These findings collectively reinforce the potential role of 5-ALA-mediated PDT in peri-implant disease management, paralleling the encouraging outcomes reported for curcumin- and riboflavin-mediated approaches. Despite the promising results, significant variability in light source parameters, photosensitizer concentrations, and incubation times across studies hinders the development of standardized guidelines [38–47]. PDT consistently demonstrated efficacy in biofilm reduction, but complete eradication was rarely achieved, highlighting its role as an adjunctive rather than a standalone therapy [38–47]. These findings underscore the potential of aPDT in peri-implantitis management while emphasizing the need for further standardization and clinical trials to establish optimized protocols and confirm long-term efficacy [38–47]. Similar research has shown comparable observations. For instance, Rahman et al. concluded that aPDT reduces bacterial loads associated with peri-implant diseases and may serve as an alternative to antibiotics, offering short-term benefits as an adjunct to mechanical debridement [49], though its clinical relevance requires further investigation and careful case selection [49]. Likewise, Fraga et al. demonstrated significant reductions in bacterial counts of *Aggregatibacter actinomycetemcomitans*, *Porphyromonas gingivalis*, and *Prevotella intermedia*, underlining PDT's efficacy in reducing microbial loads in peri-implantitis [50]. Lopez et al. reported improvements in bleeding on probing, probing depth, clinical attachment level, plaque index, gingival index, and bone level density after PDT treatment [51–54]. Zhao et al. showed that PDT and antibiotics, used adjunctively, were both effective in reducing bacterial loads [55–57]. Joshi et al. confirmed notable benefits from PDT as a non-surgical peri-implantitis management strategy [58–61]. Although PDT has demonstrated significant positive outcomes, no clear superiority of laser-based therapies over conventional peri-implantitis interventions has been definitively established, given the heterogeneity in study designs and laser parameters. Bombeccari et al. found that while PDT reduced bleeding and inflammatory exudation in peri-implantitis patients, it did not notably decrease total anaerobic bacteria compared to surgical therapy at 24 weeks [62–65]. Schär et al. reported that non-surgical mechanical debridement with adjunctive PDT was as effective as local drug delivery (minocycline microspheres) in reducing mucosal inflammation over 6 months, although neither modality consistently achieved complete resolution [66–68]. In another study, Wang et al. observed that aPDT combined with mechanical debridement significantly improved periodontal parameters in peri-implantitis patients over 6 months, surpassing mechanical debridement alone in improving clinical attachment loss [69]. Thus, aPDT shows promise as an adjunctive peri-implantitis therapy, particularly for reducing inflammation and improving clinical outcomes, though its efficacy is influenced by treatment protocols and comparative modalities [49–69].

4.2. Other Natural Photosensitisers Potentially Appropriate for aPDT Against Periimplantitis

In addition to widely studied natural compounds such as curcumin, riboflavin, and 5-aminolevulinic acid, several other naturally derived photosensitizers merit attention for their potential role in antimicrobial photodynamic therapy targeting peri-implantitis [70,71]. These compounds not only expand the photochemical toolbox but also align with the growing preference for biocompatible and plant-based therapeutic agents [71]. Among them, hypericin, derived from Hypericum perforatum (St. John's Wort), has emerged as a potent photosensitizer owing to its strong absorption in the visible spectrum and exceptional ability to generate singlet oxygen [72,73]. Beyond its antimicrobial capacity, hypericin also exhibits notable anti-inflammatory properties, a dual functionality that could be particularly advantageous in the inflammatory milieu of peri-implant diseases [25, 74]. Chlorophyllin, a semi-synthetic, water-soluble derivative of chlorophyll, is another promising candidate [75–77]. It absorbs efficiently within the therapeutic window (630–700 nm), enabling effective light activation with standard diode lasers used in dental settings [78]. Notably, chlorophyllin has demonstrated antimicrobial efficacy against both planktonic and biofilm-associated pathogens, an essential requirement in managing the complex biofilm structures on implant surfaces [79,80]. Protoporphyrin IX, an endogenous precursor in the heme biosynthesis pathway, has long been recognized for its high quantum yield in reactive oxygen species (ROS) generation [81,82]. Already used clinically in photodynamic diagnosis and treatment of neoplastic lesions, its potential for application in peri-implantitis warrants further investigation, particularly considering its intrinsic compatibility with host tissues [83]. In addition, metal-substituted phthalocyanines, such as zinc (ZnPc), aluminum (AlPc), and aluminum chloride (AlClPc) derivatives, have gained attention due to their strong absorption in the red to near-infrared spectrum (600–800 nm), which allows deeper tissue penetration [84,85]. Their excellent photostability, high singlet oxygen quantum yields, and tunable chemical structure make them compelling candidates for targeted aPDT approaches in peri-implant environments [86,87]. Although these agents were not the primary focus of this review due to the limited volume of direct evidence pertaining specifically to peri-implantitis, their well-documented photophysical properties, established antimicrobial profiles, and favorable safety data underscore their relevance. As such, their inclusion in future experimental and clinical studies may significantly broaden the scope of naturally mediated aPDT. Incorporating these compounds could enhance therapeutic flexibility, improve patient outcomes and contribute to the development of more sustainable, nature-inspired treatment strategies in peri-implant disease management.

4.3. Limitations of the Evidence

The evidence presented in this systematic review is subject to several limitations that must be acknowledged. One of the most significant challenges is the heterogeneity among the included studies, particularly regarding variations in aPDT protocols, such as light source parameters (wavelength, energy density, and fluence), photosensitizer concentrations, and incubation times. These discrepancies hinder direct comparisons between studies and limit the ability to develop standardized treatment protocols. Additionally, many studies relied heavily on in vitro models, which, while valuable, do not fully replicate the complex biological environment of peri-implantitis in vivo. The limited number of clinical trials and their relatively short follow-up periods further restrict the generalizability and long-term applicability of the findings. Furthermore, the studies often used subjective measures, such as CFU reduction or visual biofilm assessments, without integrating advanced diagnostic tools like molecular analyses or imaging techniques to provide a deeper understanding of treatment efficacy. Lastly, the exclusion of non-English articles and the grey literature may have introduced a selection bias, potentially overlooking relevant data that could have enriched the review's findings. Addressing these limitations in future research is crucial for advancing the clinical utility of PDT in peri-implantitis management.

4.4. Limitations of the Review Process

The review process faced several limitations that impacted its scope and generalizability. Significant heterogeneity among the included studies, particularly in photodynamic therapy protocols such as light parameters, photosensitizer concentrations, and incubation times, hindered the ability to conduct a meta-analysis and required a narrative synthesis of results. Language restrictions excluded non-English studies, potentially omitting valuable data, while the exclusion of the grey literature, such as conference abstracts and unpublished research, may have introduced publication bias. Some studies lacked detailed reporting of methodological aspects, including light settings and incubation periods, complicating assessments of replicability and reliability. The focus on recent publications from 2014 to 2024, while ensuring contemporary relevance, might have excluded earlier foundational studies. Although data extraction and study selection were independently performed by multiple reviewers, the resolution of disagreements through discussion introduced some subjectivity. Furthermore, the lack of uniform application of standardized quality assessment tools, such as the GRADE framework, and the reliance on in vitro studies limited the clinical applicability of the findings. Additionally, many studies featured short follow-up periods, restricting the evaluation of long-term PDT efficacy.

4.5. Implications for Practice, Policy, and Future Research

In clinical practice, curcumin- and riboflavin-mediated aPDT shows promise as a safe and effective adjunctive treatment, offering an alternative to conventional mechanical debridement and antibiotics, particularly for biofilm-associated infections. Clinicians should consider incorporating aPDT into treatment protocols, especially in cases where traditional methods are insufficient or contraindicated. However, the lack of standardized treatment parameters, including light source characteristics, photosensitizer concentrations, and application techniques, underscores the need for clear clinical guidelines. Policymakers and professional organizations should prioritize the development and dissemination of evidence-based protocols and support training programs to facilitate the integration of aPDT into routine dental practice. Future research should focus on addressing the gaps identified in this review, including the variability in aPDT protocols and the limited number of high-quality clinical trials. Large-scale, multicenter randomized controlled trials with standardized parameters are essential to establish the long-term efficacy and safety of aPDT in peri-implantitis management. Additionally, exploring the synergistic effects of aPDT combined with other therapeutic modalities, such as antimicrobial agents or nanocarriers, may enhance treatment outcomes. Innovations in photosensitizer delivery systems, such as hydrogels or nanoparticles, should also be investigated to improve biofilm penetration and stability. Furthermore, advanced diagnostic tools, including imaging and molecular techniques, should be integrated into studies to provide more objective outcome measures. These efforts will help bridge the gap between experimental findings and practical applications, ultimately advancing the role of aPDT in peri-implant disease management and improving patient outcomes. Clinicians may integrate PDT with conventional therapies, such as mechanical debridement and antiseptic or antibiotic treatments, to enhance microbial reduction and biofilm disruption, thereby potentially improving clinical outcomes. This combined approach leverages PDT's benefits, such as its non-invasive nature, reduced risk of antibiotic resistance, and anti-inflammatory effects, while compensating for its limitations in completely eradicating biofilms on its own. However, the variability in PDT protocols underscores the need for standardized parameters to ensure consistent efficacy.

In practice, this means that while PDT can bolster current treatment protocols, clinicians must carefully evaluate patient-specific factors and adhere to optimized, evidence-based protocols to achieve the best long-term results.

Our review identifies several key gaps in the current literature that warrant further investigation. First, there is significant variability in treatment parameters, including photosensitizer type and concentration, light wavelength, energy density, and incubation time, which hampers direct comparisons and calls for the development of standardized protocols. Second, the limited number of high-quality, long-term clinical trials restricts our ability to fully evaluate the efficacy and safety of photodynamic therapy as an adjunctive treatment. Future research should aim to harmonize these critical variables and implement objective outcome measures, while also exploring advanced delivery systems (e.g., nanoparticle carriers) and potential synergistic effects when PDT is combined with conventional therapies. Addressing these gaps through multicenter randomized controlled trials will be essential to refine clinical protocols and fully establish the role of PDT in managing peri-implantitis.

5. Conclusions

This systematic review shows that photodynamic therapy mediated by natural photosensitizers, particularly curcumin, riboflavin, and 5-aminolevulinic acid (5-ALA), can significantly reduce microbial loads, disrupt biofilms and improve clinical parameters in peri-implantitis. Although the findings are promising, heterogeneity in photosensitizer concentrations, light source parameters, and irradiation protocols complicates direct comparisons across studies. Additional large-scale, rigorously designed clinical trials are necessary to determine optimal treatment conditions, confirm long-term efficacy and facilitate the development of standardized guidelines. Natural-photosensitizer-based photodynamic therapy, including 5-ALA, holds potential as an effective adjunctive treatment strategy, especially in cases where conventional mechanical debridement and antibiotic therapy have shown limited success.

Author Contributions: Conceptualization, A.W., J.F.-R., R.W. and M.K.; methodology, A.W., J.F.-R., R.W., D.S. and M.K.; software, D.S. and J.F.-R.; formal analysis, J.F.-R. and A.W.; investigation, J.F.-R. and A.W.; writing—original draft preparation, A.W., J.F.-R., R.W. and M.K.; writing—review and editing, A.W., J.F.-R., M.K. and R.W.; supervision, D.S. and R.W.; funding acquisition, R.W. All authors have read and agreed to the published version of the manuscript.

Funding: This research received no external funding.

Data Availability Statement: Not applicable.

Conflicts of Interest: The authors declare no conflicts of interest.

References

1. Heitz-Mayfield, L.J.A. Peri-implant mucositis and peri-implantitis: Key features and differences. *Br. Dent. J.* **2024**, *236*, 791–794. [CrossRef] [PubMed] [PubMed Central]
2. Misch, C.M. (Ed.) Peri-implantitis. In *Misch's Avoiding Complications in Oral Implantology*; Elsevier: St. Louis, MO, USA, 2018.
3. Wada, M.; Mameno, T.; Otsuki, M.; Kani, M.; Tsujioka, Y.; Ikebe, K. Prevalence and risk indicators for peri-implant diseases: A literature review. *Jpn. Dent. Sci. Rev.* **2021**, *57*, 78–84. [CrossRef] [PubMed] [PubMed Central]
4. Smeets, R.; Henningsen, A.; Jung, O.; Heiland, M.; Hammächer, C.; Stein, J.M. Definition, etiology, prevention and treatment of peri-implantitis—A review. *Head. Face Med.* **2014**, *10*, 34. [CrossRef] [PubMed] [PubMed Central]
5. Monje, A.; Salvi, G.E. Diagnostic methods/parameters to monitor peri-implant conditions. *Periodontology 2000* **2024**, *95*, 20–39. [CrossRef] [PubMed]
6. Wilson, V. An insight into peri-implantitis: A systematic literature review. *Prim. Dent. J.* **2013**, *2*, 69–73. [CrossRef]
7. Alassy, H.; Parachuru, P.; Wolff, L. Peri-Implantitis Diagnosis and Prognosis Using Biomarkers in Peri-Implant Crevicular Fluid: A Narrative Review. *Diagnostics* **2019**, *9*, 214. [CrossRef] [PubMed] [PubMed Central]

8. Renvert, S.; Persson, G.R.; Pirih, F.Q.; Camargo, P.M. Peri-implant health, peri-implant mucositis, and peri-implantitis: Case definitions and diagnostic considerations. *J. Periodontol.* **2018**, *89*, S304–S312. [CrossRef]
9. Heitz-Mayfield, L.J.A.; Salvi, G.E. Peri-implant mucositis. *J. Periodontol.* **2018**, *89*, S257–S266. [CrossRef]
10. Berglundh, T.; Mombelli, A.; Schwarz, F.; Derks, J. Etiology, pathogenesis and treatment of peri-implantitis: A European perspective. *Periodontology 2000* **2024**, *00*, 1–36. [CrossRef]
11. Belibasakis, G.N.; Charalampakis, G.; Bostanci, N.; Stadlinger, B. Peri-implant infections of oral biofilm etiology. *Adv. Exp. Med. Biol.* **2015**, *830*, 69–84. [CrossRef] [PubMed]
12. Kruczek-Kazibudzka, A.; Lipka, B.; Fiegler-Rudol, J.; Tkaczyk, M.; Skaba, D.; Wiench, R. Toluidine Blue and Chlorin-e6 Mediated Photodynamic Therapy in the Treatment of Oral Potentially Malignant Disorders: A Systematic Review. *Int. J. Mol. Sci.* **2025**, *26*, 2528. [CrossRef] [PubMed]
13. Asa'ad, F.; Thomsen, P.; Kunrath, M.F. The Role of Titanium Particles and Ions in the Pathogenesis of Peri-Implantitis. *J. Bone Metab.* **2022**, *29*, 145–154. [CrossRef] [PubMed] [PubMed Central]
14. Kheder, W.; Al Kawas, S.; Khalaf, K.; Samsudin, A.R. Impact of tribocorrosion and titanium particles release on dental implant complications—A narrative review. *Jpn. Dent. Sci. Rev.* **2021**, *57*, 182–189. [CrossRef] [PubMed] [PubMed Central]
15. Gaur, S.; Agnihotri, R.; Albin, S. Bio-tribocorrosion of titanium dental implants and its toxicological implications: A scoping review. *Sci. World J.* **2022**, *2022*, 4498613. [CrossRef]
16. Soler, M.D.; Hsu, S.-M.; Fares, C.; Ren, F.; Jenkins, R.J.; Gonzaga, L.; Clark, A.E.; O'Neill, E.; Neal, D.; Esquivel-Upshaw, J.F. Titanium Corrosion in Peri-Implantitis. *Materials* **2020**, *13*, 5488. [CrossRef]
17. Rana, M.F.; Bukhari, J.; Idrees, E.; Akram, A.; Yousaf, L.; Anwar, A. Tribocorrosion of dental implants: A systematic review. *Pak. J. Med. Health Sci.* **2022**, *16*, 1289. [CrossRef]
18. Prathapachandran, J.; Suresh, N. Management of peri-implantitis. *Dent. Res. J.* **2012**, *9*, 516–521. [CrossRef] [PubMed] [PubMed Central]
19. Scarano, A.; Khater, A.G.A.; Gehrke, S.A.; Serra, P.; Francesco, I.; Di Carmine, M.; Tari, S.R.; Leo, L.; Lorusso, F. Current Status of Peri-Implant Diseases: A Clinical Review for Evidence-Based Decision Making. *J. Funct. Biomater.* **2023**, *14*, 210. [CrossRef] [PubMed] [PubMed Central]
20. Herrera, D.; Berglundh, T.; Schwarz, F.; Chapple, I.; Jepsen, S.; Sculean, A.; Kebschull, M.; Papapanou, P.N.; Tonetti, M.S.; Sanz, M.; et al. Prevention and treatment of peri-implant diseases—The EFP S3 level clinical practice guideline. *J. Clin. Periodontol.* **2023**, *50*, 4–76. [CrossRef]
21. Alghamdi, H.; Leventis, M.; Deliberador, T. Management of Infected Tissues Around Dental Implants: A Short Narrative Review. *Braz. Dent. J.* **2024**, *35*, e246160. [CrossRef] [PubMed] [PubMed Central]
22. Suresh, N.; Joseph, B.; Sathyan, P.; Sweety, V.K.; Waltimo, T.; Anil, S. Photodynamic therapy: An emerging therapeutic modality in dentistry. *Bioorg Med. Chem.* **2024**, *114*, 117962. [CrossRef]
23. Al Hafez, A.S.S.; Ingle, N.; Alshayeb, A.A.; Tashery, H.M.; Alqarni, A.A.M.; Alshamrani, S.H. Effectiveness of mechanical debridement with and without adjunct antimicrobial photodynamic for treating peri-implant mucositis among prediabetic cigarette-smokers and non-smokers. *Photodiagn. Photodyn. Ther.* **2020**, *31*, 101912. [CrossRef] [PubMed]
24. Anas, A.; Sobhanan, J.; Sulfiya, K.M.; Jasmin, C.; Sreelakshmi, P.K.; Biju, V. Advances in photodynamic antimicrobial chemotherapy. *J. Photochem. Photobiol. C Photochem. Rev.* **2021**, *49*, 100452. [CrossRef]
25. Łopaciński, M.; Fiegler-Rudol, J.; Niemczyk, W.; Skaba, D.; Wiench, R. Riboflavin- and hypericin-mediated antimicrobial photodynamic therapy as alternative treatments for oral candidiasis: A systematic review. *Pharmaceutics* **2025**, *17*, 33. [CrossRef] [PubMed]
26. Fiegler-Rudol, J.; Łopaciński, M.; Los, A.; Skaba, D.; Wiench, R. Riboflavin-Mediated Photodynamic Therapy in Periodontology: A Systematic Review of Applications and Outcomes. *Pharmaceutics* **2025**, *17*, 217. [CrossRef] [PubMed]
27. Hussain, Y.; Alam, W.; Ullah, H.; Dacrema, M.; Daglia, M.; Khan, H.; Arciola, C.R. Antimicrobial Potential of Curcumin: Therapeutic Potential and Challenges to Clinical Applications. *Antibiotics* **2022**, *11*, 322. [CrossRef] [PubMed] [PubMed Central]
28. Insińska-Rak, M.; Sikorski, M.; Wolnicka-Glubisz, A. Riboflavin and Its Derivates as Potential Photosensitizers in the Photodynamic Treatment of Skin Cancers. *Cells* **2023**, *12*, 2304. [CrossRef] [PubMed] [PubMed Central]
29. Aragão, M.Â.; Pires, L.; Santos-Buelga, C.; Barros, L.; Calhelha, R.C. Revitalising Riboflavin: Unveiling Its Timeless Significance in Human Physiology and Health. *Foods* **2024**, *13*, 2255. [CrossRef]
30. Schardt, C.; Adams, M.B.; Owens, T.; Keitz, S.; Fontelo, P. Utilization of the PICO Framework to Improve Searching PubMed for Clinical Questions. *BMC Med. Inform. Decis. Mak.* **2007**, *7*, 16. [CrossRef]
31. Page, M.J.; McKenzie, J.E.; Bossuyt, P.M.; Boutron, I.; Hoffmann, T.C.; Mulrow, C.D.; Shamseer, L.; Tetzlaff, J.M.; Akl, E.A.; Brennan, S.E.; et al. The PRISMA 2020 statement: An updated guideline for reporting systematic reviews. *BMJ* **2021**, *372*, n71. [CrossRef]
32. Watson, P.F.; Petrie, A. Method Agreement Analysis: A Review of Correct Methodology. *Theriogenology* **2010**, *73*, 1167–1179. [CrossRef] [PubMed]

33. Gasmi Benahmed, A.; Gasmi, A.; Tippairote, T.; Mujawdiya, P.K.; Avdeev, O.; Shanaida, Y.; Bjørklund, G. Metabolic conditions and peri-implantitis. *Antibiotics* **2023**, *12*, 65. [CrossRef]
34. Tavares, L.J.; Pavarina, A.C.; Vergani, C.E.; de Avila, E.D. The impact of antimicrobial photodynamic therapy on peri-implant disease: What mechanisms are involved in this novel treatment? *Photodiagn. Photodyn. Ther.* **2017**, *17*, 236–244. [CrossRef]
35. Cumpston, M.; Li, T.; Page, M.J.; Chandler, J.; Welch, V.A.; Higgins, J.P.; Thomas, J. Updated guidance for trusted systematic reviews: A new edition of the Cochrane Handbook for Systematic Reviews of Interventions. *Cochrane Database Syst. Rev.* **2019**, *10*, ED000142. [CrossRef] [PubMed] [PubMed Central]
36. Nejadghaderi, S.A.; Balibegloo, M.; Rezaei, N. The Cochrane risk of bias assessment tool 2 (RoB 2) versus the original RoB: A perspective on the pros and cons. *Health Sci. Rep.* **2024**, *7*, e2165. [CrossRef] [PubMed] [PubMed Central]
37. Qamar, Z.; Abdul, N.S.; Soman, C.; Shenoy, M.; Bamousa, B.; Rabea, S.; Albahkaly, H.S. Clinical and radiographic peri-implant outcomes with riboflavin loaded Poly-L-glycolic acid nanoparticles incorporated in aloe-vera gel treating peri-implantitis in chronic hyperglycemic patients. *Photodiagn. Photodyn. Ther.* **2023**, *44*, 103752. [CrossRef]
38. Higgins, J.P.T.; Thomas, J.; Chandler, J.; Cumpston, M.; Li, T.; Page, M.J.; Welch, V.A. (Eds.) *Cochrane Handbook for Systematic Reviews of Interventions*, 2nd ed.; Wiley-Blackwell: Chichester, UK, 2019. [CrossRef]
39. Etemadi, A.; Hashemi, S.S.; Chiniforush, N. Evaluation of the effect of photodynamic therapy with Curcumin and Riboflavin on implant surface contaminated with Aggregatibacter actinomycetemcomitans. *Photodiagn. Photodyn. Ther.* **2023**, *44*, 103833. [CrossRef]
40. Leelanarathiwat, K.; Katsuta, Y.; Katsuragi, H.; Watanabe, F. Antibacterial activity of blue high-power light-emitting diode-activated flavin mononucleotide against Staphylococcus aureus biofilm on a sandblasted and etched surface. *Photodiagn. Photodyn. Ther.* **2020**, *31*, 101855. [CrossRef]
41. Mahdizade-ari, M.; Pourhajibagher, M.; Bahador, A. Changes of microbial cell survival, metabolic activity, efflux capacity, and quorum sensing ability of Aggregatibacter actinomycetemcomitans due to antimicrobial photodynamic therapy-induced bystander effects. *Photodiagn. Photodyn. Ther.* **2019**, *26*, 287–294. [CrossRef]
42. Morelato, L.; Budimir, A.; Smojver, I.; Katalinić, I.; Vuletić, M.; Ajanović, M.; Gabrić, D. A novel technique for disinfection treatment of contaminated dental implant surface using 0.1% riboflavin and 445 nm diode laser—An in vitro study. *Bioengineering* **2022**, *9*, 308. [CrossRef]
43. Pourhajibagher, M.; Parker, S.; Chiniforush, N.; Bahador, A. Photoexcitation triggering via semiconductor Graphene Quantum Dots by photochemical doping with Curcumin versus perio-pathogens mixed biofilms. *Photodiagn. Photodyn. Ther.* **2019**, *28*, 125–131. [CrossRef] [PubMed]
44. Tonon, C.C.; Panariello, B.; Chorilli, M.; Spolidorio, D.M.P.; Duarte, S. Effect of curcumin-loaded photoactivatable polymeric nanoparticle on peri-implantitis-related biofilm. *Photodiagn. Photodyn. Ther.* **2022**, *40*, 103150. [CrossRef] [PubMed]
45. Wenzler, J.-S.; Wurzel, S.C.; Falk, W.; Böcher, S.; Wurzel, P.P.; Braun, A. Bactericidal effect of different photochemical-based therapy options on implant surfaces—An in vitro study. *J. Clin. Med.* **2024**, *13*, 4212. [CrossRef]
46. Rossi, R.; Rispoli, L.; Lopez, M.A.; Netti, A.; Petrini, M.; Piattelli, A. Photodynamic therapy by mean of 5-aminolevulinic acid for the management of periodontitis and peri-implantitis: A retrospective analysis of 20 patients. *Antibiotics* **2022**, *11*, 1267. [CrossRef]
47. Petrini, M.; Di Lodovico, S.; Iezzi, G.; Cellini, L.; Tripodi, D.; Piattelli, A.; D'Ercole, S. Photodynamic antibiofilm and antibacterial activity of a new gel with 5-aminolevulinic acid on infected titanium surfaces. *Biomedicines* **2022**, *10*, 572. [CrossRef]
48. Radunović, M.; Petrini, M.; Vlajic, T.; Iezzi, G.; Di Lodovico, S.; Piattelli, A.; D'Ercole, S. Effects of a novel gel containing 5-aminolevulinic acid and red LED against bacteria involved in peri-implantitis and other oral infections. *J. Photochem. Photobiol. B* **2020**, *205*, 111826. [CrossRef] [PubMed]
49. Rahman, B.; Acharya, A.B.; Siddiqui, R.; Verron, E.; Badran, Z. Photodynamic Therapy for Peri-Implant Diseases. *Antibiotics* **2022**, *11*, 918. [CrossRef] [PubMed] [PubMed Central]
50. Fraga, R.S.; Antunes, L.A.A.; Fontes, K.B.F.D.C.; Küchler, E.C.; Iorio, N.L.P.P.; Antunes, L.S. Is Antimicrobial Photodynamic Therapy Effective for Microbial Load Reduction in Peri-implantitis Treatment? A Systematic Review and Meta-Analysis. *Photochem. Photobiol.* **2018**, *94*, 752–759. [CrossRef] [PubMed]
51. A Lopez, M.; Passarelli, P.C.; Marra, M.; Lopez, A.; Moffa, A.; Casale, M.; D'Addona, A. Antimicrobial efficacy of photodynamic therapy (PDT) in periodontitis and peri-implantitis: A systematic review. *J. Biol. Regul. Homeost. Agents* **2020**, *34*, 59.
52. Wychowański, P.; Starzyńska, A.; Adamska, P.; Słupecka-Ziemilska, M.; Sobocki, B.K.; Chmielewska, A.; Wysocki, B.; Alterio, D.; Marvaso, G.; Jereczek-Fossa, B.A.; et al. Methods of Topical Administration of Drugs and Biological Active Substances for Dental Implants-A Narrative Review. *Antibiotics* **2021**, *10*, 919. [CrossRef] [PubMed] [PubMed Central]
53. Tancredi, S.; De Angelis, P.; Marra, M.; Lopez, M.A.; Manicone, P.F.; Passarelli, P.C.; Romeo, A.; Grassi, R.; D'Addona, A. Clinical Comparison of Diode Laser Assisted "v-Shape Frenectomy" and Conventional Surgical Method as Treatment of Ankyloglossia. *Healthcare* **2022**, *10*, 89. [CrossRef] [PubMed] [PubMed Central]
54. Lindhe, J.; Meyle, J.; Group D of European Workshop on Periodontology. Peri-implant diseases: Consensus Report of the Sixth European Workshop on Periodontology. *J. Clin. Periodontol.* **2008**, *35* (Suppl. S8), 282–285. [CrossRef] [PubMed]

55. Zhao, Y.; Pu, R.; Qian, Y.; Shi, J.; Si, M. Antimicrobial photodynamic therapy versus antibiotics as an adjunct in the treatment of periodontitis and peri-implantitis: A systematic review and meta-analysis. *Photodiagn. Photodyn. Ther.* **2021**, *34*, 102231. [CrossRef]
56. Jervøe-Storm, P.M.; Bunke, J.; Worthington, H.V.; Needleman, I.; Cosgarea, R.; MacDonald, L.; Walsh, T.; Lewis, S.R.; Jepsen, S. Adjunctive antimicrobial photodynamic therapy for treating periodontal and peri-implant diseases. *Cochrane Database Syst. Rev.* **2024**, *7*, CD011778. [CrossRef] [PubMed] [PubMed Central]
57. Zhao, T.; Song, J.; Ping, Y.; Li, M. The Application of Antimicrobial Photodynamic Therapy (aPDT) in the Treatment of Peri Implantitis. *Comput. Math. Methods Med.* **2022**, *2022*, 3547398. [CrossRef] [PubMed] [PubMed Central]
58. Joshi, A.; Gaikwad, A.; Padhye, A.; Nadgere, J. Overview of Systematic Reviews and Meta-analyses Investigating the Efficacy of Different Nonsurgical Therapies for the Treatment of Peri-implant Diseases. *Int. J. Oral. Maxillofac. Implant.* **2022**, *37*, e13–e27 [CrossRef]
59. Farsai, P.S. Overview of Systematic Reviews Suggests That Various Nonsurgical Therapies (NSTS) May be Effective for the Treatment of Peri-Implant Mucositis. *J. Evid. Based Dent. Pract.* **2023**, *23*, 101893. [CrossRef] [PubMed]
60. Faggion, C.M., Jr.; Chambrone, L.; Listl, S.; Tu, Y.K. Network meta-analysis for evaluating interventions in implant dentistry: The case of peri-implantitis treatment. *Clin. Implant. Dent. Relat. Res.* **2013**, *15*, 576–588. [CrossRef] [PubMed]
61. Alarcón, M.A.; Diaz, K.T.; Aranda, L.; Cafferata, E.A.; Faggion, C.M., Jr.; Monje, A. Use of Biologic Agents to Promote Bone Formation in Implant Dentistry: A Critical Assessment of Systematic Reviews. *Int. J. Oral. Maxillofac. Implants* **2017**, *32*, 271–281. [CrossRef] [PubMed]
62. Bombeccari, G.P.; Guzzi, G.; Gualini, F.; Gualini, S.; Santoro, F.; Spadari, F. Photodynamic therapy to treat periimplantitis. *Implant. Dent.* **2013**, *22*, 631–638. [CrossRef] [PubMed]
63. Aebisher, D.; Rogóż, K.; Myśliwiec, A.; Dynarowicz, K.; Wiench, R.; Cieślar, G.; Kawczyk-Krupka, A.; Bartusik-Aebisher, D. The use of photodynamic therapy in medical practice. *Front. Oncol.* **2024**, *14*, 1373263. [CrossRef] [PubMed] [PubMed Central]
64. Wu, P.; Wang, X.; Wang, Z.; Ma, W.; Guo, J.; Chen, J.; Yu, Z.; Li, J.; Zhou, D. Light-activatable prodrug and AIEgen copolymer nanoparticle for dual-drug monitoring and combination therapy. *ACS Appl. Mater. Interfaces* **2019**, *11*, 18691–18700. [CrossRef] [PubMed]
65. Yao, X.; Chen, X.; He, C.; Chen, L.; Chen, X. Dual pH-responsive mesoporous silica nanoparticles for efficient combination of chemotherapy and photodynamic therapy. *J. Mater. Chem. B* **2015**, *3*, 4707–4714. [CrossRef] [PubMed]
66. Schär, D.; Ramseier, C.A.; Eick, S.; Arweiler, N.B.; Sculean, A.; Salvi, G.E. Anti-infective therapy of peri-implantitis with adjunctive local drug delivery or photodynamic therapy: Six-month outcomes of a prospective randomized clinical trial. *Clin. Oral. Implants Res.* **2013**, *24*, 104–110. [CrossRef] [PubMed]
67. Chala, M.; Anagnostaki, E.; Mylona, V.; Chalas, A.; Parker, S.; Lynch, E. Adjunctive Use of Lasers in Peri-Implant Mucositis and Peri-Implantitis Treatment: A Systematic Review. *Dent. J.* **2020**, *8*, 68. [CrossRef] [PubMed] [PubMed Central]
68. Schwarz, F.; Schmucker, A.; Becker, J. Efficacy of alternative or adjunctive measures to conventional treatment of peri-implant mucositis and peri-implantitis: A systematic review and meta-analysis. *Int. J. Implant. Dent.* **2015**, *1*, 22. [CrossRef] [PubMed] [PubMed Central]
69. Wang, H.; Li, W.; Zhang, D.; Li, W.; Wang, Z. Adjunctive photodynamic therapy improves the outcomes of peri-implantitis: A randomized controlled trial. *Aust. Dent. J.* **2019**, *64*, 256–262. [CrossRef]
70. Wang, X.; Wang, L.; Fekrazad, R.; Zhang, L.; Jiang, X.; He, G.; Wen, X. Polyphenolic natural products as photosensitizers for antimicrobial photodynamic therapy: Recent advances and future prospects. *Front. Immunol.* **2023**, *14*, 1275859. [CrossRef] [PubMed] [PubMed Central]
71. Kashef, N.; Borghei, Y.S.; Djavid, G.E. Photodynamic effect of hypericin on the microorganisms and primary human fibroblasts. *Photodiagn. Photodyn. Ther.* **2013**, *10*, 150–155. [CrossRef]
72. Karioti, A.; Bilia, A.R. Hypericins as potential leads for new therapeutics. *Int. J. Mol. Sci.* **2010**, *11*, 562–594. [CrossRef] [PubMed] [PubMed Central]
73. Bruni, R.; Sacchetti, G. Factors affecting polyphenol biosynthesis in wild and field grown St. John's Wort (*Hypericum perforatum* L. Hypericaceae/Guttiferae). *Molecules* **2009**, *14*, 682–725. [CrossRef]
74. Theodorakopoulou, A.; Pylarinou, I.; Anastasiou, I.A.; Tentolouris, N. The Putative Antidiabetic Effect of Hypericum perforatum on Diabetes Mellitus. *Int. J. Mol. Sci.* **2025**, *26*, 354. [CrossRef]
75. Fahey, J.W.; Stephenson, K.K.; Dinkova-Kostova, A.T.; Egner, P.A.; Kensler, T.W.; Talalay, P. Chlorophyll, chlorophyllin and related tetrapyrroles are significant inducers of mammalian phase 2 cytoprotective genes. *Carcinogenesis* **2005**, *26*, 1247–1255. [CrossRef] [PubMed]
76. Nagini, S.; Palitti, F.; Natarajan, A.T. Chemopreventive potential of chlorophyllin: A review of the mechanisms of action and molecular targets. *Nutr. Cancer* **2015**, *67*, 203–211. [CrossRef] [PubMed]
77. Martins, T.; Barros, A.N.; Rosa, E.; Antunes, L. Enhancing Health Benefits through Chlorophylls and Chlorophyll-Rich Agro-Food: A Comprehensive Review. *Molecules* **2023**, *28*, 5344. [CrossRef] [PubMed]

78. Dompe, C.; Moncrieff, L.; Matys, J.; Grzech-Leśniak, K.; Kocherova, I.; Bryja, A.; Bruska, M.; Dominiak, M.; Mozdziak, P.; Skiba, T.H.I.; et al. Photobiomodulation-Underlying Mechanism and Clinical Applications. *J. Clin. Med.* **2020**, *9*, 1724. [CrossRef] [PubMed] [PubMed Central]
79. Khan, S.; Ul Haq, I.; Ali, I.; Rehman, A.; Almehmadi, M.; Alsuwat, M.A.; Zaman, T.; Qasim, M. Antibacterial and Antibiofilm Potential of Chlorophyllin Against Streptococcus mutans In Vitro and In Silico. *Antibiotics* **2024**, *13*, 899. [CrossRef]
80. Kadirvelu, L.; Sivaramalingam, S.S.; Jothivel, D.; Chithiraiselvan, D.D.; Karaiyagowder Govindarajan, D.; Kandaswamy, K. A review on antimicrobial strategies in mitigating biofilm-associated infections on medical implants. *Curr. Res. Microb. Sci.* **2024**, *6*, 100231. [CrossRef] [PubMed] [PubMed Central]
81. Kennedy, J.C.; Pottier, R.H. Endogenous protoporphyrin IX, a clinically useful photosensitizer for photodynamic therapy. *J. Photochem. Photobiol. B* **1992**, *14*, 275–292. [CrossRef] [PubMed]
82. Sachar, M.; Anderson, K.E.; Ma, X. Protoporphyrin IX: The Good, the Bad, and the Ugly. *J. Pharmacol. Exp. Ther.* **2016**, *356*, 267–275. [CrossRef] [PubMed] [PubMed Central]
83. Kiening, M.; Lange, N. A Recap of Heme Metabolism towards Understanding Protoporphyrin IX Selectivity in Cancer Cells. *Int. J. Mol. Sci.* **2022**, *23*, 7974. [CrossRef] [PubMed]
84. Gao, D.; Wong, R.C.H.; Wang, Y.; Guo, X.; Yang, Z.; Lo, P.C. Shifting the absorption to the near-infrared region and inducing a strong photothermal effect by encapsulating zinc(II) phthalocyanine in poly(lactic-co-glycolic acid)-hyaluronic acid nanoparticles. *Acta Biomater.* **2020**, *116*, 329–343. [CrossRef] [PubMed]
85. Awaji, A.I.; Köksoy, B.; Durmuş, M.; Aljuhani, A.; Alraqa, S.Y. Novel Hexadeca-Substituted Metal Free and Zinc(II) Phthalocyanines; Design, Synthesis and Photophysicochemical Properties. *Molecules* **2019**, *24*, 77. [CrossRef] [PubMed]
86. Szewczyk, G.; Mokrzyński, K. Concentration-Dependent Photoproduction of Singlet Oxygen by Common Photosensitizers. *Molecules* **2025**, *30*, 1130. [CrossRef]
87. Payne, D.T.; Webre, W.A.; Gobeze, H.B.; Seetharaman, S.; Matsushita, Y.; Karr, P.A.; Chahal, M.K.; Labuta, J.; Jevasuwan, W.; Fukata, N.; et al. Nanomolecular singlet oxygen photosensitizers based on hemiquinonoid-resorcinarenes, the fuchsonarenes. *Chem. Sci.* **2020**, *11*, 2614–2620. [CrossRef]

pharmaceutics

MDPI

Article

The Natural Anthraquinone Parietin Inactivates *Candida tropicalis* Biofilm by Photodynamic Mechanisms

Juliana Marioni [1,2], Bianca C. Romero [1,3], Ma. Laura Mugas [1,4], Florencia Martinez [5,6], Tomas I. Gómez [1,3,5], Jesús M. N. Morales [2], Brenda S. Konigheim [5,6], Claudio D. Borsarelli [2] and Susana C. Nuñez-Montoya [1,3,*]

[1] Departamento de Ciencias Farmacéuticas, Facultad de Ciencias Químicas, Universidad Nacional de Córdoba, Haya de la Torre y Medina Allende, Ciudad Universitaria, Córdoba X5000HUA, Argentina; juliana.marioni@unc.edu.ar (J.M.); bianca.romero@unc.edu.ar (B.C.R.); tomasigomez0@gmail.com (T.I.G.)

[2] Instituto de Bionanotecnología del NOA (INBIONATEC), Universidad Nacional de Santiago del Estero—CONICET, RN9, Km 1125, Santiago del Estero G4206XCP, Argentina; jesusmarcelom@gmail.com (J.M.N.M.); cdborsarelli@gmail.com (C.D.B.)

[3] CONICET, Unidad de Investigación y Desarrollo en Tecnología Farmacéutica (UNITEFA), Haya de la Torre y Medina Allende, Ciudad Universitaria, Córdoba X5000HUA, Argentina

[4] Centro de Investigaciones sobre Porfirinas y Porfirias (CIPYP), CONICET and Hospital de Clínicas José de San Martín, Universidad de Buenos Aires, Córdoba 2351 1er subsuelo, Ciudad de Buenos Aires 1120AAF, Argentina

[5] Instituto de Virología "Dr. J. M. Vanella", Facultad de Ciencias Médicas, Universidad Nacional de Córdoba, Córdoba X5000HUA, Argentina; florencia.martinez@unc.edu.ar (F.M.); brenda.konigheim@unc.edu.ar (B.S.K.)

[6] Consejo Nacional de Investigaciones Científicas y Técnicas (CONICET), Córdoba X5000HUA, Argentina

[*] Correspondence: sununez@unc.edu.ar

Abstract: Background/Objectives: Parietin (PTN), a blue-light absorbing pigment from *Teloschistes* spp. lichens, exhibit photosensitizing properties via Type I (superoxide anion, $O_2^{\bullet-}$) and Type II (singlet oxygen, $^1O_2$) mechanisms, inactivating bacteria in vitro after photoexcitation. We evaluate the in vitro antifungal activity of PTN against *Candida tropicalis* biofilms under actinic irradiation, its role in $O_2^{\bullet-}$ and $^1O_2$ production, and the cellular stress response. **Methods**: Minimum inhibitory concentration (MIC) of PTN was determined in *C. tropicalis* NCPF 3111 under dark and actinic light conditions. Biofilm susceptibility was assessed at MIC/2, MIC, MICx2, MICx4, and MICx6 in the same conditions, and viability was measured by colony-forming units. Photodynamic mechanisms were examined using Tiron ($O_2^{\bullet-}$ scavenger) or sodium azide ($^1O_2$ quencher). $O_2^{\bullet-}$ production was measured by the nitro-blue tetrazolium (NBT) reduction and nitric oxide (NO) generation by Griess assay. Total antioxidant capacity was studied by FRAP (Ferrous Reduction Antioxidant Potency) assay and superoxide dismutase (SOD) activity by NBT assay. **Results**: Photoexcitation of PTN reduced *C. tropicalis* biofilm viability by four logs at MICx2. Sodium azide partially reversed the effect, whereas Tiron fully inhibited it, indicating the critical role of $O_2^{\bullet-}$. PTN also increased $O_2^{\bullet-}$ and NO levels, enhancing SOD activity and FRAP. However, this antioxidant response was insufficient to prevent biofilm photoinactivation. **Conclusions**: Photoinactivation of *C. tropicalis* biofilms by PTN is primarily mediated by $O_2^{\bullet-}$, with a minor contribution from $^1O_2$ and an imbalance in NO levels. These findings suggest PTN is a promising photosensitizer for antifungal photodynamic therapy.

Keywords: natural anthraquinone; superoxide anion; singlet oxygen; *Candida* biofilm; photodynamic therapy; photoinactivation; reactive oxygen species; oxidative stress

https://doi.org/10.3390/pharmaceutics17050548

1. Introduction

Antimicrobial (ATM) resistance is currently a global problem that hinders the treatment of common infections, increasing the risk of serious and even fatal complications. The prolonged duration of treatment has ramifications for other domains, including the escalation of healthcare costs, both for patients and healthcare systems, due to the use of more complex and expensive treatments. Furthermore, ATM resistance reduces the safety of some medical procedures (surgeries, transplants, cancer treatments) by increasing the risk of resistant infections. This is compounded by the rapid spread of infection, which makes it difficult to control and increases the risk of epidemic outbreaks [1].

Invasive fungal infections represent a significant challenge in the clinical setting, especially those caused by species of the genus *Candida*, an opportunistic fungus responsible for most hospital-acquired infections with a high morbidity and mortality rate. The ability of *Candida* spp. to exhibit ATM resistance has been linked to their capacity to form biofilms, which are distinct in that they are formed by both morphotypes—the yeast and hyphal forms—that intertwine to create a complex three-dimensional structure. This structure affords biofilms greater resistance to traditional antifungals than their planktonic counterparts. Within this group, *Candida tropicalis* stands out for its ability to form biofilms that are highly resistant to conventional treatments, which makes eradication difficult and favors the persistence of infections in immunocompromised patients [2,3].

In the face of ATM resistance, a multitude of strategies have been proposed. Among these, antimicrobial photodynamic inactivation (aPDI) has emerged as a promising approach. This strategy involves the generation of reactive oxygen species (ROS) following the excitation of a photosensitizer (PS) with light of a specific wavelength. This approach has proven to be effective against various pathogenic bacteria, parasites, viruses, and fungi, controlling toxicity on human cells by matching the three necessary factors (PS at a non-active concentration in darkness, light, and oxygen) in the area to be treated. The triplet excited state of the PS ($^3PS^*$) may react with molecular oxygen ($^3O_2$) by two mechanisms: a charge transfer reaction to generate superoxide anion radical ($O_2^{\bullet-}$), or an energy transfer reaction generating singlet molecular oxygen ($^1O_2$), also called Type I and Type II processes, respectively. These species thus generated and the species derived from them by secondary reactions (hydrogen peroxide: H_2O_2; and hydroxyl radical: $HO^\bullet$), are ultimately those that oxidize the biological molecules in their direct environment (proteins, lipids, DNA), triggering cellular oxidative stress that eventually leads to the death of the microorganisms, which translates into regression of the infection [4,5].

In the search for new therapeutic agents, natural products have become of interest due to their structural diversity and bioactive potential [6]. Among them, lichens are an important source of secondary metabolites with antimicrobial, antioxidant, and cytotoxic properties [7–12]. These symbiotic associations between fungi and algae or cyanobacteria produce a wide variety of terpenoid and phenolic derivatives, including among the latter anthraquinones (AQs), many of which have demonstrated activity against pathogenic bacteria and fungi [7].

AQs are a family of compounds found in higher plants and lichens with photoactive properties and potential antimicrobial activity. Some AQ derivatives have shown the ability to generate ROS under irradiation, suggesting their possible application in the inactivation of pathogens. However, the mechanism of action of these molecules and their impact on the viability and structure of fungal biofilms still require further investigation [13,14].

Parietin (PTN), 1,8-dihydroxy-3-methoxy-6-methyl-9,10-anthraquinone (Figure 1), is found as orange crystals in the upper crust of lichens of the *Teloschistaceae* family, acting as an UV-B photoprotective pigment [15]. However, we have previously shown that PTN diluted in organic solvents such as chloroform is an efficient PS of $^1O_2$ with a high quantum yield (Φ_Δ = 0.69) as well as an $O_2^{\bullet-}$ photogenerator in aqueous media [16].

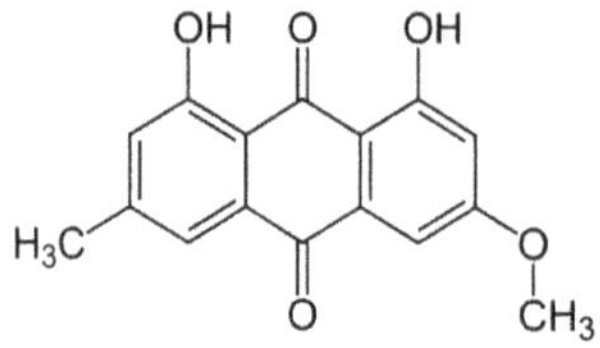

Figure 1. Chemical structure of parietin (1,8-dihydroxy-3-methoxy-6-methyl-9,10-anthraquinone, PTN).

In this work, the in vitro antifungal and antibiofilm activity of PTN was evaluated both in dark conditions and under irradiation. The aim is to determine its potential as a PS against *C. tropicalis* biofilms. The involvement of Type I and Type II photosensitizing mechanisms in the generation of ROS was analyzed; and because of this, the generation of reactive nitrogen intermediates (RNI) was also assessed, since these species can be formed as a secondary process of deactivation of $O_2^{\bullet-}$. The superoxide dismutase enzyme (SOD) activity and the total antioxidant capacity of the biological system (employing FRAP, Ferrous-Reducing Antioxidant Potency assay) were also evaluated, to establish whether oxidative or nitrosative stress would be responsible for the observed biological effect [17–19].

The results of this study indicate that the photoinactivation of *Candida tropicalis* biofilms by PTN is predominantly driven by the $O_2^{\bullet-}$ generation (Type I mechanism). Although the $^1O_2$ (Type II mechanism) also plays a role in this process, its contribution is considerably smaller compared to $O_2^{\bullet-}$. Furthermore, the study revealed an imbalance in NO levels, which likely exacerbates the overall cellular stress response, contributing to the effectiveness of the photodynamic treatment. Given these findings, PTN shows strong potential as an effective PS in antifungal photodynamic therapy (aPDT), offering a promising therapeutic approach for treating fungal biofilm-related infections.

2. Materials and Methods

2.1. Reagents and Solvents

Sabouraud dextrose broth (SDB) and Sabouraud dextrose agar (SDA) were obtained from Britania, CABA, Argentina. Sodium nitrite ($NaNO_2$), and ferrous sulfate ($FeSO_4$) were acquired from Cicarelli, Sta. Fe, Argentina. Sodium hydroxide (NaOH, Biopack, Zárate, Argentina) and Amphotericin B (AmB, Richet, Tres Arroyos, Argentina), phosphate-buffered saline (PBS) were also acquired. Roswell Park Memorial Institute 1640 (RPMI), morpholine propane sulfonic acid (MOPS), sodium azide (NaN_3), Tiron, nitro-blue tetrazolium (NBT), methionine, and riboflavin were purchased from Sigma, St. Louis, MO, USA. Water and distilled solvents (Sintorgan, Buenos Aires, Argentina) were used.

2.2. Yeast Strain and Growth Conditions

A standard strain was used: *Candida tropicalis* NCPF 3111 (National Collection of Pathogenic Fungi, Bristol, UK). It was conserved and reactivated according to Clinical and Laboratory Standards Institute guidelines (CLSI, 2002) [20]. Sabouraud dextrose broth (SDB) was used as a growth medium at 37 °C.

2.3. Natural Photosensitizer Tested

Parietin (PTN) (Figure 1) was obtained from the lichen *Teloschistes nodulifer* (Nyl.) Hillman (Teloschistáceas, identified as CORDC00005354, Museo Botánico de Córdoba, Universidad Nacional Córdoba). In the purification and identification process, the methodology previously developed was followed to obtain a purity of 95%, according to HPLC [21,22]. A hydroalcoholic solution of PTN (3.5 mM) was used as a stock solution, containing 1% ethanol (EtOH). The tested concentrations were prepared by diluting the stock with a culture medium, depending on whether the assay was carried out on planktonic yeasts or biofilm.

2.4. Irradiation System

Photoinactivation assays were carried out using an actinic Phillips 20W lamp (380 ± 480 nm, 0.65 $mWcm^{-2}$, Madrid, Spain) with an emission maximum at 420 nm, which was placed inside a black box at 20 cm above the samples [22].

2.5. Photoactive Minimum Inhibitory Concentration

The lowest concentration of the compound that inhibits the growth of the planktonic form of *C. tropicalis* was determined. The protocol described by CLSI (2008) [23] was applied to determine the minimum inhibitory concentration (MIC), adapted to be carried out under dark and irradiated conditions [24]. This allows the establishment of the photoactivated MIC (pMIC) in comparison to the MIC in darkness, suggesting the photodynamic potential of the PS. The assay was carried out on 96-well microplates (Greiner Bio-One, Frickenhausen, Germany) containing the following culture medium: RPMI 1640 with glutamine and 0.2% glucose, without sodium bicarbonate, buffered with 0.164 M MOPS and adjusting the pH to 7 with 1N NaOH. PTN solutions (100 µL) were added to each well following the additive serial double dilution method and twelve concentrations between 0.24 and 500 µg/mL were tested in triplicate. AmB was the positive control (+C), used at its MIC. The yeast suspension (100 µL) was then added to each well with a final concentration of 0.5×10^3–2.5×10^3 CFU/mL. One set of these concentrations was irradiated for 15 min at room temperature, whereas another set was shielded from light. Immediately after this time, both sets were incubated at 37 °C for 48 h. Finally, the optical density (OD) of each well was measured at 490 or 530 nm on a microplate reader (Tecan Sunrise Model, TECAN, Grödig, Austria). RPMI and yeast suspension with 1% EtOH, both without PTN, were embraced as controls (in triplicate) in both experimental conditions.

In addition, a colony-forming unit (CFU) count assay was performed. A sample (100 µL) was taken from each well, which was diluted 1:10 in PBS until final dilution 1:1,000,000. Subsequently, each suspension (100 µL) was seeded on Sabouraud dextrose agar (SDA) plates and incubated for 48 h at 37 °C. Before incubation, the CFU were counted to establish the minimum fungicidal concentration (MFC), defined as the lowest concentration of a compound that kills 99.9% of a fungal inoculum.

2.6. Photoinactivation Biofilm Procedures

Biofilms were formed in flat-bottomed 96-well microplates (Greiner Bio-One, Frickenhausen, Germany), following an adaptation from the method of O'Toole & Kolter [22]. Once a 48 h biofilm formation in SDB was achieved, the microplates were rinsed twice with PBS (200 µL × 2) at pH = 7 to remove non-adherent cells. PTN was tested on *C. tropicalis* biofilms at five concentrations in triplicate: pMIC/2, pMIC, pMICx2, pMICx4, and pMICx6, under darkness and irradiation conditions. SDB alone and SDB with 1% EtOH were included as negative controls. AmB (+C) was used as a positive control at MIC. After treatment, microplates were incubated at 37 °C for 48 h. The supernatant was replaced by PBS (100 µL per well) and sonicated (40 kHz, 60 s in Codyson CD4831, Shenzhen, China). The biofilm of each well was removed and serially diluted with PBS. Each dilution was plated (10 µL) on the SDA plate in triplicate, and the number of CFUs formed after 48 h incubation at 37 °C was counted. The counting of CFU/mL was log-transformed.

2.7. Mechanism Action Studies

To determine the mechanism of photosensitizing action, the scavenging effect of sodium azide on singlet oxygen ($^1O_2$ quencher) or Tiron on superoxide anion ($O_2^{\bullet-}$ scavenger) was evaluated in PTN-treated and untreated biofilm, both in the presence and absence of light [25]. Quencher/scavenger and PTN solutions were added on a dense biofilm (48 h) at the same time, so that the final concentration of each was 200 μM and the PTN concentrations were pMIC/2, pMIC, pMICx2, pMICx4, pMICx6. After darkness and irradiation treatment (15 min), the procedure continued as described above for CFU quantification.

Each supernatant of both microplates (dark and light) was extracted to assess the production of $O_2^{\bullet-}$, reactive nitrogen intermediates (RNI), and the activation of the antioxidant system: SOD and total non-enzymatic system using the FRAP assay.

Production of $O_2^{\bullet-}$ was determined by the nitro-blue tetrazolium (NBT) reduction method [26]. Blue diformazan formation is proportional to the generated $O_2^{\bullet-}$ in biofilms and its OD was measured at 540 nm on the same microplate reader. Results were expressed as OD_{540nm}/CFU (Superoxide anion/CFU.mL^{-1}) [22].

RNI generation was evaluated as nitrite formation, by using the Griess reaction and a calibration curve of $NaNO_2$ as the standard [27]. OD was measured spectrophotometrically at 540 nm [22] and results were expressed as the ratio between nitrite concentration values/CFU (RNI/CFU.mL^{-1}).

SOD activity was evaluated by the ability of this enzyme to inhibit NBT reduction in the presence of $O_2^{\bullet-}$, generated by the photostimulation of riboflavin in the presence of oxygen and an electron donor (methionine). Results were expressed as SOD activation (%SOD/CFU.mL^{-1}) [22,28].

FRAP assay was used following the methodology described by Benzie & Strain (1996) [29]. The absorbance was measured at 593 nm and results were expressed as the Fe^{2+} concentration values/CFU (FRAP/CFU.mL^{-1}) by using a $FeSO_4$ calibration curve [22].

2.8. Statistical Analysis

All assays were made in triplicate of three independent experiments. Data were expressed as means ± standard deviation. A p-value < 0.05 was considered statistically significant, obtained by the t-Student–Newman–Keuls test for multiple comparisons. The symbol * denotes statistical significance at $p < 0.05$ when compared to untreated biofilms and # indicates statistical significance at $p < 0.05$ when darkness and irradiation were compared.

2.9. Declaration of Generative AI–AI-Assisted Technologies

During the preparation of this work, the author(s) used ChatGPT (GPT-4 version) to improve the redaction and grammar of English. After using this tool/service, the authors reviewed and edited the content as needed and assume full responsibility for the publication's content.

3. Results

3.1. Photoactive Minimum Inhibitory Concentration (pMIC)

PTN produced most significant growth inhibition of planktonic yeasts of *C. tropicalis* at 0.98 μg/mL (≈3.45 μM) under irradiation conditions, as defined as the photoactive MIC (Figure 2). Furthermore, these values are below the cytotoxic concentration of PTN, since the cell viability of Vero cells was 80% and 60% at 100 μg/mL, under darkness and light, respectively [16]. In contrast, in the dark, PTN only produces 20% growth inhibition; therefore, it is not possible to determine its MIC.

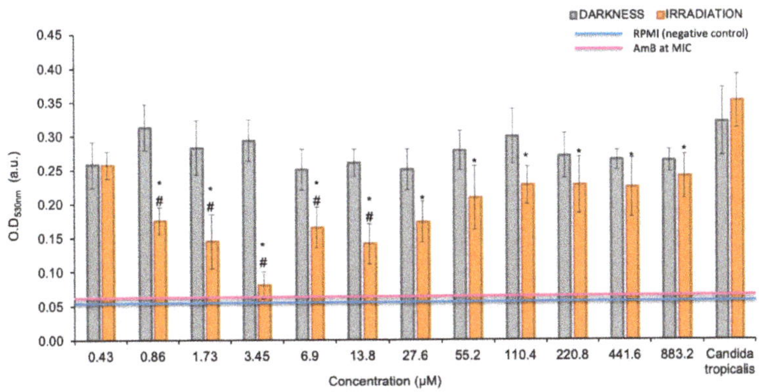

Figure 2. MIC determination of parietin (PTN) under darkness and irradiation conditions. Optical density values obtained for planktonic cells at 530 nm, previously treated with different concentrations of PTN. * $p < 0.05$ with respect to *C. tropicalis*. # $p < 0.05$ darkness vs. irradiation.

3.2. PTN Antimicrobial Photodynamic Therapy (APDT)

The antifungal activity of PTN was also tested on *C. tropicalis* biofilms at five concentrations taking as reference the pMIC value (0.98 μg/mL ≈ 3.45 μM), obtained in yeast suspensions. CFU were not affected by light conditions. Regarding the antibiofilm activity of PTN on *C. tropicalis* (Figure 3), we can state that it had no effect at the tested concentrations in the dark. On the other hand, when PTN was photostimulated, it could be observed that the photodynamic effect was concentration-dependent, starting at the pMIC and the most active concentration being pMICx2 (≈2 μg/mL), as it produced a 4-log CFU reduction. At the highest concentrations tested, no photoinactivation was observed, probably because molecular aggregates of PTN in aqueous media increase the prompt non-radiative deactivation of the singlet excited state, avoiding the generation of the ^{3}PTN* and therefore the photogeneration of ROS [25].

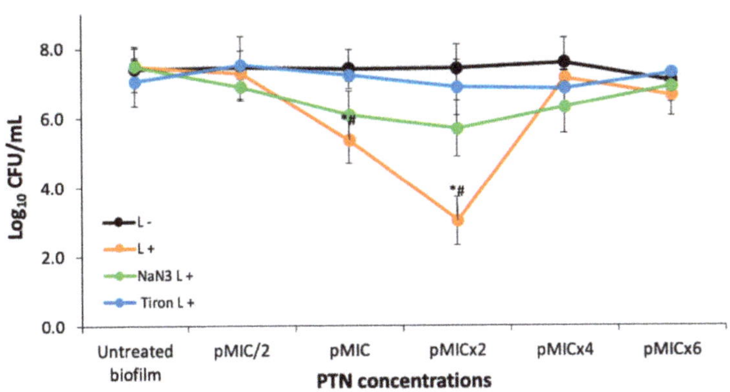

Figure 3. Photoinactivation studies and photodynamic mechanism of *C. tropicalis* biofilms with parietin at five concentrations, using pMIC (0.98 μg/mL ≈ 3.45 μM) as reference and actinic irradiation (L+) vs. darkness (L−). * $p < 0.05$ with respect to *C. tropicalis*. # $p < 0.05$ darkness vs. irradiation.

3.2.1. Photodynamic Mechanism on Analysis After PTN-APDT

To clarify the photoinactivation mechanism, the amount of photogenerated ROS was analyzed in the presence of specific ROS scavengers or quenchers. Thus, the quenching effect of 200 mM sodium azide on $^1O_2$ or the scavenging of $O_2^{\bullet-}$ by 200 mM Tiron on biofilm photoinactivation by PTN is shown in Figure 3. The addition of Tiron completely inhibited the photodynamic effect of PTN at all bioactive concentrations (pMIC and pMICx2). In contrast, sodium azide exhibited approximately half the efficacy of Tiron. Although it was unable to reverse the action of the $O_2^{\bullet-}$, sodium azide significantly increased the survival of biofilms by almost three logs at these concentrations.

3.2.2. Biofilm Stress Response After PTN-APDT

The $O_2^{\bullet-}$ generation and nitrosative metabolite production were studied for the photoinactivation process of PTN on *C. tropicalis* biofilms. An increment in $O_2^{\bullet-}$ levels was observed when PTN was photoexcited at pMIC/2, pMIC, and pMICx2 with respect to untreated biofilms (Figure 4, blue bars). In addition, at the higher PTN concentrations tested, no increase in this ROS was detected. In relation to RNI generation by this AQ when it was photostimulated on biofilms (Figure 4, red bars), the rise in RNI was greater for the most active concentration of PTN than the other concentrations tested.

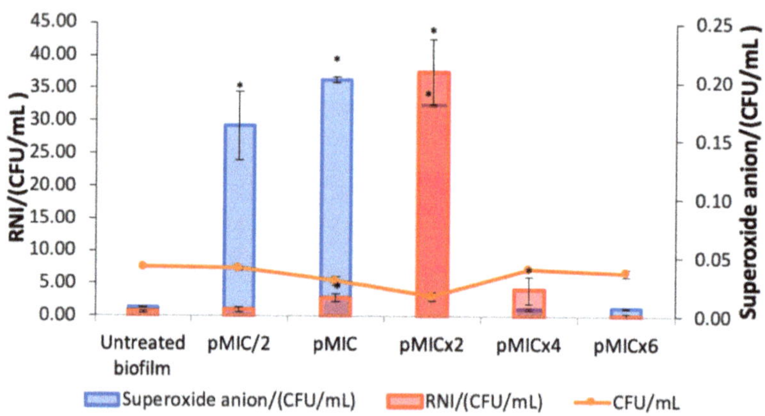

Figure 4. Reactive oxygen species (ROS) and reactive nitrogen intermediates (RNI) production on *C. tropicalis* biofilm treated with parietin and irradiation, using pMIC (0.98 µg/mL ≈ 3.45 µM) as reference. Data were obtained by the colony-forming unit (CFU) count test, corresponding to viable biofilm. * $p < 0.05$ with respect to *C. tropicalis*.

Furthermore, the stimulation of SOD activity (Figure 5, magenta bars) was observed at the photoactive concentrations of PTN (pMIC and pMICx2). The levels of total antioxidant capacity (FRAP) in the treated biofilm increased at all conditions evaluated compared to the untreated biofilm (Figure 5, green bars). Moreover, both defense systems (SOD and FRAP) were detected even in higher proportion for pMICx2.

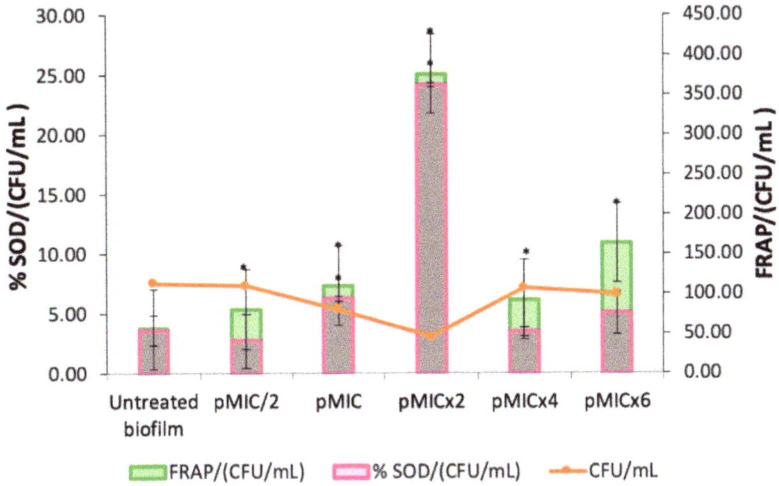

Figure 5. Activation of superoxide dismutase enzyme (SOD) and total antioxidant capacity (FRAP) in *C. tropicalis* biofilm treated with parietin and irradiation, using pMIC (0.98 µg/mL ≈ 3.45 µM) as reference. Data were obtained by the colony-forming unit (CFU) count test, corresponding to viable biofilm. * $p < 0.05$ compared to *C. tropicalis*.

4. Discussion

The treatment of candidiasis is a multifaceted process, due to the pathogenic mechanisms of *Candida* spp., particularly their ability to form biofilms and their acquired resistance or multi-resistance, which represents a significant public health concern [3]. Given this challenge, aPDI is being investigated as a possible alternative for treating fungal infections, which was the motivation for this study [30].

In this study, we started by investigating the effect of PTN-mediated PDI on planktonic yeast of *C. tropicalis*. The results showed negligible toxicity in samples treated with AQ and darkness (<20% growth inhibition). This is consistent with a previous study that reported PTN induced low cytotoxicity in Vero cells. Furthermore, in this previous work, PTN had antibacterial effect on both Gram-positive and -negative strains only after photostimulation [16]. The effect of light-activated PTN against *C. tropicalis* and other clinically relevant fungal pathogens, such as *Candida albicans*, *Candida glabrata*, and *Candida auris*, has been described using a light-emitting diode (LED) irradiation system (λ = 428 nm). Although yeast growth inhibition was achieved at a lower concentration of PTN (0.156 µg/mL vs. 0.98 µg/mL), a significantly higher irradiation dose was required (30 J/cm^2 vs. 0.59 J/cm^2) [31]. Therefore, the lower irradiation dose employed was compensated by using a higher concentration of PS, without exhibiting cytotoxic effects on normal cells. Furthermore, the irradiation system employed in our study is widely used in phototherapy for the treatment of hyperbilirubinemia in humans (https://www.lighting.philips.es/prof/lamparas-y-tubos-convencionales/lamparas-especiales/diversas-aplicaciones-uv/PHOTHER_SU/category, accessed on 7 April 2025).

Similarly, Ma et al. investigated the in vitro PDI mediated by aloe-emodin on azole-sensitive and -resistant *C. albicans* planktonic yeasts [32]. After incubation with 10 µM aloe-emodin and irradiation with 96 J/cm^2 of light, approximately 6.5 log^{10} reductions in the survival of azole-sensitive and -resistant *C. albicans* were achieved. Their findings further support the potential of anthraquinone derivatives as effective PSs against fungal pathogens, as they observed a significant reduction in yeast after light activation. In their study, a higher irradiation dose (96 J/cm^2) was required to achieve substantial antifungal effects, in contrast to the lower doses employed in our work.

Our study also evaluated the PDI of an AQ on a *Candida* spp., but this was PTN on *C. tropicalis* biofilms. In the dark, PTN showed no antifungal effect at any of the concentrations tested (up to 5.9 µg/mL ≈ 20.7 µM). However, under actinic irradiation, the antibiofilm effect increased significantly, resulting in a 99.9% decrease in viability. Our results reveal that twice the concentration of PTN was required to produce the photodynamic effect in biofilms compared to planktonic growth. This is because biofilms are more resistant than their planktonic counterparts, as they are complex three-dimensional structures; however, they appear to favor the interaction of AQ, beginning the aggregation at a high concentration (pMICx4), as observed in Figure 3. This behavior has already been observed for other AQs (rubiadin and rubiadin-1-methyl ether) in previous studies [21]. Other natural PSs that align with the blue-light emission spectrum are curcumin and riboflavin. In this sense, Quishida et al. [33] investigated the PDI of curcumin and LED light against *C. albicans*, *C. glabrata*, and *Streptococcus mutans* biofilm. The findings revealed that aPDT significantly decreased biofilm viability, metabolic activity, and biomass. However, the photoantibiofilm effect required high concentrations of curcumin (80, 100, and 120 µM). Alshehri et al. [34] examined the effectiveness of PDI using 0.1% riboflavin on *C. albicans* biofilms. Blue LED light was utilized to activate riboflavin, and fungal cell viability was assessed using 3-(4,5-dimethylthiazol-2-yl)-2,5-diphenyltetrazolium bromide (MTT) assay. Treatment with riboflavin and LED resulted in the lowest survival rate of *C. albicans*, with viability below 50%.

Furthermore, other AQs such as emodin, alizarin, alizarin red, chrysazin, quinalizarin, purpurin, and 1-hydroxyanthra-9, 10-quinone have been shown to inhibit biofilm formation of *C. albicans*. The efficacy of emodin against *C. albicans* biofilm of strains isolated from hospitalized patients was achieved in the range of 200–400 µg/mL [35]. Alizarin and chrysazin reduced the metabolic activity of *C. albicans* biofilms by >98% at 10 µg/mL and by 66% at 2 µg/mL, respectively [36]. Moreover, inhibition of *C. albicans* biofilm formation by anthraquinones-related compounds, namely pyrocatechol, alizarin red, quinalizarin, emodin, 1-hydroxyanthra-9,10-quinone, purpurin, chrysazin, and alizarin has shown to be dose-dependent [35,37]. In addition, the antifungal activity of alizarin has been largely attributed to the presence of aromatic hydroxyl groups (-OH) in its AQ core [36]. This suggests that variations in the position of the -OH groups significantly influence the antibiofilm properties. Among the AQs tested, those with a -OH group at position-1(adjacent to the carbonyl group) exhibited the highest activity in all assays. Notably, purpurin, chrysazin, and alizarin, which share an -OH group at the C1 position, demonstrated strong inhibitory effects against *Candida albicans* biofilms even at low concentrations (2 µg/mL) [36]. Therefore, the antibiofilm activity of PTN against *C. tropicalis* may be influenced by the presence of the -OH group at position-1 in the AQ structure.

Besides the AQs, hypericin (a dianthrone) and porphyrins have emerged as promising PSs with high selectivity for fungal pathogens. Hypericin-mediated aPDT demonstrated significant antifungal activity, achieving substantial reductions in *Candida* biofilm and planktonic cell viability. Furthermore, hypericin activated by yellow or orange light effectively affected fluconazole-resistant *Candida* strains with minimal cytotoxicity to host tissues [38,39].

Porphyrins are PSs with high selectivity to pathogens. Thus, the photoinactivation of different *Candida* spp. by two cationic porphyrins derived from tetra-chloride salts, meso-tetra(4-N-methylpyridyl) porphyrin and meso-tetra(3-N-methylpyridyl)porphyrin derivatives (4-H2TMeP+ and 3-H2TMeP+), and anionic porphyrin tetra-sodium salt, meso-tetra(4-sulfonatophenyl)porphyrin (4-H2TPSP−) was investigated by Amorin et al. [40].

For the irradiation process, a white-light LED and light dosage of 10.9 J/cm^2 was used. Cationic porphyrins can photoinactivate different *Candida* spp. in both planktonic and biofilm forms. *C. tropicalis* showed 35.8% interference when treated with 4-H2TMeP+, and 51.67% with 3-H2TMeP+ at 75uM for both porphyrins [40]. In addition, the tetracationic metalloporphyrin Zn(II) meso-tetrakis(N-n-hexylpyridinium-2-yl)porphyrin (ZnTnHex-2-PyP4+) was assayed against biofilms of *C. albicans* strains (ATCC 10231 and ATCC 90028) using a blue light-emitting diode. The PDI (4.3 J/cm^2) at 0.8 μM showed about 89% decrease in the cell viability as assessed by the MTT assay [41].

Therefore, PTN stands out as an effective PS against *Candida tropicalis*, displaying strong antifungal and antibiofilm activity upon light activation, whereas remaining non-toxic in the dark. As an AQ-based compound, it benefits from a well-defined photoreactive core, structural stability, and required -OH positioning, which enhances its photodynamic efficacy. Its potent effect, even at low irradiation doses, makes it a promising alternative to other natural PSs that require higher concentrations or light doses for comparable activity.

The photoinactivation mechanism of *C. tropicalis* biofilms by PTN was investigated to identify the photoprocesses occurring in PTN-PDI.

Tiron inhibits the photoinactivation *C. tropicalis* biofilm by PTN at bioactive concentration. Although Tiron is a quencher of $O_2^{\bullet -}$, it can react with hydroxyl radicals ($HO^{\bullet}$) [42]. Since $HO^{\bullet}$ production occurs after the $O_2^{\bullet -}$ generation and Tiron was added before the irradiation period, it can be inferred that Tiron acted as a scavenger of $O_2^{\bullet -}$. Thus, the Type I photosensitization mechanism would be mainly involved in PTN-mediated PDI in the biofilm. Furthermore, our previous work showed that PTN can produce $O_2^{\bullet -}$, being an efficient Type I photosensitizer [16]. On the other hand, sodium azide only has a limited protective effect on *C. tropicalis* biofilm, despite PTN being an efficient $^1O_2$ producer [16]. This type of behavior has also been reported for other AQs, such as rubiadin and its methylated derivative. For both AQs, it was shown that the main photosensitizing mechanism involved in the photoinduced antibiofilm activity is the $O_2^{\bullet -}$ formation through suppression of AQ excited states by electron transfer, whereas the role of $^1O_2$ seems to be less significant [25].

Oxidative stress is a complex process that occurs because of two main factors: an overproduction of ROS, specifically by $O_2^{\bullet -}$ levels (Type I mechanism), given the short lifetime of singlet oxygen (3 μs) [43], and a reduction in oxidative defenses. Thus, this excessive ROS cannot be compensated by the enzymatic and non-enzymatic antioxidant systems of the biofilm, which make them insufficient to remove free radicals, resulting in damage to macromolecules (DNA, protein, lipids) and cellular components (cell membrane) [44,45].

When studying the biofilm response to this oxidative burst, NO generation should also be assessed as a response to $O_2^{\bullet -}$ levels, since this occurs more rapidly than the enzymatic response of SOD, thus promoting biofilm photoinactivation [46]. Elevated levels of NO (μM concentration) can cause cytotoxicity by inducing oxidative and nitrosative stress, leading to DNA damage, enzyme modification, cellular dysfunction, inflammation, mitochondrial impairment, and apoptosis. NO can inhibit key mitochondrial enzymes, such as aconitase, and disrupt respiratory chain complexes. It also reacts with $O_2^{\bullet -}$, at a faster rate than with oxygen, to form the toxic peroxynitrite (^-OONO), which generates harmful radicals ($HO^{\bullet}$ and NO). It may react with H_2O_2 to produce $^1O_2$, further intensifying damage [47,48].

Similar oxidative and nitrosative imbalances have been reported with other AQs, such as rubiadin and its 1-methyl ether derivative, isolated from *Heterophyllaea pustulata*. These compounds also induce significant photoreductions in biofilm formation of *C. tropicalis*, likely through similar mechanisms involving the overproduction of ROS and RNI [24].

In planktonic cells, oxidative stress induced by ROS overproduction has been extensively studied. Fiala et al. (2024) [31], showed that PTN targets the cell membrane and induces cell death via ROS-mediated lipid peroxidation after light irradiation on *Candida* planktonic yeast. Aloe-emodin has also been reported to induce photodynamic damage to the cell envelope of *C. albicans* planktonic form through ROS generation [32].

All this background suggests that the oxidative burst, resulting from ROS and RNI, is a common feature in the photoantimicrobial action of AQs, as our results also show.

The study of natural PSs contributes to the development of aPDT, which has proven to be selective, fast acting and has not developed resistance to date. This selectivity is achieved through strict spatial control of irradiation on the affected area (infection), thus uniting the three agents responsible for the photodynamic effect (PS, light, and $^3O_2$). The PSs used in aPDT have not been shown to stimulate resistance mechanisms in microorganisms due to their multidimensional action, which generates a generalized oxidative imbalance that does not differentiate between resistant and non-resistant microorganisms. This photooxidation even includes the destruction of virulence factors, which are generally organic molecules susceptible to oxidation. Moreover, the PSs do not necessarily need to enter the cell to exert its action. Consequently, the pathogen cannot develop resistance through increased detoxification metabolism or export of the drug [49].

5. Conclusions

In conclusion, this study demonstrates that the photoinactivation of *Candida tropicalis* biofilms using PTN as the photosensitizer is primarily driven by $O_2^{\bullet-}$ (Type I mechanism), with $^1O_2$ (Type II mechanism) playing a secondary role. However, the photodymamic effect is dependent on the concentration of PTN, since at higher concentration PTN self-aggregation effects play a role in the prompt deactivation of the excited states of the AQ. The results also show an imbalance in NO levels, which likely contributes to the cellular stress response and enhances the effectiveness of the treatment. The dominant role of $O_2^{\bullet-}$ in biofilm inactivation highlights its significance in the photodynamic mechanism of PTN. These findings suggest that PTN ability to disrupt fungal biofilms is linked to complex oxidative and nitrosative stress pathways, making PTN a promising candidate for antifungal PDT and potential clinical applications.

Author Contributions: Conceptualization and methodology, S.C.N.-M. and J.M.; software, J.M., M.L.M., B.C.R., T.I.G., F.M. and J.M.N.M.; formal analysis, J.M., B.C.R., C.D.B., F.M. and S.C.N.-M.; statistical analysis, F.M. and B.S.K.; writing—original draft preparation, J.M., C.D.B. and S.C.N.-M.; supervision, J.M., C.D.B., B.S.K. and S.C.N.-M.; resources, supervision, project administration, and funding acquisition, J.M., C.D.B. and S.C.N.-M. All authors have read and agreed to the published version of the manuscript.

Funding: S.C.N.-M. thanks SECyT (Consolidar, tipo 2, s/res. N° 411/18 y 155/22), and Consejo Nacional de Investigaciones Científicas y Técnicas (CONICET-PIP 2021–2023, s/res. 1639/2021). J.M. thanks the Fondo para la Investigación Científica y Tecnológica (FONCyT-PICT 2018 N° 4576, s/res. ANPCyT n° 401/19). C.D.B. thanks the CONICET, projects PUE-2018-035 and PIP-2020-101043CO, and FONCyT, Project PICT-2019-02052 of Argentina for financial support. The APC was not funded.

Institutional Review Board Statement: Not applicable.

Informed Consent Statement: Not applicable.

Data Availability Statement: The original contributions presented in this study are included in the article. Further inquiries can be directed to the corresponding author.

Acknowledgments: T.I.G., J.M.N.M. and B.C.R. are doctoral fellows at CONICET. F.M. and M.L.M. are post-doctoral fellows at CONICET. J.M., B.S.K., C.D.B. and S.C.N.-M. are members of the Research Career of CONICET. ChatGPT provided assistance in proofreading the English wording.

Conflicts of Interest: The authors declare no conflicts of interest.

Abbreviations

The following abbreviations are used in this manuscript:

Φ_Δ	Quantum yield of singlet oxygen
+C	Positive control
$^1O_2$	Singlet oxygen
$^3O_2$	Molecular oxygen
AmB	Amphotericin B
aPDI	Antimicrobial photodynamic inactivation
aPDT	Antimicrobial photodynamic therapy
AQ/s	Anthraquinone/s
ATM	Antimicrobial
CFU	Colony-forming units
CLSI	Clinical and Laboratory Standards Institute
EtOH	Ethanol
$FeSO_4$	Ferrous sulfate
FRAP	Ferrous Reduction Antioxidant Potency assay
H_2O_2	Hydrogen peroxide
$HO^\bullet$	Hydroxyl radical
MIC	Minimal inhibitory concentration
MOPS	Morpholine propane sulfonic acid
NaN_3	Sodium azide
$NaNO_2$	Sodium nitrate
NaOH	Sodium hydroxide
NBT	Nitro-blue tetrazolium
NCPF	National Collection of Pathogenic Fungi
NO	Nitric oxide
$O_2^{\bullet-}$	Superoxide radical anion
OD	Optical density
PBS	Phosphate buffered saline
pMIC	Photoactive minimal inhibitory concentration
PS	Photosensitizer
PTN	Parietin
RNI	Reactive nitrogen intermediates
ROS	Reactive oxygen species
RPMI	Roswell Park Memorial Institute 1640
SDA	Sabouraud dextrose agar
SDB	Sabouraud dextrose broth
SOD	Superoxide dismutase
MFC	Minimum fungicidal concentration
MTT	3-(4,5-dimethylthiazol-2-yl)-2,5-diphenyltetrazolium bromide
-OH	Hydroxyl groups
DNA	Deoxyribonucleic acid
$^-OONO^-$	Peroxynitrite

References

1. Ahmed, S.K.; Hussein, S.; Qurbani, K.; Ibrahim, R.H.; Fareeq, A.; Mahmood, K.A.; Mohamed, M.G. Antimicrobial Resistance: Impacts, Challenges, and Future Prospects. *J. Med. Surg. Public Health* **2024**, *2*, 100081. [CrossRef]
2. Riera, F.O.; Caeiro, J.P.; Angiolini, S.C.; Vigezzi, C.; Rodriguez, E.; Icely, P.A.; Sotomayor, C.E. Invasive Candidiasis: Update and Current Challenges in the Management of This Mycosis in South America. *Antibiotics* **2022**, *11*, 877. [CrossRef]
3. Pappas, P.G.; Lionakis, M.S.; Arendrup, M.C.; Ostrosky-Zeichner, L.; Kullberg, B.J. Invasive candidiasis. *Nat. Rev. Dis. Primers* **2018**, *4*, 18026. [CrossRef]
4. Aroso, R.T.; Schaberle, F.A.; Arnaut, L.G.; Pereira, M.M. Photodynamic Disinfection and Its Role in Controlling Infectious Diseases. *Photochem. Photobiol. Sci.* **2021**, *20*, 1497–1545. [CrossRef]

5. Klausen, M.; Ucuncu, M.; Bradley, M. Design of Photosensitizing Agents for Targeted Antimicrobial Photodynamic Therapy. *Molecules* **2020**, *25*, 5239. [CrossRef]
6. Aware, C.B.; Patil, D.N.; Suryawanshi, S.S.; Mali, P.R.; Rane, M.R.; Gurav, R.G.; Jadhav, J.P. Natural Bioactive Products as Promising Therapeutics: A Review of Natural Product-Based Drug Development. *S. Afr. J. Bot.* **2022**, *151*, 512–528. [CrossRef]
7. Ranković, B.; Kosanić, M. Lichens as a Potential Source of Bioactive Secondary Metabolites. In *Lichen Secondary Metabolites: Bioactive Properties and Pharmaceutical Potential*; Springer International Publishing: Cham, Switzerland, 2019; pp. 1–29.
8. Thakur, M.; Chander, H. Potential of lichens: A Review of Bioactive Compounds with Biological Activities. *Biol. Forum Int. J.* **2021**, *13*, 39–47.
9. Poulsen-Silva, E.; Otero, M.C.; Diaz-Cornejo, S.; Atala, C.; Fuentes, J.A.; Gordillo-Fuenzalida, F. Secondary Metabolites of Lichens: The Untapped Biomedical and Pharmaceutical Potential of Antimicrobial Molecules. *Fungal Biol. Rev.* **2025**, *51*, 100410. [CrossRef]
10. Kocovic, A.; Jeremic, J.; Bradic, J.; Sovrlic, M.; Tomovic, J.; Vasiljevic, P.; Andjic, M.; Draginic, N.; Grujovic, M.; Mladenovic, K.; et al. Phytochemical Analysis, Antioxidant, Antimicrobial, and Cytotoxic Activity of Different Extracts of Xanthoparmelia Stenophylla Lichen from Stara Planina, Serbia. *Plants* **2022**, *11*, 1624. [CrossRef]
11. Kello, M.; Goga, M.; Kotorova, K.; Sebova, D.; Frenak, R.; Tkacikova, L.; Mojzis, J. Screening Evaluation of Antiproliferative, Antimicrobial and Antioxidant Activity of Lichen Extracts and Secondary Metabolites In Vitro. *Plants* **2023**, *12*, 611. [CrossRef]
12. Aoussar, N.; Laasri, F.E.; Bourhia, M.; Manoljovic, N.; Mhand, R.A.; Rhallabi, N.; Ullah, R.; Shahat, A.A.; Noman, O.M.; Nasr, F.A.; et al. Phytochemical Analysis, Cytotoxic, Antioxidant, and Antibacterial Activities of Lichens. *Evid. Based Complement. Alternat. Med.* **2020**, *2020*, 8104538. [CrossRef]
13. Christina Pires Gonçalves, L. Photophysical Properties and Therapeutic Use of Natural Photosensitizers. *J. Photochem. Photobiol.* **2021**, *7*, 100052. [CrossRef]
14. Polat, E.; Kang, K. Natural Photosensitizers in Antimicrobial Photodynamic Therapy. *Biomedicines* **2021**, *9*, 584. [CrossRef] [PubMed]
15. Fernández-Marín, B.; Artetxe, U.; Becerril, J.M.; Martínez-Abaigar, J.; Núñez-Olivera, E.; García-Plazaola, J.I. Can Parietin Transfer Energy Radiatively to Photosynthetic Pigments? *Molecules* **2018**, *23*, 1741. [CrossRef]
16. Comini, L.R.; Morán Vieyra, F.E.; Mignone, R.A.; Páez, P.L.; Laura Mugas, M.; Konigheim, B.S.; Cabrera, J.L.; Núñez Montoya, S.C.; Borsarelli, C.D. Parietin: An Efficient Photo-Screening Pigment in Vivo with Good Photosensitizing and Photodynamic Antibacterial Effects in Vitro. *Photochem. Photobiol. Sci.* **2017**, *16*, 201–210. [CrossRef]
17. Hurtado Bredda, F.J.; Nin Vaeza, N.; Rubbo Amonini, H. Estrés oxidativo y nitrosativo en la sepsis. *Med. Intensive* **2005**, *29*, 159–165. [CrossRef]
18. Baltazar, L.M.; Ray, A.; Santos, D.A.; Cisalpino, P.S.; Friedman, A.J.; Nosanchuk, J.D. Antimicrobial Photodynamic Therapy: An Effective Alternative Approach to Control Fungal Infections. *Front. Microbiol.* **2015**, *6*, 202. [CrossRef]
19. Ong, K.S.; Mawang, C.I.; Daniel-Jambun, D.; Lim, Y.Y.; Lee, S.M. Current Anti-Biofilm Strategies and Potential of Antioxidants in Biofilm Control. *Expert Rev. Anti Infect. Ther.* **2018**, *16*, 855–864. [CrossRef]
20. *M27-A2*; Reference Method for Broth Dilution Antifungal Susceptibility Testing of Yeasts; Approved Standard—Second Edition. NCCLS: Wayne, PA, USA, 2002.
21. Mugas, M.L.; Calvo, G.; Marioni, J.; Céspedes, M.; Martinez, F.; Sáenz, D.; Di Venosa, G.; Cabrera, J.L.; Montoya, S.N.; Casas, A. Photodynamic Therapy of Tumour Cells Mediated by the Natural Anthraquinone Parietin and Blue Light. *J. Photochem. Photobiol. B* **2021**, *214*, 112089. [CrossRef]
22. Marioni, J.; Arce, J.E.; Cabrera, J.L.; Paraje, M.G.; Núñez Montoya, S.C. Reduction of *Candida tropicalis* Biofilm by Photoactivation of a *Heterophyllaea pustulata* Extract. *Pharm. Biol.* **2016**, *54*, 2791–2801. [CrossRef]
23. *M27-A3*; Reference Method for Broth Dilution Antifungal Susceptibility Testing of Yeasts; Approved Standard—Third Edition. CLSI: Wayne, PA, USA, 2008.
24. Marioni, J.; Da Silva, M.A.; Cabrera, J.L.; Montoya, S.C.N.; Paraje, M.G. The Anthraquinones Rubiadin and Its 1-Methyl Ether Isolated from Heterophyllaea Pustulata Reduces Candida Tropicalis Biofilms Formation. *Phytomedicine* **2016**, *23*, 1321–1328. [CrossRef] [PubMed]
25. Marioni, J.; Bresolí-Obach, R.; Agut, M.; Comini, L.R.; Cabrera, J.L.; Paraje, M.G.; Nonell, S.; Montoya, S.C.N. On the Mechanism of Candida Tropicalis Biofilm Reduction by the Combined Action of Naturally-Occurring Anthraquinones and Blue Light. *PLoS ONE* **2017**, *12*, e0181517. [CrossRef]
26. Mattila, H.; Khorobrykh, S.; Havurinne, V.; Tyystjärvi, E. Reactive Oxygen Species: Reactions and Detection from Photosynthetic Tissues. *J. Photochem. Photobiol. B* **2015**, *152*, 176–214. [CrossRef]
27. Tsikas, D. Analysis of Nitrite and Nitrate in Biological Fluids by Assays Based on the Griess Reaction: Appraisal of the Griess Reaction in the l-Arginine/Nitric Oxide Area of Research. *J. Chromatogr. B* **2007**, *851*, 51–70. [CrossRef] [PubMed]
28. Beauchamp, C.; Fridovich, I. Superoxide Dismutase: Improved Assays and an Assay Applicable to Acrylamide Gels. *Anal. Biochem.* **1971**, *44*, 276–287. [CrossRef]

29. Benzie, I.F.F.; Strain, J.J. The Ferric Reducing Ability of Plasma (FRAP) as a Measure of "Antioxidant Power": The FRAP Assay. *Anal. Biochem.* **1996**, *239*, 70–76. [CrossRef]
30. Youf, R.; Müller, M.; Balasini, A.; Thétiot, F.; Müller, M.; Hascoët, A.; Jonas, U.; Schönherr, H.; Lemercier, G.; Montier, T.; et al. Antimicrobial Photodynamic Therapy: Latest Developments with a Focus on Combinatory Strategies. *Pharmaceutics* **2021**, *13*, 1995. [CrossRef]
31. Fiala, J.; Roach, T.; Holzinger, A.; Husiev, Y.; Delueg, L.; Hammerle, F.; Armengol, E.S.; Schöbel, H.; Bonnet, S.; Laffleur, F.; et al. The Light-Activated Effect of Natural Anthraquinone Parietin against Candida Auris and Other Fungal Priority Pathogens. *Planta Med.* **2024**, *90*, 588–594. [CrossRef]
32. Ma, W.; Liu, C.; Li, J.; Hao, M.; Ji, Y.; Zeng, X. The Effects of Aloe Emodin-Mediated Antimicrobial Photodynamic Therapy on Drug-Sensitive and Resistant Candida Albicans. *Photochem. Photobiol. Sci.* **2020**, *19*, 485–494. [CrossRef]
33. Quishida, C.C.C.; De Oliveira Mima, E.G.; Jorge, J.H.; Vergani, C.E.; Bagnato, V.S.; Pavarina, A.C. Photodynamic Inactivation of a Multispecies Biofilm Using Curcumin and LED Light. *Lasers Med. Sci.* **2016**, *31*, 997–1009. [CrossRef]
34. Alshehri, A.H. Mechanical and Antimicrobial Effects of Riboflavin-Mediated Photosensitization of in Vitro C. Albicans Formed on Polymethyl Methacrylate Resin. *Photodiagnosis Photodyn. Ther.* **2021**, *36*, 102488. [CrossRef]
35. Janeczko, M.; Masłyk, M.; Kubiński, K.; Golczyk, H. Emodin, a Natural Inhibitor of Protein Kinase CK2, Suppresses Growth, Hyphal Development, and Biofilm Formation of Candida albicans. *Yeast* **2017**, *34*, 253–265. [CrossRef]
36. Manoharan, R.K.; Lee, J.-H.; Kim, Y.-G.; Lee, J. Alizarin and Chrysazin Inhibit Biofilm and Hyphal Formation by Candida Albicans. *Front. Cell. Infect. Microbiol.* **2017**, *7*, 447. [CrossRef]
37. Tsang, P.W.-K.; Bandara, H.M.H.N.; Fong, W.-P. Purpurin Suppresses Candida Albicans Biofilm Formation and Hyphal Development. *PLoS ONE* **2012**, *7*, e50866. [CrossRef]
38. Galinari, C.B.; Biachi, T.D.P.; Gonçalves, R.S.; Cesar, G.B.; Bergmann, E.V.; Malacarne, L.C.; Kioshima Cotica, É.S.; Bonfim-Mendonça, P.D.S.; Svidzinski, T.I.E. Photoactivity of Hypericin: From Natural Product to Antifungal Application. *Crit. Rev. Microbiol.* **2023**, *49*, 38–56. [CrossRef]
39. Łopaciński, M.; Fiegler-Rudol, J.; Niemczyk, W.; Skaba, D.; Wiench, R. Riboflavin- and Hypericin-Mediated Antimicrobial Photodynamic Therapy as Alternative Treatments for Oral Candidiasis: A Systematic Review. *Pharmaceutics* **2024**, *17*, 33. [CrossRef]
40. Amorim, C.F.; Iglesias, B.A.; Pinheiro, T.R.; Lacerda, L.E.; Sokolonski, A.R.; Pedreira, B.O.; Moreira, K.S.; Burgo, T.A.L.; Meyer, R.; Azevedo, V.; et al. Photodynamic Inactivation of Different Candida Species and Inhibition of Biofilm Formation Induced by Water-Soluble Porphyrins. *Photodiagnosis Photodyn. Ther.* **2023**, *42*, 103343. [CrossRef]
41. Souza, S.O.; Raposo, B.L.; Sarmento-Neto, J.F.; Rebouças, J.S.; Macêdo, D.P.C.; Figueiredo, R.C.B.Q.; Santos, B.S.; Freitas, A.Z.; Cabral Filho, P.E.; Ribeiro, M.S.; et al. Photoinactivation of Yeast and Biofilm Communities of Candida Albicans Mediated by ZnTnHex-2-PyP4+ Porphyrin. *J. Fungi* **2022**, *8*, 556. [CrossRef]
42. Bors, W. Pulse-Radiolytic Investigations of Catechols and Catecholamines II. Reactions of Tiron with Oxygen Radical Species. *Biochim. Biophys. Acta BBA Gen. Subj.* **1979**, *582*, 537–542. [CrossRef] [PubMed]
43. Snyder, J.W.; Skovsen, E.; Lambert, J.D.C.; Poulsen, L.; Ogilby, P.R. Optical Detection of Singlet Oxygen from Single Cells. *Phys. Chem. Chem. Phys.* **2006**, *8*, 4280. [CrossRef] [PubMed]
44. Vatansever, F.; De Melo, W.C.M.A.; Avci, P.; Vecchio, D.; Sadasivam, M.; Gupta, A.; Chandran, R.; Karimi, M.; Parizotto, N.A.; Yin, R.; et al. Antimicrobial Strategies Centered around Reactive Oxygen Species—Bactericidal Antibiotics, Photodynamic Therapy, and Beyond. *FEMS Microbiol. Rev.* **2013**, *37*, 955–989. [CrossRef] [PubMed]
45. Elian, C.; Méallet, R.; Versace, D. Photoactive Dye–Loaded Polymer Materials: A New Cutting Edge for Antibacterial Photodynamic Therapy. *Adv. Funct. Mater.* **2024**, *34*, 2407228. [CrossRef]
46. Wink, D.A.; Mitchell, J.B. Chemical Biology of Nitric Oxide: Insights into Regulatory, Cytotoxic, and Cytoprotective Mechanisms of Nitric Oxide. *Free Radic. Biol. Med.* **1998**, *25*, 434–456. [CrossRef] [PubMed]
47. Fraix, A.; Sortino, S. Combination of PDT Photosensitizers with NO Photodononors. *Photochem. Photobiol. Sci.* **2018**, *17*, 1709–1727. [CrossRef]
48. Zhao, Z.; Li, H.; Tao, X.; Xie, Y.; Yang, L.; Mao, Z.; Xia, W. Light-Triggered Nitric Oxide Release by a Photosensitizer to Combat Bacterial Biofilm Infections. *Chem. Eur. J.* **2021**, *27*, 5453–5460. [CrossRef]
49. Tavares, A.; Carvalho, C.M.B.; Faustino, M.A.; Neves, M.G.P.M.S.; Tomé, J.P.C.; Tomé, A.C.; Cavaleiro, J.A.S.; Cunha, Â.; Gomes, N.C.M.; Alves, E.; et al. Antimicrobial Photodynamic Therapy: Study of Bacterial Recovery Viability and Potential Development of Resistance after Treatment. *Mar. Drugs* **2010**, *8*, 91–105. [CrossRef]

MDPI AG
Grosspeteranlage 5
4052 Basel
Switzerland
Tel.: +41 61 683 77 34

Pharmaceutics Editorial Office
E-mail: pharmaceutics@mdpi.com
www.mdpi.com/journal/pharmaceutics